Advance Praise for Love Me, Fee

"A must-read for families—especially adoptive ones—but really everyone, because food issues are so rampant today. Rowell tackles the tough issues, and they would have helped my parents when I was adopted and are already helping me with my foster children now . . . This information is desperately needed to help families deal with common challenges that come up involving food. This book shows parents how to build trust and relationships, while avoiding conflict and power struggles."

— Ashley Rhodes–Courter, bestselling author of *Three Little Words*

"There are few relationships more important or more complex than the one between child and parent over food. When children are eating well and growing and developing normally, parents feel validated. However, when feeding becomes an unpleasant chore, parents question their abilities and self-worth. Much of our contact with young children occurs in conjunction with food and without confidence and pleasure in this interaction, the process of mutual attachment is stilted. *Love Me, Feed Me* is designed to help families understand and rectify feeding problems commonly encountered in children who suffered early deprivation and is one of the best sources of coherent information on this extremely important topic."

— Dana E. Johnson, MD, Ph.D, Professor of Pediatrics, International Adoption Medicine Program, University of Minnesota

"Understanding and tuned-in feeding is a powerful way for you to show your foster or adoptive child that you love her and understand how she feels, and s/he can trust you to take care of her. Katja Rowell's book will show you how."

— Ellyn Satter, MS, RD, LCSW, BCD, author of *Child of Mine, Your Child's Weight* and *Secrets of Feeding a Healthy Family*

"In her book, *Love Me, Feed Me*, Dr. Rowell offers parents a deeply complex, loving, and effective plan of action for resolving feeding problems. She skillfully introduces the reader to the Trust Model, then builds the reader's skill in applying the model in even the most extraordinary circumstances. Throughout, she pays careful attention to the issues of attachment that are entwined with feeding. I recommend this book to community-based programs and providers serving parents of adoptive children. They will find a new treatment paradigm that I hope transforms their program policies."

— Carol Danaher, MPH, RD, Public Health Nutritionist

"This may be the most important book you read about attachment and feeding with your foster or adopted child. Wherever you are in your parenting journey, this essential guide will equip you to handle common feeding challenges and build trust and attachment with your child. Difficulties around feeding and eating are often more intense with the foster or adopted child, and the conventional wisdom about how to address these problems may just do more harm than good. If meal times are a constant power struggle and you are weary from the battle, this revolutionary approach will allow you to reclaim joy and freedom at the family table. You will learn to trust your instincts, and more importantly, your child, so that you can *support* his innate ability to eat well. You may even find some healing from your own long-standing struggles with food. Whether you have been struggling with feeding for what seems like an eternity or you simply want to anticipate and prevent common problems with eating and weight concerns in your child, this is a must read."

— Katherine Zavodni, MPH, RD, LDN

"I wish I had read *Love Me, Feed Me* before we had our son with us. It would have saved us so much worry and heartache. Our family has been transformed by the Trust Model and Dr. Rowell's practical advice. It felt like she was describing our situation to the letter, when we felt like we were the only ones. This book has helped more than I would have imagined, both with our biological son's picky eating and our adopted son's intense interest in food. As a bonus, the practical, science-based information will help me take better care of my patients."

— Ruth Coffman, mother and Family Nurse Practitioner

"As a dietitian specializing in eating disorders and working with children with all kinds of feeding problems, I've also earned my stripes personally as a picky eater and a stepmother of picky eaters. Dr. Rowell's advice is right on target for all of the above. It's time to replace the "obesity crisis" paradigm with a focus on developing competent eaters."

— Jessica Setnick, MS, RD, CSSD, CEDRD, International Federation of Eating Disorder Dietitians, author of *The American Dietetic Association Pocket Guide to Eating Disorders*, National Director of Training and Education for Ranch 2300 Collegiate Eating Disorders Treatment Program

"As someone who works with families fighting life-threatening eating disorders, I see this as essential reading for parents who are feeling challenged by feeding issues. This well-researched guide gives parents a foundation for raising children who can learn to trust their bodies to guide their eating, even if there are significant feeding challenges."

— Becky Henry, CPPC, author of *Just Tell Her to Stop: Family Stories of Eating Disorders*

"This book is a blueprint for adoptive and fostering parents on how to achieve a healthy feeding relationship, written with clarity and compassion."

— Ines M. Anchondo, DrPH, MPH, RD CSP, Certified Specialist in Pediatrics Nutrition

"So little information is offered to parents pre-adoption regarding how to feed a child in a way that encourages trust and attachment. A stress-free, pleasant family meal is essential in the attachment process with adoptive and foster children. Dr. Rowell's spot-on advice in *Love Me, Feed Me* has truly been a key to the attachment process with my adoptive son. The Trust Model has also helped me deal with feeding challenges with confidence when they come up. I love that this book goes into so many of the day-to-day feeding challenges as well as the bigger picture topics. I recommend this book highly."

— Margo Johnson, mother to a son adopted at 8 months of age

Nicole Stanton

Love Me, Feed Me

THE ADOPTIVE PARENT'S GUIDE
to ending the worry about
WEIGHT, PICKY EATING, POWER STRUGGLES
AND MORE

KATJA ROWELL, MD • THE FEEDING DOCTOR

With foreward by Deborah Gray, MSW, MPA, Nurturing Attachments

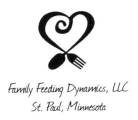

Family Feeding Dynamics, LLC
St. Paul, Minnesota

Nicole Stanton

ISBN-13: 978-0615691312
LCCN# 2012-948112

First Edition

Printed in the United States of America

© 2012 by Katja Rowell, MD.

Published by Family Feeding Dynamics, LLC

Saint Paul, Minnesota

Book design: Stephanie Larson
Proofreader: Rhiannon Nelson
Indexer: Top Hat Word and Index

14 13 12 11 10 / 10 9 8 7 6 5 4 3 2 1

Disclaimers and Terms of Use:

Privacy

To protect the privacy of the children and their families who have generously consented to share their experiences for this book, I have changed individual identifying details, such as a specific person's name, gender, country of origin and, in some cases, age. Rarely, to illustrate a point or further protect a family's identity, an anecdote or quote may be a composite of one or more family's experiences.

Financial and Conflict of Interest

At the time of writing, I am an advisory member of the SPOON Foundation and of the Midwest Dairy Association's Health and Wellness Council. I receive no financial reward from any of the books or products mentioned in *Love Me, Feed Me*, including Ellyn Satter's works, which I frequently recommend.

Medical

This book and the information it contains are provided for educational purposes only. The text of this book is not meant or intended to replace careful observation, evaluation, diagnosis, or ongoing medical or nutritional care for a child, and the text of this book should not be used in place of such careful observation, evaluation, diagnosis, or ongoing care. The author has provided general information in this book and cannot make any assurances in regard to the applicability of any information to any particular person in any particular set of circumstances. The reader assumes all risk of taking any action or making any decision based on the information contained in this book. The author shall have no liability or responsibility for any such action taken or decision made by any reader of this book, and no liability for any loss, injury, damage, or impairment allegedly arising from the information provided in this book.

Table of Contents

Dedication

For the children, who deserve health, happiness, and our trust.

Acknowledgements

Thank you, dear husband, for your unwavering support, patience, and being my IT department and so much more. You are a great dad, and I'm so lucky that you like everything I cook—and you do the dishes! A big "thank you" to my daughter for being a delightful dinner companion, and a sweet, smart, and funny person whom I get to share my life with.

Thank you, Mom. You cooked every night for your family, giving me wonderful memories of delicious and happy family meals that I am passing on to my daughter. It's the heart of what I hope to share with families who have lost their joy at the table.

Thank you, the parents who open your homes to me, sharing your pain and triumphs. I have learned more from you, with your strength, passion, and dedication to helping your children, than you will ever know.

Hydee Becker, RD—thank you, thank you, thank you! Your experience, wealth of knowledge, and good sense around feeding is critical to the work I do with families. Thank you for your support and generosity and for reading drafts of this book! Thank you for being my friend.

Thank you, my draft readers Margo, Becky, and Jenny, and my editor and graphic designer Stephanie, for your support and handholding. I couldn't have done this book without you! And thank you, Connie, for getting me started, often the hardest part.

Thank you, Michelle and Michele. Our discussions over the years helped me rewire some of my neural pathways as I wrapped my head around these difficult issues.

To my blog readers: your stories and kind words teach and inspire me, and make me think and smile.

Thank you also to 16-year-old Yiseth, adopted from Guatemala, who gave me the title for this book during our interview. At the time, I was winnowing down several choices for the title. When I ran them by Yiseth, a mature and thoughtful young lady, she pondered: "Why not just call it 'Love Me, Feed Me?' That's what it's about, right?" So true. Thank you, Yiseth, for breaking it down to its most essential.

Finally, I want to thank Ellyn Satter for her work that has so enriched my life personally and professionally. I am grateful to my colleagues in the Ellyn Satter Institute who have shared their wisdom and experience: Ines, for her research help and expertise, and Clio, Patty, Pam, and Carol for their mentoring and encouragement.

Foreward

Katja Rowell, MD has written a sensible, healthy, and emotionally intelligent guide to feeding children—even when feeding issues are complex. The book teaches a "trust model" that succeeds in encouraging parents as it educates them.

I learned so much from this book. The book gently helps us to see our inconsistent beliefs in feeding our children and feeding ourselves. Using a multitude of examples, Dr. Rowell helps parents to identify and take the responsibilities necessary for good nutrition in children. She steers parents away from nonproductive control battles or manipulation over food. Instead, she outlines ways to shift the responsibilities of knowing their bodies back to children. Her description of the Division of Responsibility is advice that all of us will be better following. The outcome is a dramatically healthier, happier family with pleasant mealtimes. I have rarely learned so much valuable information in one book. This will be on my recommended list for all families.

— Deborah D. Gray, MSW, MPA, Nurturing Attachments
    Author of *Attaching in Adoption: Practical Tools for Today's Parents* and *Nurturing Adoptions: Creating Resilience after Trauma and Neglect*

Part 1:

What Are You Worried About? Learning How to Feed Your Family

Introduction

The Cry for Help and the Beginning of Understanding

"We've spent so much money on attachment therapists, and I feel like all I do is fight with Mari about food. If I can't feed her, if all I am told to do is to deny her constant requests for food, I feel like she can never really trust me…"
— Carol, mother of Mari, age 2½, adopted from Ethiopia

It was the second such call in one day from one of two moms on opposite sides of the country, both anxious and desperate to do the right thing for their little girls.

I had been working one-on-one with parents as a childhood feeding specialist for a few years, when these cries for help reached me. Over time, they have become more frequent, and ultimately motivated me to share what I have learned with a wider audience. My clients' initial goals usually sound something like this: *"I want Sam to eat more vegetables,"* or *"I want Lilly to learn portion control so that she will lose weight,"* or *"Tanya is so small that every calorie counts, and I have to get her to eat more protein,"* and finally, *"I just want her to be healthy and happy."*

Deep down, what these parents desperately want is to stop worrying and fighting about food—and to bond with their children. They want to:

- Have a family table where everyone wants to be together.
- Look forward to, and not dread, family meals.
- Have kids who are happy and healthy.

The good news is that realizing the short-term goals of having a more pleasant table and enjoyable family meals is what leads to the long-term goal of raising a happy, healthy, competent eater—that is, a child who eats a variety of foods in the right amounts for him or her. The reality is that this takes time and patience. The bad news is that up until now, many parents have felt unsupported with their feeding challenges, and there is a lot of *misinformation* for the most common feeding concerns that adoptive and foster families might face—from power struggles and selective eating to nutrition and weight concerns, and more.

In fact, in my research on adoption resources, the topics of food issues, feeding, or selective eating typically get a paragraph or two in a standard book, a line in an article or Website, or maybe a list of helpful tips like serving breakfast for dinner or providing sweets to aid with attachment. Rarely is there mention of the interactions around food beyond the bottle.

> The terms "feeding" or the "feeding relationship" throughout this book describe the interactions between a parent and child around food. It is what happens when the parent offers food, how the child reacts, and how the parent in turn responds. Feeding goes far beyond bottle or spoon-feeding, and encompasses all that goes on in a family around food.[1]

Feeding Is Central to Parenting and Attachment

"Knowing deep within us that someone is going to feed us when we are hungry is how trust and love begin..." — Mister Rogers, *Mister Rogers' Neighborhood* [2]

Lara, mother of two adopted school-aged children, agreed: *"Feeding was absolutely essential to attachment."* Feeding is unique because it provides daily opportunities for completing the "attachment cycle," where the parent meets the child's needs. Lara adds, *"We follow the advice that bonding activities ideally should have a sensory piece and be repetitive, pattern-based, and relationship building.[3] What better meets those criteria than feeding your kids—with the smells, colors, tastes, and routine of meals and snacks."*

> **The sad thing is, when feeding is not going well, not only is the opportunity for bonding lost, but the troubled feeding relationship becomes a source of conflict that can put up additional barriers to trust and attachment.**

The Worry Cycle

Sue, another mom, knows all too well how a difficult feeding relationship can take its toll. She recalls how unprepared she felt for feeding challenges with her children from Kazakhstan: *"Despite having read a TON in preparation, I wish I had known how much feeding is a key for attachment, even for older children. I wish I had had more information that there was a good chance that the table could be a very difficult place for a while, and some of the reasons for that—that is, the possibilities of chewing/swallowing/sensory issues. I may have been better able to stay calm and let some things slide if my expectations of a happy family meal had not been met with such a slap in the face."*

More than one client has likened feeding difficulties to a "black hole" that they are circling, then falling in, deeper and deeper—and the harder they try to scramble out, the worse things get. Research backs this up:

- Surveys show that almost one-third of internationally adopting parents identifies significant feeding and weight worries.[4]

- In the general population:
    - One in three parents ask a health care professional for help with feeding.[5]
    - One in five children may qualify for a feeding disorder.[6]
    - Up to 80 percent of children with developmental issues or autism spectrum diagnoses will struggle with food.[6]

> If you have feeding or growth concerns, it may feel like feeding, and thinking about feeding, is all you do. It affects how you feel about yourself as a parent, how you feel about your child, and your ability to attach and enjoy your time together. Through no fault of their own, many parents struggle with feeding. Adopted or foster children often have additional challenges with complex feeding histories as well as medical, developmental, and nutritional or weight concerns. Parental worry, coupled with a lack of information and support, often invites counterproductive feeding practices, such as pressure put on the child to eat more, less, or different kinds of foods than she would willingly eat.

As one feeding expert put it, "Ensuing parent-child struggles around feeding may consequently increase parental distress and worry, leading to further attempts to make the child eat that cause further disruption to the feeding relationship."[7] It's a vicious cycle, as this diagram illustrates:

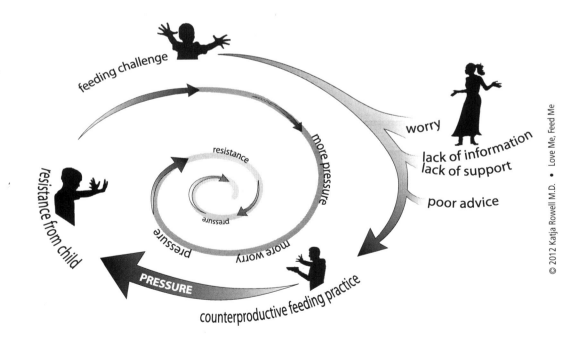

© 2012 Katja Rowell M.D. • Love Me, Feed Me

Trust Yourself, Trust Your Child

This book is not about pointing fingers or blaming parents. Families need sound feeding information before their children arrive; they need help at the first signs of conflict, anxiety, or worry over growth or eating. Sadly, most of my clients have struggled for years. Well-meaning but untrained experts, from family doctors and pediatricians to gastroenterologists and even feeding therapists, may give families feeding advice that makes matters worse—not better.

Parents say, *"I've been doing everything they told me, and it's getting worse,"* or *"She keeps getting bigger,"* or *"He seems to want to eat even less now."* One mom told me, *"Everything I've done with feeding has gone against every one of my instincts, but when you have a nutritionist, gastroenterologist, and even an international adoption doctor telling you the same thing, you go along with it. It has been torture."* This is wrong. And it makes me sad and angry on behalf of the families and children who have been so poorly served.

Part of turning this around, or preventing feeding problems in the first place, is to give yourself permission to trust your instincts. As Dr. Spock famously said, "Trust yourself. You know more than you think you do." If it feels wrong, look further. If your family is being negatively impacted (I've heard "destroyed," "torn apart," and "ruined") by food battles, get help. I'm not saying that feeding kids well isn't hard work, because it is. It's not easy to plan and serve balanced meals and snacks or arrange your lives to prioritize family meals, even without the added challenges faced by so many adoptive and foster families.

The difference between the Trust Model and the "feeding and worry cycle" is the difference between being tired but satisfied that you are doing the right thing at the end of the day, versus chronic confusion, second-guessing yourself and the experts you rely on, anxiety, and stress surrounding meals—and probably in the middle of the night, too. Listen to that inner voice.

> You know your child better than any therapist or doctor does, so if you're doing everything you are told, and it's making things worse, not better, trust yourself and look further for the right help for your family.

This book is intended for parents who are waiting for their children to arrive, parents who share their lives and love with foster children, and adoptive parents who already have their children with them, whether it's been two days or ten years. If, as the parent, you have personally struggled or still struggle with food, or are recovered from an eating disorder, it may be more difficult to trust your instincts around feeding, so this book may be especially helpful.

In presenting common concerns, I hope to help you address and let go of your worries and fears, and give you practical information on how to begin, or how to heal the feeding relationship you have with your child. You *can* have a peaceful family table and raise competent eaters.

A Humbling Journey

Years ago, I didn't know I would become a feeding specialist. I trained at a top-ten medical school, and time and again as a family doctor, I saw the physical and emotional burden that children and families dealt with when they struggled with eating, weight, or body image issues—*caused by broken relationships with food and their bodies.*

I counseled parents and children when the child was "overweight," and I nagged and cheered my "overweight" adult patients as well. But following the standard of care and "evidence-based guidelines" for weight loss simply didn't work. I figured it was because my patients, or the parents of my patients, simply weren't doing what I recommended. I never asked myself if what I was telling them to do was actually helping. In addition, I saw the devastation that anorexia and other eating disorders brought to my patients and their families. Very few people, from clients to friends and colleagues, actually felt good about food and their bodies.

When my daughter was born, a healthy dose of humility came home with me from the hospital. As all parents do, I suddenly realized how much I didn't know. It shook my identity as a mother and as a doctor. I had been giving feeding advice all along, *but wasn't really trained to do so.* I knew *what* I was supposed to feed my daughter, but not *how.* By age fourteen months, following the standard practice, my child was preoccupied with food—and therefore, so was I. And sadly, my anxiety was ruining our time together. *I needed to learn how to raise a healthy, happy child.*

A Model of Wellness

I am grateful that I found renowned childhood feeding expert, therapist, dietitian, and author Ellyn Satter's Division of Responsibility, which is the core of her Trust Model of feeding. Within a few weeks of instituting the model, my daughter's inborn abilities with eating were emerging, and she was eating the amounts that were right for her. She enjoyed meals, but wasn't constantly wondering when she would eat next, and she was happier. The transformation in my own home was life changing. I literally left the anxiety and worry behind, felt confident again, and could enjoy my family more fully.

I read everything I could about weight, growth, and feeding. To round out my training, I learned about and attended conferences in feeding-clinic therapies for children with feeding disorders; read books about intuitive eating, eating disorders, and binge eating; and collaborated with colleagues working in the field. The more I learned, the more I realized that this Trust Model and information about the importance of the feeding relationship were the missing pieces. **Helping a child have a healthy relationship with food and his or her body is at the core of health and happiness. It is preventive medicine at its most powerful.**

Ellyn Satter's feeding and eating models (the Trust Model for children and Eating Competence for adults) are models of wellness and healthy eating. Her institute members have more than 100 years of combined clinical practice, and the research on Eating Competence is compelling. In essence, adults who are eating competently have a healthy relationship with food. Studies show they tend to have a more stable weight, less disordered eating and dieting, and enjoy better nutrition. Even those tests that doctors love—blood sugar, cholesterol, and blood pressure—are better in adults who are eating competently.[8,9,10,11] The other component is that these folks also do better socially and emotionally.[11] There it is, exactly what my clients tell me they want for their children—*healthy and happy*. The Trust Model of feeding is a way to raise your child to be a competent eater.

Soon after I left family medicine behind and devoted myself to helping families struggling with feeding and weight concerns, I began to get calls from adoptive parents. I wanted to help. I was pleased to see leaders in the field of international adoption (IA) medicine recommending Ellyn's books, and I dove into research about adoption, attachment, and feeding. I grilled my friends with adopted children about their experiences, and when asked, I doled out free advice and saw encouraging results. I realized: If there is a model of wellness for eating, why shouldn't it work with *all* children?

Transitioning to the Trust Model

The adopting and fostering parents who came to me knew what they were doing wasn't helping with their feeding struggles. Many had heard about the Trust Model of feeding, and even tried out some of the strategies, but could not trust the process or even envision what it might look like without help. Understandably, parents who have tried everything from feeding clinics to negotiation and bribes, sometimes for years, were skeptical and scared. I heard, *"But my daughter was starving,"* or *"We tried it for three days, but he ate only bread. It won't work for us."*

I was finding that on their own, many families with deeply entrenched feeding problems and worries struggled to transition to the Trust Model. Essentially, my role has been one of supporting families through that transition.

It is not an easy process. It involves a leap of faith, acquiring knowledge, consistency and effort, and often nothing short of a major shift in thinking from: how can I *get* my child to eat a certain amount of certain foods, to how can I *support* my child so that her natural capabilities with eating can emerge? This book can help guide you through the process for your particular worries.

I have been overjoyed when so many of the adopting families I worked with were resolving long-standing battles over selective eating, or children who had never had a "stopping place" were saying, "I'm full," and running off to play. My hope is that by sharing the experiences of families with children who came from severe neglect, starvation, or other challenges, and who *thrived* with the Trust Model, you will gain inspiration and confidence that this can work for you, too.

"We worked so hard to have our daughter with us, and I hated to admit that I wasn't enjoying her, and our other kids were really suffering. Our lives revolved around what

she was or wasn't putting in her mouth. I finally feel that we are moving in the right di-
rection. Our stress at mealtimes is way down, she's happier at the table, and we can see
her eating slowly starting to improve. I am beginning to enjoy my family again, and it
feels great." — Kelly, mother of three-year-old Bailey, adopted from China

Every experience and interaction I have had, every interview with a parent or professional for this book, has strengthened my belief in the Trust Model as a way to help adopting families who are so desperately looking for a helping hand out of that feeding problem spiral.

How to Use This Book

Though primarily intended for parents or anyone doing the work of parenting and fostering, this practical guide is useful for extended family, caregivers, and professionals working with adopting and fostering families. Ideally, this information will be part of the adoption process, like learning about discipline, trauma, attachment, and routine. Families need to learn about feeding so they can anticipate common challenges, and start off on the right foot. Remember, feeding is fundamental to attachment.

> This book is about *how* to feed. I am limiting the information on what parents choose to feed their children to the basics of food groups and balance in terms of fats, proteins, and carbohydrates. What families put on the table is personal, with cultural, and financial factors playing a role. Excellent resources abound on cooking and more, if you are interested. In Chapter 8, "What About the What," I will briefly discuss dietary changes, including gluten- and casein-free diets, and touch on nutrition fears that come up repeatedly with my clients. While I don't endorse any particular diet or eating style, I will review how you can support a healthy feeding relationship, which is essential no matter what you feed your family.

As a feeding specialist, many families who come to me may be experiencing typical food battles, or may find themselves in real crisis. We will explore in depth the most common concerns, from underweight, overweight, and picky eating to oral-motor (mechanical or anatomical problems with chewing and swallowing), sensory system issues, and more.

Many of you aren't currently struggling or won't struggle with feeding, and I don't want this book to frighten you. Even if things are going relatively well, being able to anticipate and get through common feeding challenges will help you feel more confident as you deal with the limit-testing and food quirks that every family inevitably faces.

If you are considering adopting or fostering, or are waiting to welcome your child home, I suggest you read this book from beginning to end to cover most scenarios.

If you are already in the thick of it, you know who you are; you can use the index or table of contents to find the topics that relate to your situation, and learn as much as you can. Start the feeding and intake journal in the addendum and work through "Taking the Lead" (Chapter 9) to explore how your own history with food might make interpreting your child's signals more difficult.

What You Will Learn

This book is divided into two parts. Part I, "What Are You Worried About? Learning How to Feed Your Family," covers an introduction to the Trust Model, where we are now, and how we got here with feeding, as well as a comprehensive look at the main feeding and weight worries I see, which are:

- Special Needs and Feeding—including oral-motor and sensory concerns (Chapter 3)
- Low-Weight Worries, Picky Eating, and Power Struggles (Chapter 4)
- Food Preoccupation and Concerns About Weight Gain (Chapter 5)

Each of these three chapters will walk you through a process similar to what I do with clients:

- Address the underlying worry through a general review of terms, relevant research, and background, as well as share stories from families who have been there.
- Review how and why parents usually get stuck.
- Describe what transitioning to the Trust Model and healing the feeding relationship looks like, including preparing you for common stumbling blocks.

Part II, "Making It Work: There's More You Need to Know" (Chapters 6–10), covers topics ranging from eating disorders to common nutrition worries, as well as how to help children learn the difference between emotions and the physical feelings of hunger and fullness. These chapters are less linearly organized and are meant to address a wide array of topics and challenges you might face, including the questions that came up most frequently with my clients or tripped up families with their transition to the Trust Model.

You will see some overlap and repeated themes throughout the book. For example, if you are struggling with selective eating, the chapters on picky eating and power struggles, oral-motor, and "underweight," may all be relevant, and some of the experiences, worries, and themes are similar.

This book is not organized by age, as many feeding books are. For one thing, the information needs to be accessible to families with infants, teens, and every age in between. Happily, the basic feeding philosophy is the same. Also, some children can have significant developmental delay, so chronological information may not be helpful.

As you read, feel free to take notes in the margins. Observe what is working—and what is not—for *your* family right now, and what does and what doesn't feel good with feeding. Some ideas for note taking include:

- Does a story remind you of your child or another child you know? *"I see my niece begging for food all day long, and my sister is constantly trying to get her to eat less."*
- Do any parts resonate with you? *"That was me. I was forced to eat sweet potatoes, and I won't touch them to this day."*
- Do some parts upset you, or is there advice you think you *know* won't work for your family? *"If we serve dessert with the meal, he'll never eat a vegetable."*
- Are there stories or tips from parents that give you hope?
- Pay particular attention to the sections or recommendations that make you upset or uncomfortable, that resonate with you, or make you say, "Yes!" or "Ah-ha!"

Families have graciously shared their stories. More than one parent has said, *"This has been so awful; please share our story so that other families won't go through what we did. If this can help someone, it will mean so much to me."* The parents interviewed for this book say that support from other parents who have been there is most inspiring, so I have tried to include as much of their wisdom as possible.

I hope that you might recognize your own children, families, and struggles in the stories on these pages, and get inspiration and practical advice.

Let this resource be your welcome to the world of the Trust Model of feeding, and perhaps be a companion book to Ellyn Satter's comprehensive feeding book, *Child of Mine*, which is recommended by many international adoption and feeding clinics, or Satter's *Secrets of Feeding a Healthy Family*.

I will recommend books, articles, and DVDs throughout the text and on my Website under "Resources" at www.thefeedingdoctor.com.

Special Notes

Health at Every Size

I work from a "Health At Every Size" (HAES) approach, which means I accept that children come in a range of shapes and sizes. This is especially true for children who may have experienced severe malnutrition or neglect with feeding. A child can be healthy, happy, and thriving at a range of weights, just as parents can also be healthy at a range of weights. Therefore, this book is a safe resource for parents of small or large children. When I write "obese" or "underweight" in quotations, it indicates that this is a label given to the child based on growth chart cutoffs, and may or may not have any clinical relevance.

The Sensory Symbol

Look for this symbol for specific sensory tips or stories, but know that all the information in the book can help children with sensory concerns. (Chapter 3 deals more thoroughly with sensory processing and integration challenges; therefore, you will not see the symbol in that chapter.)

When I think of sensory processing challenges, the image of a computer processor comes to mind, like the intricate neural pathways that process incoming sensory information. The reality, though, is more hopeful. Brains are "plastic," meaning they can change and grow, with new neural pathways laid down over time.

Gender References
I will alternate "he" and "she" throughout.

Let's get started!

Chapter 1

Where Are We, and How Did We Get Here?

When your child is first home with you, you may feel like you live in a bubble. You might marvel over little toes or admire the older child's skill with a baseball or her quick wit. You may be struggling with developmental delays or behavioral outbursts. Extended family comes to visit, you go back to work—or not—and life goes on, but at the end of the day, it's you and your child: your family.

It is with intention that I say this book is to help you feed your adoptive or foster *family*, rather than only feed your adopted or foster *child*. She is fed, and eats best, within the context of your family, whether that includes you and your child, a partner, biological children, extended family, etc. The beauty of the Trust Model of feeding is that it works for families. It works for adopted and biological children, and adults also do well with feeding themselves this way. (See "Eating Competence" in Chapter 6, page 165).

The adoptive and fostering families I work with may have special challenges, but surprisingly, all of the families who come to me with feeding and weight concerns are more alike than different. For example, Jennifer, a mother of two girls adopted from Guatemala, was relieved to hear that it is common in all families for struggles with selective eating to begin or worsen during major transitions, such as when a new sibling enters the picture. *"I'm so glad to hear that other families went through this, too. I always worried I screwed her up somehow, or because of the adoption that things were especially bad."*

Regardless of your child's history with food, her genetic makeup, malnutrition, weight, or catch-up growth, no family lives in a bubble. The culture your children live in affects how you feed and how your children feel about food and their bodies. In Chapter 9, Taking the Lead, you will also be asked to examine your own feeding history, how it affects your own eating, and how you feed now.

From the outside world of schools, doctor's offices, and women's magazines to the familiar world of your kitchen, what are you and society bringing to the table? In this chapter we start with where we are culturally with food and look back at how we got here in order to understand why parents and their kids get stuck in unhelpful feeding dynamics. In the next chapter, I will introduce the Trust Model of feeding to help you overcome your feeding worries and challenges.

Where We Are Now

In spite of what the current national focus on children and weight would lead us to believe, we are not facing an "obesity" crisis, we are facing a *feeding* crisis.

Consider:

- Almost half of parents prepare separate meals for their grade-school children.[1]
- One in three parents will seek help with feeding from a child's physician.[2]
- Roughly 80 percent of kids with developmental problems will have trouble with feeding.[3]
- Early feeding problems correlate with accelerated adolescent weight gain[4] and an increased risk of the onset of eating disorders.[5,6]
- Parental worry about obesity, even in a "normal" weight child, correlates with accelerated adolescent weight gain.[4]
- Parents who pressure with feeding—and 85 to 95 percent of American parents do—tend to have kids who are more picky and struggle with weight. [7,8,9,10]
- Eating disorder diagnoses are on the rise, and in ever-younger children.[11,12]
- One in three preschoolers eats no vegetables, and one in four eats no fruit on any given day.[13]
- Two-thirds of teens diet, with half of those using extreme measures like vomiting, fasting, and laxatives.[14]
- Roughly half of nine-year-olds wish they were thinner, and about half of the nine-year-old girls in an American study said they felt better about themselves when they diet.[15]

The vast majority of family doctors and pediatricians receive no training in feeding and don't understand, nor are they aware of, the relevant research.

There is plenty of discussion on TV, parenting magazines, and blogs about how to get kids back to good nutrition and health habits. Most of the focus is on *what* kids are eating, with ideas like banning chocolate milk in schools or taxing sugar-sweetened drinks. What you might not hear is information about the feeding relationship and how we can raise kids to feel good about food. But *how* we feed our kids matters—a lot.

I don't know of any parent who is not aware that children should eat more fruits and veggies or drink milk or water instead of soda. I hear health teachers bemoan the fact that kids "know" carrots are healthier than chips, but they "always choose the chips." Parents know roughly what kids "should" be eating but can't figure out how to make it happen, and they get stuck in frustrating battles that most often make kids eat less variety and too much or too little.

**How you feed is the key to what kids eat,
and how they grow up feeling about food.**

Why Are We Here?

Based on my clinical experience, interpretation of the research, and interactions with parents and professionals, it seems that a basic lack of knowledge and misperceptions around nutrition, growth, and development are at the root of most counterproductive feeding practices. What we don't know or understand can hurt us.

> To help you approach this information with an open mind, take the brief True-False quiz in Appendix 1: Fact or Fiction. You may be surprised that some or much of what you think you know about feeding, food, and weight is wrong, as was the case for me years ago.

The key knowledge gaps, misunderstandings, and worries that affect feeding are:
- Misunderstanding and worry about eating patterns and how kids learn to eat.
- Misunderstanding and worry about growth and development of the child.
- Belief that pressuring a child to eat more or less will work to:
  - determine weight, either up or down,
  - increase intake of fruits and vegetables, and
  - get kids to try new foods.

Let's review these three areas to prepare for the more in-depth application of the principles of the Trust Model in Chapters 3, 4, and 5.

Misunderstanding and Worry About Eating Patterns

Eating capabilities are inborn[16,17] and cover two basic areas: self-regulation and food acceptance.

Self-Regulation

Self-regulation is the ability to eat the amount of food needed to grow at a steady rate. Infants are born with this skill, which they can retain if parents do a good job with feeding and parenting.

Standard nutrition education and resources imply that a child of a certain age or weight should eat a certain amount or eat certain portion sizes at meals and snack times. That's simply not how young children eat.

Rebecca recalls that when eight-month-old Adina arrived from Ethiopia, she was told that Adina had been "overfed" in the orphanage, as her weight-for-length was close to the 80th percentile. The result of the pediatrician's worry over size and subsequent recommendations to limit formula meant that even though Adina screamed after every bottle and seemed clearly interested in eating more, her mother still thought it best to limit her to the amount the doctor told her was healthy. Rebecca's trust in Adina was undermined right from the start.

Tamara, mom to three-year-old Alvin, adopted from Haiti, asked, *"Does malnutrition in-utero mean my son can't self-regulate? If I don't limit him, he won't stop eating."* If your child isn't self-regulating—which means to eat the right amount for healthy growth—many other factors may play a role, including medical issues, feeding practices, attachment concerns, and the impact of his feeding history. Children who were malnourished in-utero may have also experienced early growth delay due to poor feeding. Many of these children do catch up and eat large amounts initially. (See Chapter 5 on catch-up growth and food insecurity.) Your son may have stabilized at a higher-than-average but healthy-for-him weight. If the rate isn't continuing to accelerate (assuming he is done with catch-up growth), he is probably fine. I am not convinced that children are incapable of regulating intake due to in-utero conditions. While there is some correlation between in-utero malnutrition and later health problems, the research on this topic is not conclusive. Many who experienced in-utero malnutrition do just fine with self-regulation. Trust that your son can do it. Assume that his experience of food scarcity means that attempts to limit his eating may worsen his anxiety and actually contribute to what seems like overeating.

Adina is now two and a half years old, and the family is transitioning to the Trust Model. Rebecca says, *"I did what the doctor told us to do. Now I wonder: If I had given her a few more ounces here and there and let her decide when she was done, maybe she wouldn't have developed such a serious food obsession."*

Children do very little "by the books," including how they eat. The amounts and types of food young children eat vary greatly any given day or week. A healthy child might eat half of a cracker and a bite of banana for lunch one day but consume two bananas and an entire piece of bread with three slices of lunchmeat the next. This is normal. In addition, one child may eat far more than another, and both can be healthy. We all know adults who eat large amounts and stay lean, or relatively fatter adults who eat little.

"My children have very different body types—Fannah is much more "solid" than her brother Beckett, who is like a little bird—and she has much more of a need to burn off energy than he does. Clearly their bodies ask for different things. They are both growing steadily, though she is on the high end of the curve and he is on the low end."

— Elsa, mother of Fannah, age six, adopted from Ethiopia, and biological son Beckett, age eight

"Breakfast the other day consisted of one Greek yogurt, a decent-sized bowl of raisin bran, a whole banana, and half a grilled cheese sandwich. Lunch was less impressive, but he can put away a surprising amount of food."

— Molly, mother of Colin, age 18 months, who is growing steadily at about the 50th percentile

This normal but seemingly erratic eating pattern can confuse and worry parents, especially if they are also concerned about a child's size. The parent of a small child will often try to get the child to eat more, while the parent of a large child may feel alarmed by a hearty appetite and try to get the child to eat less. **Knowing that normal patterns of eating can mean a lot of food for one meal or one day and less the next will help you trust this process.** Note: A child who has experienced severe food restriction or unreliable feeding or starvation will often eat very large amounts for some time.

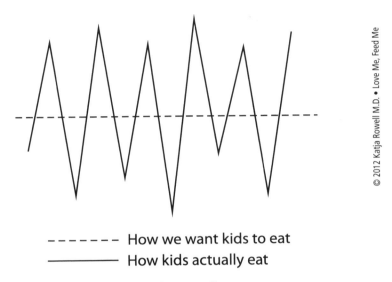

© 2012 Katja Rowell M.D. • Love Me, Feed Me

- - - - - - - How we want kids to eat
————————— How kids actually eat

1.1 Schematic of how we want kids to eat, and how they actually eat

Food Acceptance

Food acceptance refers to the innate human drive to seek out a variety of foods. Kids want to grow up to eat a variety,[17,18] but *what* a child chooses to eat from one day to the next is as unpredictable as how much. Trying to predict what a child will eat will make you crazy. Even if they make a special request, they are still bound to reject it. If you like bananas and you want to provide the opportunity for your little one to grow up learning to like them, you need to keep serving them. One day out of the blue, she will probably enjoy bananas again.

"Well, it took two years, but over the last week Cori has started eating cucumbers, and just tonight, finally tried eggs! Two years of waiting patiently, not forcing, just offering... and we still see it pay off!" — Alicia, mother of Cori, age four

"Since he's developed an opinion about what he eats, green foods are out. It's so curious to me. He calls broccoli "trees" and puts them in his mouth, but promptly spits them out.

Until two days ago he had been a savage for broccoli. He has also hated hummus since day one—until today. I fear the diaper after all those heaping spoonfuls."
— Molly, mom to Colin, age 18 months

Children do not eat by rules such as the U.S. Department of Agriculture's (USDA) Food Pyramid or the newer USDA "Myplate,"[19] or even eat from all the food groups at every meal or snack. Often, children pick and choose one or two things from what is offered. At the end of the day—or even the week—it tends to even out.[6,17,21]

Nutrition Evens Out: Three Examples From Parents

"One day my toddler ate apples for breakfast, sour cream and chives for lunch, brown rice with tamari for snack, and roasted chicken for dinner. It was wild. But after three years of this, I know I can relax because she knows what she needs. Her preschool teacher tells me she is the best example of mindful eating she has ever seen. Take that, USDA food pyramid or plate or whatever you are these days!" — Hillary, mother of a two-and-a-half-year-old

"One day last weekend my daughter ate four slices of toast for breakfast. At lunch I made her a quesadilla (a usual favorite) and she had two bites, but ate about a cup and a half of cottage cheese. I trust her now to take in what she needs." — Meghan, mother of an 18-month-old

"I see patterns with my six-year-old son; in fact, there still is the occasional day where he eats very little (calorically) and then he eats a lot on a different day, similar to when he was much younger." — Chloe, mother of a six-year-old boy adopted from Guatemala at eight months

What parent hasn't heard, "It takes 10 times of trying a new food for a child to learn to like it?" It would be nice if it were so simple. Children who are slow to warm up, have a troubled feeding past, or have developmental or neuromuscular or sensory issues may need from dozens to *hundreds* of exposures. Those exposures also need to be pleasant and free of pressure. And of course, ice cream and other easy-to-like foods usually take one try before they are enthusiastically accepted.

Even the "neurotypical child," with no oral-motor or other identifiable feeding challenges, can take a long time to learn to like new foods. Hydee Becker, RD, a pediatric dietitian who has consulted with our families, served chicken in every possible preparation to her son for more than two years before he ventured to try a drumstick. By age four he was eating and enjoying chicken prepared in a variety of ways.

Misunderstanding How Kids Learn to Eat

Learning to like new foods is not a logical, linear process; it is experiential. To like a new food, your child first has to see others enjoy it, ideally at a family meal; then she might smell it or touch it, put it in her mouth and spit it out, and eventually swallow it. Parents often have trouble interpreting signals from the child and confuse the process of learning to like new foods with rejection. Many infants squint and frown with new foods, but with repeated exposures they learn to like them. In one example, although the infants studied accepted and were eating green beans after eight exposures, the mothers' perceptions were that the children didn't like them. [20]

The process of learning to like new foods goes quickly for some children and very slowly for others. One of my early clients was a dietitian whose toddler, Chelsea, only ate plain pasta and rice, crying for them first thing every morning. On our second call, Mom was discouraged because Chelsea had chewed a blueberry but spit it out. I, on the other hand, was elated. Chelsea had never put a blueberry in her mouth before. In addition, the crying for pasta first thing in the morning had stopped. Chelsea and her parents were on their way.

Underestimating what a child will like is common. On one grocery run, I was behind a man in the frozen fruit section. As his daughter toddled along, pointing to and reaching for various bags, he scolded, "No Sophie, you don't like raspberries, no Sophie, you don't like blueberries, no Sophie, you don't like mangos." Dad was doing two things that will make it harder for Sophie to expand her tastes. First, I assume he is not buying foods she doesn't readily accept, thus missing out on exposing her to a variety of foods; and second, he is cementing her identity as the "picky eater" and giving her the message that she *can't* learn to like new foods. Similarly, another mom—this time standing in line at an Indian restaurant buffet—said to her daughter, "Well, you probably won't like anything here, but they do have rice."

Yiseth, adopted from Guatemala as an infant, is a 16-year-old member of her school's tennis team and less than a year into the transition to the Trust Model with her family. She says, *"Sometimes as my mom started making more recipes again, a food would come up, and I'd say, 'Oh my gosh, I love that,' and my parents would say, 'Really? You do?' It might be something we hadn't had for years because they thought I didn't like it."* (To be fair to Yiseth's mom and dad, she had probably rejected that very same food multiple times.)

Another client with three boys was worried about protein. I asked if she had tried shrimp, and Mom said, *"Oh no, they don't like shrimp."* Dad looked at her, then me, and said, *"We haven't had shrimp since we moved into this house—five years ago."*

Misunderstanding Growth

Currently, our nation is intensely focused on childhood obesity, and we have seen increased rates of "overweight" and "obese" kids in the last 30 years. However, many parents, and even health care professionals, misunderstand normal growth—with harmful consequences. According to the Centers for Disease Control and Prevention and the National Institutes of Health, body mass index (BMI) is not a diagnostic tool but rather a preliminary screen, and it is certainly not meant to diagnose a health problem.

Experts and scholarly articles, including one on the American Heart Association's Website, acknowledge that BMI is not a reliable predictor of health for the individual.[22,23] Many children who are labeled as "overweight" or "obese" or "underweight" based on the BMI-chart percentile are actually growing in a normal and healthy way—for them.

> Interpreting growth can be far more complex for the adopted or foster child for various reasons:
> - The height and weight of the biological parents is often unknown.
> - The height and weight of the biological parents is known, and the worry that a biological parent is "obese" affects feeding.
> - Early feeding in an institutional or neglectful home can have profound consequences on growth and initial eating behaviors.[24,25,26]
> - Stress and growth are intimately related. Research shows that children who have spent time in an institutional setting have prolonged hormonal variations, including growth hormones, cortisol, and others, which affects both catch-up growth and, for some, the timing of the onset of puberty.[27] For example, children from neglectful or traumatic situations have higher cortisol levels.

Faith in Numbers?

BMI is not a reliable proxy for health, even though it is most often viewed that way in conventional wisdom. Much of the standard medical advice in the last few decades has focused on encouraging individuals to fit into the "normal" weight range as currently defined in adults by a BMI of 18.5–24.9. What this advice ignores is that not all bodies were meant to be in this range and that many bodies can be bigger or smaller and be healthy.

> "Normal" BMI was originally up to 28 for women and 27 for men until the cutoff was lowered in 1998. As a result, millions of Americans went to bed "normal" and woke up the next morning "overweight."

This concept is illustrated by the bell curve for a population, with most people's weight falling around middle or average and fewer people on the lower or higher ends. BMI approximates this Bell curve distribution, and while most people are around the middle or average weight, there will always be those who are leaner and those who are fatter. They are not *abnormal* by default; there are just fewer of them in the population as a whole. The current standard arbitrarily defines 85th percentile as "overweight" and mislabels many people who are healthy in this weight range. I've always wondered why 24.9 is considered "healthy" and 25.0 is "overweight." Do those few ounces confer the risk implied by the label?

Arbitrary cutoffs and weight goals are not innocuous, as trying to force the broad range of healthy human bodies into only the middle part of the curve actually drives more people to the extremes through dieting, disordered eating, and other practices that fight physiology and psychology.

There have always been, and will always be, healthy "skinny" and healthy "chubby" kids and adults.

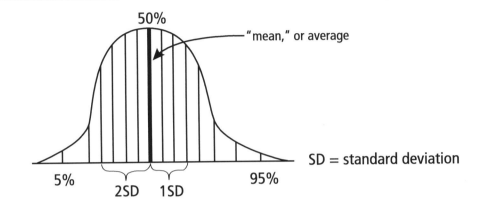

1.2: Bell Curve

Following Growth Over Time

What matters most is the pattern of growth. If a child has always been big and the relative percentile is tracking about the same, that is a reassuring growth pattern. However, if the rate of weight gain increases or decreases over time, that is more likely to indicate a problem and should be looked into.[28] Also keep in mind the possibility of catch-up growth, which is easy to misinterpret.

Relying on BMI alone as an indicator of health not only leads to the mislabeling of many healthy and larger-than-average children, but also misses a significant portion of children in the "normal" weight range who may have higher fat-to-lean-body-mass ratio or have unhealthy habits.[29] Most adults who struggle with weight were "normal" or "underweight" as children.[30] If we want to raise happy and healthy adults, we need to look at the whole picture and not be falsely alarmed or ignore poor health in "normal" weight children based on BMI alone.

When a health care provider sees a growth deviation, either up or down, the question must be: *What is happening that this child is no longer able to eat and grow at a steady rate?*[31] This evaluation is complex, with multiple possible contributing factors, such as medical issues, a history of malnutrition or unsupportive feeding, current feeding practices, and social, nutritional, or behavioral influences. Alas, most clinicians only think to ask, "What and how much is that child eating?" No matter what other factors may be playing a role, the feeding relationship must be supported and can't be separated from other concerns.

Interpreting Growth Curves

Because growth is an important indicator of a child's overall well-being and health and may be the main focus of your visits with your child's health care provider, you need some understanding of the uses and limitations of growth curves and the labels doctors use. Parents are often confused by growth curves; therefore, I will spend some time on this discussion and include some weight-for-length charts for further explanation. (When there is a significant crossing of percentile lines on the weight-for-length chart as in cases B and D below, it is important to look at both height-for-age and weight-for-age, and Z-score calculations may further help to clarify the situation.)

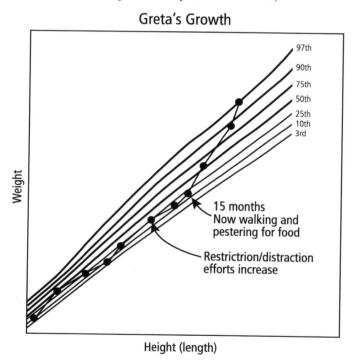

1. 3: "Steady" growth doesn't mean your child's growth must plot exactly along a percentile line. There is usually some variation around a general area on the curve, as seen on Greta's growth chart. As children grow, weight often increases first, followed by height, which results in a wavy pattern on the weight-for-height chart. Rapid catch-up growth may look like a tidal wave but is not problematic for the growth-delayed child. Concerning patterns that require investigation include steep ups or downs, as in the Greta's growth after 15 months of age. (Sustained gradual deviation may be normal, but screening for healthy feeding and behaviors is in order.)

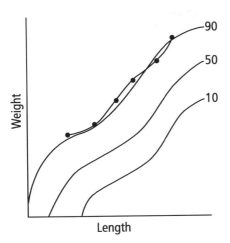

1.4: Chart A—High and Steady. This child is large compared to the overall population but is growing at a steady rate. If the child has healthy eating patterns and behaviors, this is probably healthy growth. Efforts to reduce weight, such as calorie or portion restriction, are likely to backfire. Parents should continue supporting healthy behaviors.

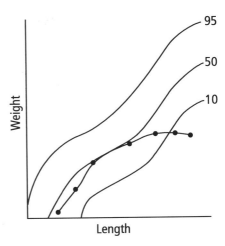

1.5: Chart B—Growth Deceleration. Note the clear deceleration in this pattern. This child is rapidly crossing percentiles and needs further evaluation.

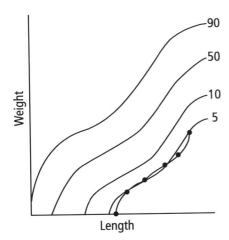

1.6: Chart C—Low and Steady. This child is small but growing at a steady rate. If an evaluation of feeding and health behaviors doesn't indicate a concern, this is probably healthy growth. Parents should continue monitoring and supporting behaviors that support good health.

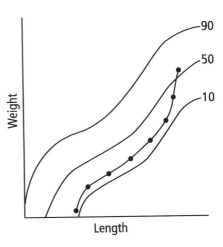

1.7: Chart D—Growth Acceleration. Note the dramatic shift across percentiles. Further evaluation is needed to determine why this child is growing at such a rapid rate. Timing and history helps determine if this is catch-up growth. Medical and nutritional issues, as well as a thorough understanding of the feeding relationship, must be considered.

Body Type and BMI

Many parents and clinicians don't take into account that there are ethnic differences in terms of body type. On the standard American growth charts, the current definition of "overweight" is a BMI above the 85th percentile. However, for Navajos[32] and some Central or South American populations, the mean BMI is close to the 85th percentile, [33,34] meaning that roughly half the population may have a BMI below this number and half above. Most pediatric offices would therefore label half the population as "overweight" with current cutoffs. Is it clinically meaningful to label children who are about average for their ethnicity as "overweight?" Similarly, some ethnic populations have less dense body types; therefore, children from these groups may appear "underweight" when plotted on the standard charts, when in fact their weight is healthy—for them.

There is some controversy around using growth charts from the country of origin, but it is something to consider. Growth charts from many countries are felt to be outdated and may reflect a state of general low growth for a population that was undernourished at the time the data was collected. Your international adoption doctor or adoption agency may be a good resource for these questions. The Center for Adoption Medicine has a discussion and set of charts available online. Go to their general Website and click on "Topics" and "Growth Charts." (Accessed 2012.)

Parents can avoid a lot of the worry and confusion about the role that ethnic background might play if the child's growth is tracked and he is compared only to himself.

Tracking growth matters because it is a good overall indicator of nutrition status and well-being. I spend a lot of time explaining growth because in my observation, *worry about growth* is the number one reason why parents get into feeding problems. Parents of big kids are often told to worry that their child is fat and will be unhealthy, even though the child is healthy and growing consistently or is having a period of accelerated, but unproblematic, catch-up growth. Conversely, parents of small children are also told to worry and are encouraged to try to get the child to eat more.

Growth must be assessed as accurately as possible. One mother told me about how her "failure-to-thrive" daughter, who was being considered for a feeding tube, was weighed. Mom was incredulous when one visit her daughter was weighed in her underpants and the next visit she was weighed in shoes, jeans, and T-shirt. Clearly this was not a helpful comparison and would tell little about the child's nutrition or health. I have also seen growth charts where height was documented as *less* from one visit to the next, and the resulting "weight-for-height" measure, when added to the growth chart, distorted the picture. Advocate for accurate measurements, using the same scale and experienced staff.

If your child is new to your family, ideally you would have two measurements at least two months apart to assess a pattern of growth. It is not okay to label a child as "overweight" or "obese" if their weight is healthy and normal for that child. The same holds true for children on the lower end of the growth curve. (Clearly, if your child is nutritionally compromised or there are weight worries, do not wait two months to follow and assess weight. You don't want to miss a problem or let them decline in health or growth. Follow up with your child's doctor or RD.)

What Factors Play a Role in Weight?

Unhealthy weight patterns often have multiple contributing factors. We need to start asking:

- *How* is the child fed, not just *what*?
- What else is happening in the child's life that is not allowing him to eat and grow in a healthy way?

It turns out that *how* a child is fed impacts weight. Restricting (calories, portions, kinds of foods), allowing grazing, pressuring with feeding, and having a parent who diets and binges are all factors associated with unhealthy eating and weight patterns in children.[35,36,37] Other factors associated with unhealthy weight patterns are:

- Stress or chaos in the home
- Poverty and food insecurity—not having reliable access to enough food
- History of dieting, restriction, or neglectful feeding
- Lack of adequate sleep[38,39,40]
- Lack of family meals[41]
- Excessive time in front of the TV[39]
- Certain medical conditions such as thyroid problems or cystic fibrosis, to name a few
- Medications that influence appetite
- Parenting style. Authoritative parenting, which is parenting with the appropriate balance of love and limits, is associated with healthy weight, while neglectful or authoritarian (think drill sergeant) parenting styles are associated with less healthy weight patterns.[42]

I would venture a guess that the majority of foster children have experienced many of the above risk factors, which may help to explain why as a group, foster children have higher rates of "obesity."[43]

Some children will naturally be small, but that might not be a problem. Others, who have experienced growth delay due to malnutrition or poor early care, might never catch up with the population average, but again, if they are growing at a steady rate, there may not be a problem. As Sue says about her daughter Mary, *"She's settled on her own line below the growth charts, but she's growing steadily."* If the child is otherwise healthy and thriving and growing steadily, even at or below the third percentile, it is likely healthy growth for her, and a label of "failure to thrive" is then inaccurate.

As you can see, weight and growth are complex, but understanding growth and labels will help you avoid counterproductive feeding. This brings us to our final knowledge gap: The belief that pressure with feeding helps.

The Belief That Pressure With Feeding Helps

Parents use different feeding tactics because they "work"—in the short term. Bribing with dessert or the "two-bite rule" might work to get a child to eat two bites of broccoli tonight, or it might lead to a 90-minute standoff. Your daughter may eat a little more if her favorite DVD is on or if you hand her a toy with every bite, but do these tricks teach your child to eat and enjoy these foods?

If you have tried these strategies, you are not alone. The norm for feeding in the United States does not seem to help children learn to eat the variety and the amount needed for healthy growth. Studies show that 85 to 90 percent [44,45,46] of American parents feed in what some refer to as a "control model" where kids are pressured, pushed, begged, and bribed to eat more or less, which is not consistent with the Trust Model.

You're probably doing it or heard others pressure, "Come on Timmy, you need to have two more bites of chicken before you can have dessert," or "You have to try two bites of everything before you can have more chicken nuggets." Or it's those tips you learned to get the baby to finish the bottle when you were babysitting: tickle her cheek, jiggle the bottle, and other tactics.

Here's a rundown of tactics from one study. "Typical negative food-related behaviors of parents with two- to five-year-old children: bargaining, bribing, and forcing; promising a special food, such as dessert, for eating a meal; withholding food as punishment; rewarding good behavior with food; persuading children to eat; playing a game to get children to eat; taking over and feeding children who refuse to eat; threatening punishment for not eating; and making children clean their plates." [44]

Pressure doesn't always appear negative; even the subtle disguise of "encouragement" can still feel like pressure to many children. Some examples include:

- Praise
- Rewards (stickers or toys)
- Letting kids watch TV or play with toys at the table so they eat
- Letting children sit on parent's lap to eat more
- Letting children leave the table and then come back for food handouts
- Overselling food (going on about how great it is)
- Going to the store to buy five different kinds of pesto after your daughter tried it once at a restaurant
- Excessive attention

One client's selective son had some early success with the Trust Model, and provided an example of excessive attention as a form of pressure. Mom complained during a call that her son Benji wouldn't even try a hot dog. When we delved further, she realized that while he was sitting at the table—the only one with a hot dog—Mom, Dad, Grandma, Grandpa, and brother Jim were staring at him. She laughed when she realized that as Benji was about to take a bite, he looked up to see several expectant sets of eyes. He simply looked around, put the hot dog down, and refused to eat anything more. Even nonverbal cues can pressure.

Why Do Parents Pressure?

Parents pressure because they love their children and because they want to be good parents. The worry is the fire, pressure is the smoke, and our culture around food, including advice from parents and professionals, fans the flames.

Parents pressure with feeding for the following reasons:

- Concern about the child's size.
- Nutrition concerns, including wanting the child to eat certain food groups such as protein, dairy, fruits, and veggies.
- It seems to work in the short-term.
- Sleep. Parents often want the child to finish a bottle or eat more at the last meal or snack of the day so they don't wake up "hungry" in the middle of the night.
- Financial concerns. Formula is expensive, and wasting food feels wrong.
- Habit. It's how the parents were fed.
- It's the cultural norm.
- "Experts" advise pressure tactics ranging from "two-bite rule" to the ominous, "Do whatever you have to, just get food into that kid."
- Using food for behavior control in the form of punishment, reward, or a way to keep a child calm.

When I consult with parents struggling with feeding, we need to uncover and address the worry that motivates the feeding behaviors. Is it a valid fear? If not, how can we reassure parents? If it is valid, is the current approach helping or harming, and is there a better way?

Labels Lead to Worry, Which Leads to Pressure

Kids grow in a variety of shapes and sizes that can be healthy. Labeling a large, healthy, growing child as "overweight" or "obese" or a small child as "underweight" will not make him or her healthier. Studies support what my clients tell me, which is that labeling a child *increases* parental worry, which often leads to harmful interventions and unnecessary pressure on feeding. Remember the cycle of worry, pressure, and worsening feeding problems parents get stuck in? (See page 3 for a refresher.) It is common for families to get started on the cycle due to the relentless worry sparked by labels like "failure to thrive" and "obese."

This worry makes it harder to follow the Trust Model. If parents are told their child is "too big" or "obese," the knee-jerk reaction is to try to get him to eat less, while parents who are told their child is "too small" will try to pressure her to eat more. Studies show that neither works; pressure tends to backfire.

Why Does Pressure Backfire?

Think of it in terms of a child's development. Your child will need to learn to trust you to attach. Once he is securely attached, eventually the job of the adopted and foster child, like anyone else, is to become a separate individual from the parents. This leads to the natural and necessary tension, and even open conflict, around autonomy such as the stereotypical "terrible twos." The child wants control and will fight for it, refusing to put on a coat or shoes or to brush her teeth. Simple tasks can become monumental battles.

What if you are dealing with a child who has experienced significant trauma, abuse, or neglect, or has attachment difficulties? It is invaluable to anticipate that the child may seek out opportunities for conflict, and you need to be prepared to neutralize power struggles over food.

According to Gregory Keck and Regina Kupecky, authors of *Parenting the Hurt Child*, these children are often "afraid to be cooperative, compliant, and receptive. To them, such behavior represents giving in, which translates to losing . . . Consequently they choreograph battles over the most insignificant issues."[47] One bite of rice can seem like an insignificant issue, but to a child who will not lose, it is anything but.

It's Just One Bite, or Is It?

Two popular pieces of feeding advice: The "no thank you" and "two-bite" rules result in some of the more serious, frequent, and avoidable battles I see. In the first instance, the parent is told to require that the child take one bite before he is allowed to reject a food, or say, "no, thank you." The "two-bite rule" means the child is required to eat two bites of everything at the table or on his plate.

I often hear variations on this theme, *"Our older son is a great eater, and we use the 'no-thank-you bite' rule for him. That rule helped him learn to eat with no problems, so we've been using it on our younger son, but he's really picky and we argue over that one bite for most of the meal."* Indeed, the easygoing, eager-to-please, or fearful child may go along with the rules for now, but what happens if you try these methods on the persistent or sensitive child, or the child who is locked with you in a power struggle, or the hurt child who is anxious and desperate for control? These seemingly innocuous rules can result in impressive battles, and are not consistent with the Trust Model. Parents forget that it's not about one bite—it's about control.

If what you are doing—for example, the "two-bite rule"—is working for your family and you are happy, your kids eat a good variety, and meals are pleasant, then by all means continue. Connie, mother of Ric and Alicia, relates that both of her adopted children didn't seem to mind being encouraged (not forced) to try a few bites of food and that it didn't lead to battles. In other words, it worked for her family and with her children and their temperaments. But for many clients, this tactic backfires, and they don't know any alternative.

Why Can Pressure, Both Positive and Negative, Distort the Feeding Relationship?

When you are locked in conflict over food, predictably strong emotions arise in you and your child. Stress hormones flood his system. Think about when you are upset or stressed. Are you able to tune in and listen to your body? When the child is upset or anxious or waging war at the table, the last thing he can pay attention to is the food. He is locked in battle with you, and the food is forgotten.

When you, the parent, ignore cues coming from your child and try to get him to eat more or less than he wants, that pressure and conflict compromises his trust in you. As one research paper put it, not feeding in a responsive way "has the potential to undermine the child's trust in an otherwise responsive parent."[48] This can hinder the attachment process.

That is why pressure does not help, and in most cases, worsens feeding and growth issues. In essence, you unwittingly contribute to the very outcome you are working so hard to avoid. Stress kills the appetite for the anxious child who has been pressured, causing him to eat *less*. The child who has experienced food insecurity, restriction, or neglectful feeding is prone to overeat in times of stress. Like quicksand, the more you fight and struggle, the more stuck you become.

> **Stress and mealtime battles make it hard for children to tune in to hunger and fullness cues coming from their own bodies and makes it more likely they will eat more or less than they otherwise would.**

Another anxious parent told me: *"But we don't pressure, we praise and encourage. That's what we were told to do."* Pressure sounds negative, like "push," "force," or "threaten." Many parents don't pressure in these negative ways, but they still pressure. Praising Bobby for trying a new food can feel like pressure to Bobby. Giving Suzy a sticker or a toy for eating her veggies is pressure. Clapping wildly and commenting about how brave Timmy is to try a food may feel like pressure to Timmy. Going on about the nutritional benefits and how it will make him strong is also pressure. Don't forget, if you are locked in a power struggle over food and you make a big deal of Bobby eating a piece of broccoli, you have now handed him control. He has a little green power chip.

Ashley Rhodes–Courter, author of *Three Little Words,* lived for 10 years in foster care, which included experiences of severe neglect and abuse around food. She describes the significant and lengthy conflict she had with Gay, her adoptive mother, over food. *"I knew Gay was trying to please me, but for some reason, I resisted every attempt she made. She made chicken nuggets in the oven so they'd have the KFC flavor, but not as much fat. They were quite good, although I was annoyed by the way she preached to me about eating healthy foods."*[49]

What Kids Think About "Positive" Pressure Like Praise and Rewards
- "Hmm, Mom really cares about me eating broccoli, and I want to annoy Mom." (You see where this is going.)
- The persistent or independent child who wants it to be *his* idea; he wants to be in control and may feel robbed of that feeling if he is encouraged or praised.
- "This stuff must taste really bad if I need a reward to eat it."
- "They must not think I can do this if they are buying me a present."
- "Will they love me if I don't eat this tomorrow?"

Iris homeschools her two daughters: Ali, her biological daughter, and her youngest, Bea, who is thriving in an open, transracial adoption. Iris notes that with their schoolwork, Ali shuts down completely with any praise or direction, while Bea responds to some direction and is more eager to please adults. When she connected their learning styles to their eating, she says it was eye opening. *"I realized we had been subtly trying to get Ali to eat more foods. We knew outright pressure didn't work, so we tried games, talking up the nutrition, or praising when she tried something. Like with her schoolwork, any attempt to steer Ali toward something backfired. Bea, on the other hand, enjoys food and is more easily encouraged, but that can be a downside, too. She might finish her plate to please an adult rather than listen to her body."*

From my reading of the research, and my clinical experience, it boils down to this:
- Children who are pressured to eat more tend to eat less (Chapter 4).
- Children who are pressured to eat less tend to eat more (Chapter 5).
- Children who are pressured to eat fruits and vegetables tend to eat fewer (Chapters 4 and 6).

What matters is your child's attitude toward food. Your child doesn't have to be eating squid by age two, and you don't have to make yourself crazy exposing him to every imaginable food out there to try to train his tastes. I didn't try sushi or Thai food until my twenties, but I approached it with curiosity and a positive attitude and enjoyed them both. Kids who feel good around and about food in general will move themselves along to try and enjoy a greater variety of foods.

Think of raising a healthy and happy child as if you are planting tulips. The bulbs are planted in the fall, and it's a leap of faith that something will come up after the long, hard winter. First you prepare the soil in the garden plot. Next you lovingly mulch and compost, then you find your bulbs, plant them at the right depth, give them the right amount of water—and you wait. In the spring, the first green shoots emerge.

Even with weeds, and maybe mosquitoes, you are excited—but then you grow impatient. You've been waiting months for those flowers. You continue to water and watch. But you can't wait any longer, so you start pulling on the stems and peeling the buds apart to get at the flower faster. You can probably guess the results.

Raising a healthy eater is similar. You put in a lot of work, time, and patience, and you can do a lot to slow down the process, but not much to speed it up.

So if you can't bribe, praise, or threaten, how will your child learn to eat? How do you optimize your chances of raising a competent eater who enjoys a variety of foods and knows how much to eat based on internal cues of hunger and fullness? How do you nurture your family when it comes to food? The answer is the Trust Model of feeding.

Chapter 2
Trust Is the Goal

"Feeding was REALLY important for attachment with our daughters. For the first two months, we ate every meal possible together at the table. It really cemented us as a family of five." — Kim, mother of two adopted daughters

The Trust Model Is Healthy Feeding

The Trust Model of feeding is a way to feed well—a model of healthy feeding and of wellness. If we restore or establish structured, reliable, rewarding, and healthy eating strategies for the whole family, we allow children to rely on messages of hunger and fullness that come from *inside* their bodies, which helps them grow up to be competent eaters. Perhaps most importantly, when we feed our children reliably and with love, we teach them they can trust and rely on us as parents.

Amy tells a poignant story about her teen foster son who had a habit of running away. Early on, he disappeared for 36 hours. Amy explains that when he returned, *"… we made sure he was okay, then we threw a box of mac-n-cheese on the stove to get him some comfort food. That floored him, because it turns out he'd been denied food in his home after his running. I think this gesture ended up bonding him to us much more than anything else could have."*

The beauty of the Trust Model of feeding is that it nurtures and provides. It is a way to feed your whole family—yourself included. You can feed your biological children, your toddler, and your teen with the same underlying strategy. Your lean, lithe, labeled-as-underweight child and your stocky, muscular, labeled-as-obese soccer player are fed and loved the same way. You don't have to make yourself and your kids crazy trying to feed them differently. It doesn't matter what your child's chronological or developmental age is—you feed in a reliable and responsive way without ricocheting from one strategy to the next. Bottom line: You can feed with confidence *and* joy.

Consider Lila's dilemma. Lila adopted two half-sisters from foster care. Her four-year-old daughter Martha was growing steadily at around the 10th percentile. At seven, her older sister Julia, who had grown steadily at around the 75th percentile for years, had recently experienced weight acceleration into the "obese" category at the 90th percentile. Almost a year ago, alarmed by the large portions Julia was eating, Lila started using "green-light/red-light" food rules, which meant Julia could eat as much fruit and vegetables (green-light foods) as she wanted but was limited on everything else (red-light foods). Julia was also not allowed to have juice or any treats or desserts unless they were sugar-free. Almost every meal ended in tears.

Lila complained, *"I'm shoving ice cream and milk shakes at Martha and keeping them out of Julia's hands. My husband gets angry if he finds out Julia had a treat. He blames me for not controlling her. Julia is totally obsessed with dessert and candy. When we go to a friend's house she hounds them for all the stuff we can't let her have. It's embarrassing, and I'm worried Julia is heading for an eating disorder!"*

Julia and Martha can both be trusted with eating. In fact, trying to feed children differently doesn't work. Trying to get Martha to eat more causes conflict, and trying to get Julia to eat less isn't working either. The message they both get is that they aren't okay as they are, they can't handle eating, and they can't trust their bodies when it comes to food. Also, when parents are locked in conflict around food or when parents are told to deny their child food, attachment and trust are challenged on a most fundamental level. Everyone is miserable.

Or consider Sue. Her adopted daughter Mary had been part of their family for more than a year, and her eating issues—primarily oral-motor delay and possible sensory concerns—were largely resolved. When her son Marcus arrived, he seemed to want to eat only cheese and bread. His tantrums ruined meals for the whole family. Sue recalls, *"I did not know how to get out of the tantrum cycle without simply letting him eat whatever he did or didn't want. And to do that felt too lacking in parental boundaries for me. I did not know how to maintain expectations for my daughter at the table, but I set entirely different expectations of my son."*

> **Parents know intuitively that using opposing strategies to feed children in the same family doesn't work, but don't know how to handle the different challenges and temperaments at the table.**

The answer: Feed them the same way. The principles in this book can be applied to both your adopted and biological children, including children with special needs.

"We were desperate for help for our food-obsessed son. That dynamic was completely taking over our family. Unexpectedly, this Trust Model is helping our older son too, who is pretty picky and on the small side. A week into this and our 'food-obsessed' son is breaking free from his food anxieties, and our picky eater actually helped himself to some chicken the other night with no prompting. All of this is beyond our expectations."
— Anneliese, mother of two boys, one adopted, one biological

Temperament refers to the characteristics of the child, how calm or reactive she is. A less precise way to think of it is personality traits or how she approaches the world in general. Is your child boisterous or more of a quiet observer? Is she sensitive and cautious or easy-going and able to let things roll off? Temperament and personalities play an important role in the feeding relationship.

The Trust Model and the Division of Responsibility in Feeding

A central theme in the Trust Model is to follow your child's cues with feeding. You may not know his history and you certainly can't change it if you do, but you will be far better off if you follow his cues, consider things from his perspective, and then take the lead as the parent. In other words, this is a parent-led, child-responsive way of feeding. As one mom shared, *"When I learned to look at this all from my daughter's point of view, from her past and current experiences, things got so much better."*

The Trust Model works with children big or small, cautious or adventurous. With the right support and structure, children can be trusted to:
- Grow up to eat the foods the family eats
- Grow in a way that is healthy for their bodies
- Eat the amount of food that is right for them

This model looks at every child as having capabilities with feeding—knowing how much to eat and the drive to eat a variety of foods. Some children have lost touch with these skills due to unsupportive or pressured feeding. But make no mistake: those skills are there. The delayed child has skills—maybe a year or two behind his peers, but they are there. The child with a neuromuscular disorder or a genetic syndrome also has skills. If we approach children from the viewpoint of building on what they *can* do, rather than focusing on what they *can't*, it helps us recognize that our role is to optimize the environment so our children can do their best with eating.

A Shift in Thinking

I wish the "answers" to feeding and weight worries were as simple as making the child take one "no-thank-you" bite before she is allowed to turn down a food item, a system of "red-light and green-light foods," or making smiley faces out of raisins and peanut butter. In fact, feeding in the Trust Model usually means nothing short of a complete shift in the way you think about food, weight, your child and his capabilities, and your role as a parent. Here are a few examples of this shift:

From: How far can I push (encourage, get) my son to eat more (less, different foods)?
To: How can I give him the best feeding environment and support so that his natural capabilities with eating can emerge?

From: What is wrong with my son?
To: What are my son's capabilities? What can he do? How can I support him?

From: How do I get more calories in her?
To: How can I offer appetizing foods at her skill level in a pleasant, stress-free environment so she can be allowed to eat the amount she needs?

From: How can I feed him so he will be smaller (bigger)?

To: How can I feed him so he grows to have the body that is right for him? (With the understanding that if there has been significant malnutrition or growth disturbance, that may not mean an "average" outcome.)

Or, as 16-year-old Yiseth, adopted from Guatemala, says with a twinkle in her eye, *"Think of it from the kid's point of view. What is the kid thinking? It shouldn't be 'how can I get her to try this,' but 'how can I help my child do this at her own pace.'* Yiseth, the "picky eater" of the family, likes the changes as her family has switched to the Trust Model and family meals.

Do you see the difference? It is huge.

What Can I, the Parent, Do?

The Division of Responsibility (DOR), the rock-solid basis for the Trust Model of feeding, was pioneered by dietitian and therapist Ellyn Satter. It is the feeding strategy endorsed by the American Dietetic Association[1] (now the Academy of Nutrition and Dietetics) and is used by federal programs from Women, Infants, and Children (WIC) supplemental nutrition to the USDA and Head Start in guiding feeding intervention and policy.

Essentially, the DOR says that you and your child have separate responsibilities when it comes to feeding and eating.

- *Parents decide* three things: the when, where, and what of feeding. (Infants are fed on demand, so they decide the when. Deciding *when* transitions to the parent through late infancy and toddlerhood.)
- *Children decide* how much and if they will eat from what is provided.

Remember, these stages are not as clear-cut with children with developmental delays and are based on what the child can do, not his or her age (see page 319).

One mom at a workshop on starting solid foods said, *"This is my ah-ha moment. I thought I'd come in here and you'd tell me what to feed him and how much, and make me feel bad about not making my own organic baby food, but you're saying I don't have to worry about how much he eats; that it's his job. This feels so good."*

This approach is based on permission, nurturing, and providing. It specifically rejects that children should diet or worry about weight. It does not focus on avoidance, "shoulds," or "shouldn'ts," but rather starts from where you are as a family and moves forward with changes that feel good and are therefore sustainable.

It sounds simple, but it is not *easy*. Feeding well is hard work that you get to do for years, but struggling with feeding is even harder and the outcomes are worse. Most people who struggle around food issues mix up their jobs. That is, they let the child do the parent's job of selecting foods and deciding when and where to eat them, and/or the parents try to do the child's job of deciding how much to eat.

With the impressive list of agencies and professionals who recommend the DOR, why does the concept still seem so revolutionary? For one, most doctors and even many feeding therapists you may encounter haven't heard of the DOR.

And then there are those professionals, from feeding therapists to dietitians, who have heard about and even recommend the DOR, but don't really practice it. They talk about the DOR, but then advocate portion control and red-light/green-light foods, encouraging or pushing children to eat more or less to influence weight. In effect, they are not "all in," and the stumbling block seems to be that they can't trust the child to self-regulate.

During a feeding therapy training session I attended, the trainer came right out and said, "We believe in the Division of Responsibility," but minutes later, "Humans can't self-regulate, so someone has to teach kids portion control." No wonder this is confusing.

Self-regulation does seem more elusive in today's day and age with ready access to every imaginable food, a loss of family meals and structure, food insecurity, and the pervasive dieting culture. While supporting self-regulation may take a little more effort than 50 years ago, people can and do self-regulate. In the end, it comes down to trust. If you don't believe that humans can self-regulate with supportive feeding, then you will need to teach portion control and have rules about eating. Even if someone says they are practicing the DOR, if their approach is trying to get a child to eat more, less, or different foods, then they are not using the Trust Model. Don't be fooled.

Feeding your malnourished infant with the DOR will feel very different than with a teen you are fostering, for example, but the underlying trust and division of responsibilities are the same. The DOR changes and grows up along with your child (see Chapter 8). Being responsive to your child will help you figure it out.

The following three-step review includes goals to work toward in your jobs with feeding:

1. When to Feed, or Structure

"My personal perspective as an adoptive and foster mom is that you have meals and snacks at a set time, and everyone eats together."
— Linda, caseworker and foster and adoptive mom

Reliable structure is one of the most important ways to help children with eating. Structure allows children to tune in to internal cues of hunger and fullness and to not worry about them between meals and snacks.

- Younger children usually eat every two to three hours, or roughly three meals and two to three snacks a day.
- Older children usually do well with eating every three to four hours, at about the same time every day. This adds up to three meals with one to two snacks a day.

- Note that if a child is new to you or there are significant nutritional or growth delays, you may need to offer food more often at first until you learn to read your child's cues and he learns to trust that he will be taken care of.

Many foster and institutionalized children have extreme anxiety around food. They may have come from chaotic and unsupportive homes in terms of feeding. Being absolutely reliable about structure is critical. Don't forget a snack because you are going to the park. As Deborah Gray says in *Attaching and Adoption*,[2] "Successful parents have seen how much better their child performs with high structure. They work hard to provide that structure." The Trust Model fits well with the "high structure/high nurture" thinking around attachment. Feeding well *is* hard work.

What is so wonderful about structure is that a child who eats a small meal or snack— which he will—soon has another opportunity to eat, so the parent can relax, too. Parents can also have flexibility within the structure so families can eat together. Plan for a snack after school with foods that are balanced and filling and make dinnertime later or, if it works better, have dinner early and then plan on a snack before bed.

Structure also means no grazing. Often parents of small children are instructed to follow the child around with food and high-calorie drinks at all times. This is a common counterproductive feeding practice. Allowing only water between meals and snacks helps kids have an appetite so they will be more open to trying new foods, but they won't come to the table starving and perhaps eat more than they need. Regular meals and snacks also help balance blood sugar, which improves energy and behavior. Avoiding grazing also lowers the risk of dental problems, because frequent eating is a major risk factor for cavities, which are more common in children in foster care and children who are adopted.

The Appetizer: There will be times when waiting the full two to three hours between eating is not what your child needs. You will learn this as you go. A helpful stopgap is the appetizer, where you offer a small snack (this is different than a regular snack where the child is allowed to eat as much as he wants). You might use the appetizer if dinner will be later than usual or if the planned snack was at a park, pool, or other place where your child may have been too excited or distracted to pay attention to eating. I advise making a distinction from a normal snack, such as: "Here is an appetizer; dinner will be really soon." Or "Here is a little something until dinner." I use, "We'll save some hungry for dinner." Examples of appetizers are a small bowl of crackers, or cut up fruit or veggies. It doesn't need to be a mini-meal, but it should take the "edge" off the hunger. My daughter's favorite appetizer for years was a little bowl of frozen peas.

2. Where to Feed (and With Whom)

Family meals are very important. You have to eat, and it's better when you do it together. Ideally, meals would be with the whole family around a table. However, one supportive adult eating with the child is a family meal. Children do best with eating when they sit down for meals and snacks and are free from distractions like TV, phones, toys, and books. Meals can be a fun and pleasant time to connect.

Eating with the family:
- Helps kids tune in to "hungry" and "full" cues
- Helps kids eat the right amount
- Lowers the risk of choking
- Helps children learn to like new foods. Remember it's a process, and seeing someone they trust enjoy a food is the best first step
- Aids attachment and helps children feel they are part of the family
- Is the best predictor of overall success in life, more than the socioeconomic or educational milieu and after-school activities[3,4]

> **Siblings Adopted Together.** Ivan, age 14, was adopted from Romania with his younger sister. They were taken from their parents when Ivan was found begging for food with his little sister. Ivan was feeding his younger sister, Marina, who was attached to Ivan as his caretaker.
>
> When the siblings came to live with their new family, their mother was very deliberate about feeding both children. Being clear that food came *from Ruth and her husband* allowed Ivan to be nurtured and to attach but was also critical for allowing Marina to transfer her attachment to her parents. Both needed to be cared for, nurtured, and free to be children. The repeated bonding cycles of feeding and meeting their needs helped them feel safe.
>
> Kim, mother to sisters adopted at age three and six from Eastern Europe, agrees: *"Preparing and giving both girls food helped them see that they do need me."* Kim did not follow the advice in the books she read to have food available to the girls at all times. She felt it was critical to be very deliberate that the food came from her and that *she* would meet their needs. She offered and maintained eye contact during meals and snacks.

3. What to Feed

Notice that I put this last, but most folks who work with kids and food issues start here. Have a selective eater? The default in most articles is how to disguise veggies or get in more protein. Without steps one and two in place, step three is more of a struggle, because the key to improving *what* kids eat boils down to *how* they are being fed—that the child can count on enjoyable, no-pressure family meals that include a variety of tasty foods.

> In this book, you will not find graphs of calorie counts or charts with portion recommendations. Plenty of resources already do that, and in my opinion, most of them are *not* helpful. This book is about the *how* of feeding—what happens when you offer food, how your child reacts, and what you do from there—otherwise known as the "feeding relationship."

Good nutrition depends on eating a variety of foods. Parents have heard a lot about the USDA Food Pyramid over the years—and MyPlate more recently—but for many parents, trying to get their children to eat by prescriptive rules brings pressure into feeding and feels overwhelming. Remember how young children tend to eat: lots for lunch, almost nothing for snack, and most often picking and choosing one or two food items from what is available. Kids who are offered a variety of foods without pressure tend to consume a balanced diet over several days.

The key with meals and snacks is to plan ahead to offer carbohydrates, protein, and fat. Think of it in terms of the food groups if that is easier. (See the Snack and Meal Ideas Appendix as well as "Snack Ideas" on the Feeding Doctor Website: www.feedingdoctor.com.)

At meals, try to offer:

- One or two grains, one being bread or cultural equivalent (carbohydrate)
- Two fruits/veggies (carbohydrate and fiber)
- One dairy or dairy substitute if there are allergies (protein and fat and carbohydrate)
- One meat or bean source or nuts like peanut butter (protein and fat)

Classic snack mistakes parents make is to give a small amount to "not spoil dinner" or offering only treat or snack foods without balance. With the Division of Responsibility, parents have to recognize that they can't decide when a child is hungriest. Often children have a large appetite right after school. You can plan for a balanced and filling snack and move dinner later into the evening or plan for an early dinner and offer an appetizer beforehand. What most parents I work with do is try to offer a small amount of food and then ask the child to wait up to three hours for dinner. Some of the "witching hour" effect (as many parents call the whiney and restless after-school, pre-dinner time) is due to hunger and low blood sugar. For a child with poor impulse control or behavioral issues, these blood sugar dips can trigger major meltdowns.

Offering fat, protein, and carbohydrates is essential for stable blood sugar levels and energy. Many snacks today are basically simple carbohydrates or quick energy. I've seen too many intake analyses (daily recordings of what a child is eating) that show a snack of Goldfish crackers and juice or peeled apple slices and juice. Often this is followed about an hour later with a child's meltdown or constant whining for more food. Carbohydrates offer quick energy and are certainly necessary and favored (particularly by small, growing children), but protein and fat (and fiber) are also needed to help the child feel full and satisfied and to give him extended energy to make it until the next meal or snack.

Notice I did not say, "*Get* the child to eat fat, protein, and carbohydrates;" rather, *offer* them.

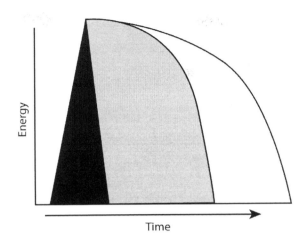

3.1: Black = simple carbohydrates like juice, candy, and Goldfish crackers. Gray = protein like meat, beans, and dairy. White = fat.

While it's a lot of work to put all these options on the table, it can also save time and aggravation. A parent's food prep job is done when the food is on the table. There are no separate meals for the kids and no need to argue or negotiate over food.

So we've covered the basics. Are you inspired or tired? You may be thinking, "Yes, but…" If so, keep reading. The next three chapters will delve into the most common feeding and weight topics and lay the groundwork for transitioning to the Trust Model.

Chapter 3

Pieces of the Puzzle: Oral-Motor, Sensory, Special Needs, and More

"While I chose not to pursue therapy, I had an understanding of Jack's needs and I knew what NOT to do. It helped me relax and worked well for our family as Jack learned to eat." — Lucy, mother of Jack, age two

"These are complicated kiddos who come home with puzzle pieces scattered all over the place—feeding is one of them, and this involves gaps in fine motor skills, the inability to regulate emotions, the hyper-aware state, the band of sensory components, etc. It all affects what happens at the table."
— Sue, mother of Mary and Marcus, adopted as toddlers from Kazakhstan

If you have a child with special needs, or aren't sure if your child's eating may be affected by oral-motor or sensory issues, this chapter is for you. If your child is "neurotypical," with no obvious challenges or diagnoses, this chapter is also for you. Because if you are adopting or fostering, there is a good chance you are dealing with a child whose early feeding was less than ideal, which can greatly affect how much your child eats, her attitudes toward food, and the variety she will eat.

> "Neurotypical" was a term first coined by the autism community to refer to people who were not on the autism spectrum. It has become more widely used to describe people with what is considered "normal" brain functioning and development.

I have chosen this chapter as the first of the three main topics because it includes a discussion of how your child's feeding history affects the feeding relationship; that is, how she reacts when you offer food, your response to her reaction, and so forth. If there are concerns, delays, or challenges with the physical skill set and experience of eating and digesting, it will impact every other issue you may face around food, from selective eating to food preoccupation, which are covered in the next chapters.

My intention is not to scare you. On the contrary, I hope to prepare and support you for possible feeding challenges so you can meet them more competently and with confidence. My goal is to offer that helping hand from the outset, rather than after months or years of turmoil living in the "worry cycle," when turning a difficult situation around is much harder. To refresh your memory, here it is again.

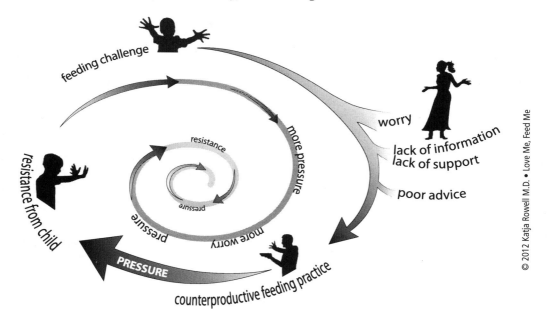

Many of you will not have to deal with therapists or developmental delays. Still, having a basic understanding of some of the challenges you might face, as well as observing your child and following her lead, will serve you well.

What You Will Learn

This chapter begins with an overview of some of the factors that could play a role if your child has feeding or growth challenges: from physical development and medical conditions to feeding history, temperament, and attitude toward food. The chapter then reviews how feeding problems might be evaluated and diagnosed and describes various interventions from individual therapy, to feeding teams, to supporting healthy feeding in the home with the Trust Model. For some of you, this chapter will be an introduction to new ideas; for others, this will be a review of the therapeutic scene you have been immersed in for years. (See Appendix III: Tips for Dealing With Health Care Providers.)

> Most parents today with feeding concerns are offered a feeding therapy referral and little else. As this chapter will show, it is not just a choice between formal therapy or "doing nothing."

Background

Briefly:

- **Oral-motor** challenges include problems with the anatomy, muscles, or nervous system involved in mouthing, chewing, and swallowing food—in other words, getting it past the lips, and into the stomach.
- **Sensory** concerns include a spectrum of experiences related to the senses and nervous system, including touch, taste, sound, etc. Challenges in this area may present as avoiding certain textures, not wanting to get messy, or seeking extreme input like hot sauce, carbonation, or crunch.

Every child and family is unique, and a variety of approaches deal with feeding challenges; some are helpful, others are downright harmful. Lara is the mother of two biological children and two half-siblings adopted from foster care who struggle with the effects of fetal alcohol spectrum disorder (FASD). Lara warns, *"Bad therapy is worse than no therapy."* Parents tell me they wish they had known that the approach they were advised to use would set them back, or that when they force-fed with a bottle or spoon, it would backfire. A major goal for this chapter is to empower you to recognize when an approach is not helping your child so you can advocate for the support you need.

Knowing what *not* to do is step one.

> The vast majority of professionals working with children care deeply and are doing what they believe is in the best interest of the child. I think that suggesting/recommending therapies that are counterproductive is not willful, but instead is largely due to inadequate training and understanding.

The Trust Model is not just for "neurotypical" kids. With its emphasis on following the child's lead and avoiding pressure, the Trust Model may be even more imperative when feeding and trust challenges are present and may help rather than exacerbate other challenges you are facing, from malnutrition to power struggles.

> Remember, the Trust Model says that if you do your jobs with feeding, your child can be trusted to eat the right amount for his body and he can learn to enjoy a variety of foods. The Division of Responsibility (DOR) defines your job as providing the *what, when,* and *where* to eat, and your child decides *how much* to eat from what you provide.

It's Complicated

This is a fairly lengthy chapter for two reasons: 1) It covers complex material and 2) there is no agreed-upon standard of care, with little research to guide specific intervention recommendations. Even among experts, there are differences in treatment philosophies and protocols. Parents experience this first-hand, trying to reconcile the different approaches of the occupational therapists (OTs) and speech and language pathologist (SLP) or speech therapist (ST) involved in the care of their children—even how differently one OT may treat the same child compared to another OT.

I recognize that parents who seek me out tend to be a skewed population; that is, I often see children who have already "failed" feeding-clinic therapy or whose parents have unsuccessfully tried other interventions. I do not often hear from families for whom these therapeutic options went well, though I know they are out there. The client stories, as well as my insights from my reading, training, and interviews included in this chapter, were selected based on what I believe will be the most helpful to parents who are wondering how to help their child.

Again, clients tell me that other parents are an invaluable resource. Consider reaching out to find support forums in your area or ask your social worker to connect you to helpful resources or groups. To further build your support, try asking your trusted health care provider whom he or she works well with. Beverly, whose son Danny has complex medical needs and developmental and feeding delays, gushes about his lung specialist (pulmonologist) who seemed to provide the most help with her son's complex medical care. Beverly asked their pulmonologist to recommend therapists and other specialists and has been pleased with the referrals overall.

Finally, I am not a speech or occupational therapist, but I can provide an overview of what parents might encounter as it relates to feeding. This chapter is not meant to replace careful observation and evaluation or diagnosis of your child. If you are struggling, please get support and don't stop looking until you get the right help for your family. I hope that by the end of the chapter, as you ponder your options, you will realize that having a healthy feeding relationship at home is critical to helping your child be the best eater she can be.

What Are "Feeding Problems?"

Surveys from the Minnesota International Adoption Clinic show that feeding and growth worries are a concern for many parents.[1] Even in the general population, one in three parents wrestle with picky eating or worry that the child isn't eating enough. With so many families struggling, it may be hard to know if what you are experiencing is run-of-the-mill or something more. In general, if you feel significant anxiety, worry, and conflict around food and weight, and the advice you have been given isn't working, then you could use some support.

Why is this so complicated?
- The act of eating involves so many physical and emotional inputs, such as sight, touch, smell, taste, core muscle strength for holding the body upright to eat, muscle tone around the jaw and tongue, and coordination needed for swallowing.
- Both gross and fine motor skills, from pincer grasp to holding a spoon to getting food from hand to mouth, play a role.
- The internal experience of swallowing and the gastrointestinal (gut) experience are involved, and if infection, allergy, or constipation is present, this may be downright painful (see Appendix II: Medical Issues Than Can Affect Feeding).
- Anxiety issues around trust and behavioral or cognitive challenges impact feeding.
- Past feeding experiences and trauma also come into the mix.

Phew—and I've probably missed some.

Where Can Oral-Motor and Sensory Challenges Start?

It might help to think about this complex question this way: oral-motor and developmental/sensory concerns can have a "primary" origin, meaning the child presents with a challenge so that, even in the best environment, feeding may be more difficult. This could include a child born with:
- A chromosomal abnormality or genetic syndrome
- A neuromuscular condition
- Drug or alcohol exposures
- An anatomic abnormality such as cleft palate, airway or swallowing tube malformations
- Heart defects, lung problems, or other major medical conditions that increase calorie needs
- Severe reflux, constipation, or other gastrointestinal (GI) issues

Or the problem may emerge because of environmental factors, meaning how the child was cared for, including unsupportive or understimulating caretakers, environment, or feeding.

The World Health Organization says this about the role of feeding: "Inappropriate feeding practices are often a greater determinant of inadequate intakes than the availability of foods in the households." [2] I hope to assist you in recognizing if unhelpful feeding practices are contributing to your feeding and weight struggles and lay out responsive and supportive feeding practices that can turn things around.

Within adoption and foster care, many children who struggle with feeding have a combination of primary and environmental factors. A child may have been born prematurely or is weak due to low birth weight, poor prenatal growth, heart or lung defect, or in-utero exposures. But what happens after birth also affects feeding and can lead to or worsen sensory and oral-motor issues. Lack of nutrition and poor quality of food can also affect feeding and development if there are deficits of critical nutrients during certain developmental windows.

Challenges with feeding may be due to primary, environmental, or a combination of factors:

- Low overall muscle strength (tone) and coordination.
- Difficulty regulating the nervous system and states of alertness, sleep, and appetite (known as homeostasis and regulation).
- Increased sensory integration problems due to early deprivation, drug, or alcohol exposures.
- Behavioral challenges, also more common with FASD, including inflexible thinking and poor impulse control, temper tantrums, etc.
- Neurological conditions with a genetic component, like anxiety, depression, bipolar depression, ADHD or obsessive-compulsive disorder (OCD). (For example, OCD may manifest as pica—the eating of nonfood items—and may run in families. One foster child frequently ate nonfood items, and the family was intrigued to learn that a biological cousin had eaten a glove.)
- Generalized anxiety or heightened arousal states from history of trauma or neglect.
- Genetic syndromes affecting muscle tone, coordination, and digestion.
- Allergies.
- GI pain/discomfort from infection, food intolerance, etc.

Nutrient deficiencies can affect feeding in the following ways:

- Iron deficiencies can cause weakness, anemia, and sleep difficulties.
- Severe vitamin D deficiencies lead to rickets, which can be a painful condition, as well as perhaps behavioral and mood consequences (the research is ongoing).
- Inadequate calories and fat can lead to fatigue.
- Vitamin deficiencies can lead to mouth sores and more.

Inappropriate practices where the parent or caretaker was unresponsive, neglectful, or coercive:

- Poor attachment leading to apathy and disinterest in food. Studies show that children with poor caretaking, even with enough calories, often fail to take in enough food to grow normally.[3]
- Feeding exclusively from a bottle beyond what is developmentally appropriate.
- Forceful feeding; hand and spoon feeding is faster than allowing the child to learn to feed herself.[4]

- Feeding a fixed amount on a strict schedule, where the child may have been coerced to eat more or less than she wanted.
- Not advanced in terms of texture, such as giving only thickened liquids when the child should have moved on to purees and then mashed table foods.
- Limited in terms of exposure to a variety of flavors.
- Lacking the opportunity to explore different shapes and textures by mouth, which helps oral-motor and sensory development.

Jenny McGlothlin, speech-language pathologist/faculty associate (SLP) at a university-based center for communication disorders, says it often comes down to trust and early feeding experiences. "Parents need to trust their child. Whatever the child's behaviors are, there is a reason behind it. Be careful about labeling the child as having a behavioral problem (or letting someone else label them). The child has so much history that parents don't know about that goes into trust. If the child doesn't yet trust caregivers, much of what is going on is probably due to the inability to trust."

Medical Issues That Contribute to Feeding Challenges

In an article about feeding disorders, the authors explained the myriad factors that contribute to feeding problems: "Organic, medical, neuropsychiatric, or neuromuscular problems may impair the child's ability to feed, affect the feeding dynamics, and heighten parental anxiety and concern."[5] It is critical to rule out and address any medical conditions that can adversely affect hunger, appetite, digestion, and general well-being. Whether you are dealing with multiple medical complications or just a routine, occasional ear infection, if your child doesn't feel well or his body is stressed from illness, it will impact his eating, growth, and development. (See Appendix II for a brief list of medical conditions that influence feeding.)

Many children who are internationally adopted initially see a specialized international adoption (IA) doctor, but are then followed by a primary care physician. If an IA doctor or clinic is not an option, there are resources for families and clinicians that provide information about the common medical and nutritional problems children experience from different countries, including Websites for the Center for Adoption Medicine, the International Adoption Clinic at the University of Minnesota, SPOON Foundation Adoption Nutrition, and the American Academy of Pediatrics online resource for providers and parents.

If you are adopting domestically, you may not have access to specialized services. However, at least one study has shown that for children in foster care, standard community-based services missed diagnoses and had worse follow-up care versus evaluations with a multidisciplinary team.[6] If you are caring for children in foster care and you feel that your concerns are not being adequately addressed, you may be right. Children in foster care, with their higher rates of mental and behavioral problems, medical and dental problems,[7] benefit from more coordinated care.

Defining Typical or Problematic Eating

This section reviews common criteria used to label and diagnose feeding challenges. (See the "Toddlers" section in Chapter 7, page 196, for a discussion of normal finicky eating.) Part of this diagnostic focus is a practical consideration, as a diagnosis is needed for insurance to cover treatment and to access early childhood services. However, a simple label for the child can be problematic because by necessity, relying on a list of the child's characteristics will miss significant opportunities to help the child and family. Look back at the previous list of contributing factors with feeding struggles and you will see why I hesitate to include the following narrow criteria for "picky" versus "problem" eaters.

> The term "picky" eater can bring up negative feelings and implies blame. Using words like "selective" or "choosy" may help parents feel more empathy toward the child, which may be particularly helpful if the child's early feeding and care was less than ideal. I will use "picky" at times as it is widely used in the research and when it reflects parents' own words and conflicted feelings around feeding. I will also use the term "selective" in the text when possible. In addition, words like "problem" feeder or even "feeding disorder" can contribute to feelings of hopelessness. Consider feeding "challenges" or "learning to eat" as alternatives.

I include the loose "definitions" of picky versus problem eaters that are broadly agreed upon in the therapeutic community because this is what you may encounter with your child. The list can help you observe your child. Consider these two questions as you read the criteria:

1. Should the child eating 30 foods be considered "normal" and offered no support when he may be battling at the table or losing weight?
2. Should a child who eats only 15 foods but is thriving and progressing begin "treatment?"

A "picky eater:"
- Accepts 30 or so foods.
- Eats at least one food from all texture groups.
- Often picks up a rejected food again within a few weeks.
- Generally tolerates foods put on his or her plate.
- Will often touch or even taste a new food.

A "problem" feeder:
- Eats fewer than 20 accepted foods.
- Stops eating a certain food and never picks it up again.
- Refuses to eat whole categories of foods.
- Eats only one texture, such as all soft or all crunchy.
- Reacts strongly to new foods.

Even defining food "rejection" is problematic. Most parents give up on offering a food after only a handful of tries, and studies show that parents aren't always able to distinguish the process of learning to like new foods from rejection. In one study introducing green beans, babies squinted and frowned with the new food, but with repeated no-pressure exposures, most were eating the green beans after about a week. Interestingly, though the infants were eating the beans, the authors wrote, "Mothers were apparently unaware of these changes in acceptance."[8] Clearly, quantifying rejection is tricky, and the quality of the feeding relationship plays a role in the apparent traits of the child.

Some in the field use even broader criteria, potentially mislabeling many children. For example, one Website claims that a child who is unwilling to try a new food after 10 exposures is a "problem feeder." Given a child's history, many of these traits may be a perfectly healthy stage in the process of learning to eat.

Childhood feeding expert Ellyn Satter focuses on the child's attitude to help parents know if what they are experiencing is typical or not: "…your child has gone past ordinary picky eating if she gets upset when she sees unfamiliar food, only ever eats her few (and shrinking list of) favorite foods, and worries she will be unable to eat away from home."[9]

Looking at the child as part of the picture, and not separating her eating from her medical or developmental concerns or from the feeding relationship, leads to a more complete and accurate understanding that is critical to help the child and family succeed in moving forward.

What About "Sensory" Issues?

Selective eating issues are the largest part of my practice. Through workshops, phone and in-home consults, and email, I have interacted with thousands of parents who are concerned about the variety of foods their child will eat. Increasingly, parents tell me, "He has sensory issues," even when the child eats an impressive variety of textures, temperature ranges, and flavors and is neurotypical.

I've heard experts in the field claim that somewhere in the range of 90 percent of behavioral and feeding problems are due to the child's sensory system. This implies that "desensitizing" the child will solve the concerns. Again, it is more complicated than that:

- The child who is challenging to feed is vulnerable to counterproductive feeding practices that often worsen the initial presentation.
- A child who presents delays and difficulty with the mechanics of eating is harder to feed.
- Combine the parent's desperate need to make up for real or perceived malnutrition and growth delay, with a lack of understanding on the part of their health care providers, and here we are again in the worry cycle. (See page 3.)

Sensory processing disorder (SPD) and sensory integration challenges are more common when a child's formative months lack the rich sensory environment ideal for the developing brain. If a child lived in an institutional setting staring at the ceiling with little stimulation, think of all she has missed out on. This early deprivation effects neurological development and may predispose the child to learning and behavioral difficulties, as well as fine and gross motor, balance, auditory, speech, language, and feeding delays. [10]

Lara, mother of Brian, adopted at age two, notes that Brian had severe sensory issues, due largely to his FASD. She explains, *"His brain is misreading cues."* When he has helped her cook over the years, he often had a handkerchief tied over his mouth and nose to make odors more tolerable. While sensory processing disorders present a challenge, they do not mean the child is incapable of learning to expand tastes and tolerate different sensory inputs. Lara notes: *"Brian is almost 13, and in the last year we have seen incredible improvements with the variety he will eat."*

Other parents tell of children complaining about smells or refusing to eat next to someone eating a "squishy" food. In my experience, for many children—when all the pressure is off and they can trust that no one will try *to make them touch or taste* those squishy foods—their tolerance to being near them immediately improves. Carla, nanny to four-year-old Paul, explained with excitement that within days of instituting the Trust Model, for the first time he was content to sit next to her while she ate oatmeal.

Extreme cases like Brian's sensory issues are easy to spot, and are part of a complex behavioral and developmental picture. In terms of feeding, when there aren't oral-motor issues and there is a question of possible sensory concerns, it can be tricky to understand. The following list is meant to be a general guide, as all too often, simply relying on a list of possible symptoms prompts a rush to label and diagnose. Many children who have a history of unsupportive feeding may have traits from this list, but I do not imply that a diagnosis or specific therapeutic intervention is necessarily in order.

Pediatric Registered Dietitian (RD) Hydee Becker, who has worked with a children's hospital feeding team, comments on lists like these: "In different stages, these can be issues all children have."

Some possible signs of sensory issues with eating:
- Sensitivity to temperature, texture, or smells
- Increased awareness of flavor
- Difficulty manipulating utensils
- Spills a lot

- Chews with mouth open
- Bites tongue and fingers when eating
- Dribbles
- Drops food often
- Fidgety and unable to sustain attention to eat adequate amounts
- Frequent wiping of hands and mouth
- Prefers carbonation or high sensory-input foods, for example with crunch or intense spice
- Accepts only smooth or uniform textures

Many of the items on a sensory checklist are understandable if a child has experienced unsupportive, coercive, or violating styles of feeding. If a child has a tantrum or panic response to a food being placed on the tray or plate in front of him, he has almost certainly been pressured or coerced to eat it.

Yes, feeding challenges make it more difficult for children to eat, but extreme reactions to foods are often the result of anxiety, pressure, previous painful experiences, and forcing, not the fact that a bowl of applesauce is on the table.

A 2012 policy statement from the American Academy of Pediatrics on Sensory Integration Treatment helps explain why diagnosis and treatment is so confusing. "Because there is no universally accepted framework for diagnosis, sensory processing disorder should generally not be diagnosed. Other developmental and behavioral disorders must always be considered, and a thorough evaluation should be completed." They further explain that sensory processing difficulties are present in many developmental behavioral disorders, including the autism spectrum disorders, ADD/ADHD, anxiety disorders, and developmental coordination disorders. With significant "overlap" of symptoms, and no evidence showing "sensory integration dysfunction exists as a separate disorder" they caution the use of the label. What they recommend is a careful evaluation by appropriate specialists, including a developmental pediatrician and a child psychiatrist or psychologist, to be sure that other disorders are not present that have more tested therapies. They also state that while a trial of integrative therapies may be in order, the evidence to support sensory therapies "is limited and inconclusive."[11] My interpretation is, as ever, you know your child best, and you will need to trust your gut as to whether or not sensory integrative therapies, or behavioral therapies, or a combination, are best for your child.

Sensory Problems or the Spectrum of Human Experience?

Over the years, our five-year-old nephew, who is a competent eater, has preferred foods at room temperature; reacted strongly to smells (balking at any fish smell, though he occasionally eats it); refused mixed foods (typical of the finicky phase of the toddler); and bitten his fingers and, not infrequently, his tongue while eating. He also hates auto-flushing toilets; will not use the air hand dryers in the public restrooms; cries when hearing loud, startling noises; does not like tags in his clothes; and wants to only wear socks pulled up past his knees. All of these reactions have been included on various lists as indications of sensory disorders. My friend Dana is also sensitive to loud noises and doesn't like crowds. But both my nephew and Dana are happy and thriving with their unique ways of experiencing the world around them.

In general, if your child is doing well, progressing, and settling in with your family, and these traits do not interfere with his overall happiness and development, you could choose to think of it as part of the spectrum of human experience.

> Kids often prefer foods that are barely above room temperature. Consider adding ice cubes to soups or putting some food out on a plate to cool it down faster. I've heard of infants from baby homes (orphanages) where they were fed hot formula, who cried unless their formula was quite warm—warmer than parents might feel comfortable serving. Following the child's lead will help.

Temperament Plays a Role

The temperament aspect is often missing in the discussion about feeding. Your child's temperament will affect how he approaches life experiences in general, and that includes food. An easygoing or eager-to-please child who is up for adventure may happily try a new food the first time he sees it—and like it! A child with this temperament often goes along with "two-bite rule" with no fuss.

On the other hand, a cautious or anxious child, or one with sensory aversions or a history of trauma, may be suspicious of new people and experiences in general, including food. This child may react strongly to pressure or even the suggestion to try a new food. It may take dozens to hundreds of exposures before a cautious child decides he likes a new food. He may have to see others enjoy the food many times before he even can think about trying it himself. And then there are children who fall somewhere in between adventurous and cautious. Throughout this book, I have tried to illustrate how a child's temperament, among other factors, plays a role in his reaction to new foods and to pressure.

Keeping in mind that children approach foods differently from infancy on[12,13] might help you relax and resist pressure. Observing and understanding your child's traits, such as extrovert to introvert, what kinds of sensory experiences he can enjoy or tolerate, and his overall approach and temperament will help you be responsive to your child. If your child doesn't like loud noises, bright lights, or crowds, perhaps it is best to avoid the State Fair or even Target on a Saturday morning. Understanding that you have a cautious child may reassure you and help you avoid pressure and counterproductive feeding.

How Are Problems "Diagnosed?"

With up to 80 percent of children with developmental concerns having feeding issues, accompanied by the increasing attention to and diagnoses of spectrum disorders, we've seen a remarkable increase in the last fifteen years in the number of individuals and therapeutic settings that evaluate and address feeding.

Diagnosing and addressing feeding problems is not easy. Remember the lists from the beginning of the chapter on pages 45–47 and all the factors that come to play? There is a lot to know and consider, and some who do feeding work with children neither have a broad understanding of feeding issues nor adequate experience.

During medical training, doctors have so much to learn that normal feeding and development, and certainly feeding challenges, are simply not on the curriculum.

While some children would benefit from specialized evaluation, I fear that many primary-care physicians aren't aware of even basic interventions to help families with feeding. Any challenge, from a normal developmental stumbling block to a serious oral-motor delay, is referred for evaluation.

For example, I have had several calls from frantic parents of older infants transitioning to solids, and their feeding clinic appointment is still weeks away. The parent worries, *"He isn't taking the spoon anymore. I can't get him to eat, and he isn't gaining enough weight!"* After briefly detailing what I do and what is involved in my evaluation, I often suggest in the meantime: "Hand him the spoon, load another one, let him have control, and by all means, do not force or pressure." About half the time, I hear from the parent a few days later saying that all is resolved; the child is eating a variety of foods again and doing well.

During a workshop I attended on feeding therapies, I watched a poignant video where a mother tells her story about the years she agonized over feeding her twins. She lamented, *"No one told me not to force-feed my children."* Here it is: Don't force-feed your children.

How else might this scenario play out? With a feeding clinic referral, the parents may worry that something is seriously wrong. It isn't far-fetched to think the parent might panic and begin pressuring and forcing food. Then when the child shows up for her feeding evaluation, she may be diagnosed with an "oral aversion" because the spoon has been repeatedly forced into her mouth. Was the oral aversion there in the first place, or did it develop because of forceful feeding?

For example, a father I worked with had been given particularly harmful advice: "Do whatever you have to, just get food into her." Dad forced the bottle repeatedly into baby Frieda's mouth, even at times holding her head in place. When Frieda was then evaluated by speech therapy and diagnosed with a "nipple aversion," it begged the question: Was the nipple aversion there initially, or did it develop because of forceful feeding fueled by Mom and Dad's desperation and a lack of support?

Frieda had been seen twice by speech therapists for slow growth and feeding concerns before she was five months old, although she was growing steadily at around the 10th percentile. When speech therapists diagnosed an "oral aversion," Dad was advised to put an oral stimulation brush into her mouth several times a day, which she didn't like. By the time I saw them, her intake was down and Dad had resorted to giving Frieda the bottle while she slept, which was the only time she took anything in. Dad was told not to make eye contact while feeding to avoid "overstimulation."

With two home visits, I was able to observe feeding and saw a gorgeous little girl who, once awake, cooed and smiled at her father, pushing the bottle out of her mouth to get his attention while he stared straight ahead. Frieda was more interested in him looking at her than eating. When Dad's fears were addressed, he was able to trust that his daughter would be okay, and they worked on figuring it out together. He learned to watch for and respond to her cues by offering and not forcing the bottle, talking and interacting when she initiated, and offering the bottle again a while later. Within three days, Dad was able to feed Frieda while she was awake and look at and talk to her while she drank—and her intake was up as well.

Several years ago, most patients in feeding clinics had anatomical or feeding-tube challenges. Today, the scope of children included in the intensive treatment model has widened. In my interactions with several feeding therapists, I have learned that a growing number of children in feeding clinic therapy are neurotypical "problem eaters," like Frieda and several of the other children described in this book.

In addition to the knowledge gaps with primary-care and specialty physicians, some feeding therapists also lack broad experience and perspective. McGlothlin agrees: "Some don't get much training. They may be doing speech therapy, and they are encouraged by an employer to do feeding work. So they attend a conference and then begin doing feeding therapy."

What Are Some Red Flags That Might Indicate a Need for Evaluation?
- Frequent choking, gagging, or vomiting
- An abnormal chewing pattern; for example, chewing only with the front teeth well past 12 months of age
- Food frequently tucked into cheeks long after mealtime and snacks are over (pocketing)
- Uncoordinated suck/swallow
- Anatomic abnormalities like cleft palate
- Slow weight gain
- Failure to do catch-up growth in a growth-delayed child
- Apparent pain or discomfort with eating

- Formula or liquids lost frequently or continually from the mouth
- Behavioral problems such as appearing anxious or stressed by eating
- Breathing problems or frequent lung infections such as pneumonia, a possible sign that food or liquids are getting into the breathing tubes (aspiration) or that there is a swallowing problem
- When you, the parent, are concerned

> All parents should get CPR training and know what to do if their child chokes. This is particularly true if your child has oral-motor or swallowing problems.

Who Might Evaluate a Concern?

Speech–language pathologist or speech therapist (SLP, ST): 1) Observes the child eating and swallowing a variety of liquids and food textures to assess oral-motor skills, 2) looks into pharyngeal (swallowing tube) dysfunction, and 3) should recommend ways to improve safety with eating by matching foods with mouth and swallow skills.

- Occupational therapist (OT): Assesses sensory, gross, and fine motor skills as well as core strength, body positioning, and feeding skills, and may recommend oral-motor techniques, adaptive seating, utensils, and other equipment.
- Pediatric Registered Dietitian (RD): Should assess growth patterns, intake and nutritional status, energy needs, and macro- and micro-nutrient intake and deficiencies. Should be able to assist with tube feeds, including timing and management, and recommendations for making up gaps in intake.
- Pediatric gastroenterologist (GI doctor): Diagnoses and treats medical conditions of the upper and lower gastrointestinal tract, including the esophagus (swallowing tube), stomach, and intestines.
- Pediatric ear nose and throat (ENT or otolaryngologist): Evaluates concerns with anatomy and infections of the ears, nose, and throat.
- Pediatric dentist: Addresses concerns if poor dental health is playing a role.
- Behaviorist or psychologist: Evaluates the quality of the feeding interaction within the context of the family dynamics. They are preferably familiar with the Division of Responsibility or the Trust Model. If attachment concerns exist, or a therapist is involved for any reason, communication is needed between the mental health provider and those involved in the evaluation.

As you can see from this list, it is possible that each professional is focused on his or her own area of expertise and, at times, the feeding context and history falls through the cracks. Ideally, your ST or OT, or the main person you are working with, will gain a thorough understanding of all relevant factors, including exploring the feeding relationship. Communication between the specialists involved is essential.

The Pressure of Reimbursement: Is it Influencing Your Child's Diagnosis?

Diagnosing sensory concerns around food may be straightforward in some cases but can be difficult to diagnose in others. Other factors that may influence diagnoses *don't* involve the child or feeding. Pam's interaction at daughter Sara's initial evaluation illustrates a scenario I have heard from more than one client. Sara was adopted from China at 11 months and Pam was doing a great job with feeding. Sara enjoyed a variety of foods, was not food preoccupied, and ate the amount of food that supported stable and healthy growth.

When Sara was evaluated by the team for general sensory concerns and anxiety, Pam was asked repeatedly about feeding, "Are you *sure* there isn't a feeding problem?" When Pam reassured the team that Sara ate well and consumed a variety of foods with no concerns, they explained, "Well, if we can diagnose a feeding problem, then all the other sensory services are paid for." (Remember there is no accepted diagnosis for SPD yet.)

Sara's other services were necessary, but I do want to caution the reader that there may be an incentive to *find* a feeding problem—perhaps where it might not merit intervention. Hopefully, this billing quirk will change in the future.

Pursuing intensive feeding therapies means a huge amount of effort and possibly money (depending on your insurance coverage or government assistance). As such, parents need to carefully consider all options when intensive, out-of-home services are recommended that may occur twice a week for months or years. When I review the OT and ST evaluation and treatment plans of my clients, they are usually several pages long, but most include only a few sentences or a paragraph or two about feeding before recommending feeding clinic intervention. Critical aspects of relevant history and context are often missing.

Increasingly, I am getting calls from families who have been in various feeding therapies for two, three, and even four years with no improvement, and even worsening of the initial concerns.

I do not want to diminish serious problems, and know that many children who could use support are not getting it, but I did want to bring to light the fact that a diagnosis is not always straightforward, correct, or even desirable.

The right speech therapist or feeding team evaluation can be incredibly helpful. Identifying your child's baseline skills with eating, including chewing and tongue lateralization (the ability to move food from the front teeth to the sides and place in the correct position for chewing with molars), can help you provide foods that are safe, help your child progress with her eating, and help you feel confident and supported at home.

Questions to Ask a Feeding Therapist
Qualifications/training:
- How long have you worked with feeding?

- Have you completed your training and are you certified? (I added this to the list after reading about a feeding clinic staffed entirely by OT *students*.)
- What extra training or certification do you have with feeding?
- Are you aware of the Trust Model of feeding, the Division of Responsibility, or Responsive Feeding? (See sidebar below.)
- Are you aware of the "Get Permission" approach from Marsha Dunn Klein? (Dunn Klein is a pediatric occupational therapist, author, and founder of Meal-time Notions.)
- Were you exposed to a variety of feeding therapies in your training?

Treatment Philosophies:
- How do you help families integrate your advice in the home?
- Will you separate me from my child or ask me to use my attention or lack thereof to motivate my child to eat?
- What do you consider "successful" treatment? What criteria determine when treatment is "over?"
- What resources do you recommend?
- What can you offer if "therapy" meals or other suggested techniques result in conflict or a power struggle?
- Do you show disapproval or hold food in front of the child's mouth until she gives in?
- Do you use external rewards like stickers or toys to motivate my child to eat?
- Can I observe a treatment session or watch a video?

"Responsive feeding" is a term often used in malnutrition, famine, and childhood feeding research and outreach that describes the feeding interaction, including recognizing and responding to cues from the child. In a 2011 review of responsive feeding for the journal *Nutrition,* the authors state that Ellyn Satter "operationalized" responsive feeding.[14]

What Satter did was create the feeding dynamics (or Trust) model for feeding, which is "responsive" in that it follows the child's lead, is developmentally appropriate, and does not pressure. But the Trust Model goes further by stressing family meals and structure (what, when, and where), thereby providing a comprehensive framework for feeding from birth through adolescence.

A Brief Review of Intervention Options

Working with an ST or OT to address feeding challenges and advance volume and variety is often referred to as "feeding therapy" or "feeding clinic therapy." I have read about and attended training for various therapeutic approaches, but I've learned most from the parents and children I've worked with. Parents describe various treatments, with most accounts telling of therapists using a mix of behavioral modification and desensitization techniques (described below).

General Approach

Here are three (somewhat artificial) categories parents I have worked with have experienced:

- The most common scenario I hear about is the therapist and child work on "desensitization" during sessions, like the "sequential oral sensitization" (SOS) approach for kids with sensory or oral-motor concerns. The OT, SLP, or ST works with the child alone or with the parent. The basic idea is to take a child who might cry at the sight of applesauce or a puree and desensitize his response by decreasing pressure and anxiety, allowing the child to have a positive experience—to first see the food, smell it, play with it, and eventually eat it. This is often high-energy, with play and praise and without negative reinforcements or specific physical rewards. In the words of a therapist teaching the SOS approach, the therapist "works kids up the hierarchy." Parents are expected to do therapy meals with desensitization techniques and move kids up the hierarchy at home, in addition to regular therapy appointments. This "hierarchy" might look something like this basic list (from bottom to top), with some lists having more than 30 steps:

and eventually to eating the food

to putting the food in his mouth and then spitting it into a bowl or garbage can

to blowing the food into a bowl or garbage can

to licking it

to getting the food near the face

to touching his arms with the food

to touching the food with a utensil or other item like a lollipop

to tolerating small exposures to the smell of a food

tolerating the food on the table

- Parents and child work with a therapist. The therapist evaluates the child and educates and supports parents with specific oral-motor skills and food preparation ideas in the clinic as necessary, setting up the parents to help the child at home.

McGlothlin explains this approach: "We help the parent in essence become the 'therapist.' I have many clients that I touch base with by phone or email but see only occasionally in the clinic setting to gauge their progress and help problem solve." Jenny describes hands-on training such as modeling strategies that show a child how to use her molars or "chewing teeth." Families may be educated with the Trust Model for feeding at home. Groups of families may go through a feeding program together. As McGlothlin explains further, "I run 10-week sessions with three or four families. They support each other and are able to see that they aren't alone. They also share what helped, such as booster chairs, utensils, etc." Each program setup may look different, but this is the general flow.

- Behavioral modification programs are largely run by psychologists who oversee the treatment plan while therapists and therapy technicians provide the meals. In a classic behavior modification approach, the therapist works with the child using negative and positive reinforcement (punishment and rewards) to motivate the child to eat. Initially, children are often separated from the parent; then the parent is brought in and trained in the techniques. The child is generally in a high chair or chair where she can't get down, and she may be upset during sessions, which can be very distressing for parents. One parent described the first day of a behavior modification program as "the worst day of my life." Parents often share that this approach "works" initially to increase volume and even texture, but over time, the rewards lose their power and the negative consequences are increasingly painful to enforce.
  - Positive reinforcements include: verbal praise, attention from the parent or therapist, stickers or other small rewards for reaching a goal, play time with a special toy, or video time for each completed task.
  - Negative reinforcements include: ignoring or not making eye contact with the child, withholding favorite toy, or time-outs.

Behavior modification programs are intended to transition children from needing continuous reinforcement to intermittent reinforcement, and finally no reinforcement. However, parents and therapists alike have observed that not all programs provide specific training to parents on how to do this, and the families wind up stuck in the stage of providing continuous reinforcement. In the end, the child may have significant difficulty learning to be self-motivated to eat.

Team-Feeding Clinic Approach

The team often includes a dietitian, GI doctor, an ST, OT, or a physical therapist (PT)—sometimes all evaluating and working with the child. An advantage to an approach like this, which may happen at a children's hospital feeding clinic, for example, is that the child has a thorough evaluation and testing in one place, with the shared results and cooperation with treatment. The team may or may not include a behaviorist or psychologist, and sometimes includes a social worker.

Cindy recalls that when her 18-month-old daughter Marissa's growth slowed, it was reassuring to have a team assessment saying there was nothing of concern in terms of anatomy or development. When she was given the "all-clear," however, and handed a sheet of tips and a recommendation to read Satter's books, she felt let down. *"We were still circling that black hole. I desperately needed more than a handout to help us figure this out."*

Another option is group intervention, where a handful of children participate in therapy together with one or more therapists. The idea is to use positive motivation and peer influence to make eating fun, decrease stress and anxiety, and help children feel safe to explore food—perhaps biting bologna into a moon shape or wiggling a noodle up the child's arm. This is often used with the SOS approach.

Parents may be asked to do "therapy meals," where they prepare foods that are similar in shape or color and try to move a child to accept increasing variety. They are told to focus on the food, talk about the flavor, praise the food, and reward the child with big smiles and gestures. "Spit" bowls, or blowing food into the trash at the end of a meal, is encouraged to try to get the child to put food into or near the mouth without the pressure of swallowing it.

> **You will know in your gut if a therapy is helping your child. Some children respond well to peer groups and praise and may enjoy "spit" bowls, gaining confidence and skills that transfer into the home.**

Therapeutic feeding clinic treatment for picky or problem eating has not been tested in a controlled way. (For fairness, neither has the Trust Model.) At a cost of between $9,000 and $12,000 a year, this is expensive care. Many children are also reported to need repeated courses of therapy.

Successful Therapy Journeys

"We only saw our therapist a handful of times. Most of the work was what we did at home applying the tools we learned. The little nubby stick that she could dip into food was a big help. She liked feeding herself with that, and the nubs helped with desensitization. The support was so helpful, knowing it wasn't something I had done wrong. She improved pretty quickly with the help we got."

— Kelsey, mother of Madison, who wasn't eating any solids at age one

Sue, who adopted two children from Russia, experienced major struggles around food. Mary was adopted first and had significant growth delay and selective eating. She came home at 13 months with poor strength in her cheeks, tongue, and jaw muscles (low tone), as well as obvious difficulty with liquids. Mary had probably been coerced to drink or possibly aspirated (fluids into the breathing tubes), which was surmised because she was afraid of and refused liquids. She was also behind in terms of chewing skills.

Initially, through her state's early intervention program, the OT who came to her home twice a week tried to help Mary with her eating. Sue remembers laughing about a report that stated, "…by 18 months, Mary should be proficient with utensils." Sue says, "*I'd be thrilled most nights if my husband would be proficient with utensils. They didn't seem to get how her history affected things and that her delay was normal, given where she had come from.*"

The OTs tried to get Mary to eat meat. "*Mary was really averse to meats. I knew in my gut that it was plain uncomfortable. The OT was prompting her with harder foods. I backed off. I figured, she's going to eat meat eventually; maybe we're pushing too much. I'm going to keep offering it, but I won't push it, even with a game. She's smarter than that.*"

Meats can be difficult for children, as the grinding molars don't come in before 18-24 months, with all 20 baby teeth in by around age three. Thus, chewing meat is a "late" skill. Consider grinding meats and spreading them on toast or teething biscuits, using a slow-cooker, or serving ground meats in sauces as ways to provide more manageable textures.

Sue didn't feel confident in this OT, who also recommended a swallow study where Mary would be expected to swallow a variety of textures while being filmed by a special X-ray machine. Mary had undergone several surgeries, and Sue knew that her terror in the medical setting would make the test almost impossible. "*Our OT didn't seem to know what to do beyond the basics and had little experience with adopted children. She suggested sticking a toothbrush in Sue's mouth before meals, which was really unpleasant.*" The fact that the technique of pushing a brush into Mary's mouth resulted in a battle was a clue that it was not the right approach for them. Sue was feeling nervous, doubting herself and the therapists who were trying to help, but not sure what else to do.

Sue found a better fit when her international adoption (IA) pediatrician recommended Paula, an SLP who had experience working with adopted children. Simply put, Mary's problem was that she couldn't really tell where food was in her mouth and what to do with it once it got there, a problem that McGlothlin calls a "blip in the sensory motor connection." Sue felt she could trust Paula and that she was learning a lot about the process. "*I had a gut feeling that she would be a great match for my daughter. Paula really listened and agreed that a swallow study wasn't immediately necessary, so we tried other interventions first and had a plan if they didn't work."*

Beverly, mother to Danny, who has complex medical needs and developmental and feeding delays, found her trusted OT through her local school system. *"Our OT was great. She offered so many suggestions and was open to finding something we could integrate as a family. If Danny wasn't game for something, we didn't fight it. Frankly, I didn't have the nerves for fighting it with all his other needs."* This was the second therapist for Beverly as well, since the first one they worked with was not a good fit. *"I learned to get over worrying about hurting someone's feelings. Our current therapy center is a godsend. Everyone is interested, and it feels right."*

SLP McGlothlin explains, "Because of unsupportive early feeding with some of the children adopted internationally, there are often delays in oral skills, so most of these kids have a normal, but deprived, system and progress goes pretty quickly once they get the skills. Usually the biggest issue is helping the parent understand that we might have to go back to the beginning, like using mouthing, purees, or textured foods. If they understand that their child won't eat like a two-and-a-half-year old right away, it really helps." Of course, children with underlying neurological or anatomical issues may take longer to advance with feeding skills and may reach a different final skill set with eating.

Some time after Mary's mother Sue began working with Paula, she brought Mary's half-brother Marcus home at age 13 months. Marcus was having a rough time with eating from the start and Sue was relieved to have Paula to turn to for help. Sue agrees that it is critical to listen to your gut, but admits, *"Relying on my gut didn't always help. When Paula said, 'Forget trying to get veggies in and serve dessert with the meal,' that went against how I was raised. But I realized that though my gut didn't feel good with this, what we were doing wasn't working with Marcus, so I had to try it, and I trusted Paula."*

Home was the place where these children made the most progress and where eventually, that "blip" in the sensory-motor system worked itself out. *"Mary's real growth and mastery happened in the home, not in the clinic. When we did our 'homework,' she never realized there was therapy going on at home. However, when the OT would push Mary during sessions, with 'here, try a piece of pepperoni,' her response was 'no.' She would get irritated, might agree at first, and then push back."*

Sue's experience with her son Marcus shows that trying to pin down a diagnosis may not really matter. Sue shares that Marcus had only one visit with Paula, who watched him pick up, mouth, and swallow various foods and textures. Marcus was believed to have some mild chewing delay, as sometimes he'd hold food in his mouth. Paula helped primarily by ruling out serious issues, reassuring about nutrition, and suggesting appropriate foods, but mostly by helping Sue trust the Division of Responsibility.

Sue continues, "*We did have a question about sensory issues, as he primarily ate bread and cheese when he came home to us. We never entirely got to the bottom of how much of his stuff was sensory. Again, to go with that gut feeling, it felt more like his behavior had to do with stubbornness and/or fears and mistrust. We did not do anything particularly sensory-related for him other than continuing to introduce a variety of textures and stay the course of reintroducing periodically, whether he liked a food or not.*"

A theme I hear over and over when talking with parents is:

Don't underestimate your crucial role in helping your child learn to eat.
Most progress occurs at home, with the family.

Sue got the information and support she needed with her children's feeding challenges, and the family thrived. Though she met with her feeding therapist only once a month, they made progress. Their "homework" took place during meals and snacks. Paula skillfully explained how to prepare a variety of foods so they were safe for Mary and Marcus. Sue appreciated specific advice on appropriate cups and utensils, and the recipes and food prep ideas helped support the children's nutrition while they gained skills. All of this specific direction helped Sue do her best job with feeding.

Mom Beverly notes how helpful it was to bring Danny in for his visits mostly because the ST was able to observe his progress, such as his lip closure or decreased size of pocketed food, which Beverly might not have otherwise noticed. Beverly discovered that having progress pointed out, even though it was slow, helped her continue her efforts at home.

Harmful Interventions

As you can see, many therapies are successful; however, some have the potential to do more harm than good. How will you know the difference?

Watch for the following warning signs:
- Any time food is forced or placed in the child's mouth against his will
- Making a child take more bites after vomiting or gagging, sometimes multiple times during a therapy session
- Putting food in front of the child's mouth or on his lips until he gives in
- Eating is visibly upsetting to the child
- Holding, shaming, or punishing the child
- Bribing the child
- Keeping the child apart from the parents unless she eats
- Not allowing parents to make eye contact or interact with the child unless she is eating

Adoptive father Dan says, *"Our OT insists that our son, who is on the (autism) spectrum, has to eat two bites of a non-preferred food before he can have a preferred food. Every single meal and snack, we end up yelling at our son. The worst part of my day is coming home for dinner."* Clearly this approach is not working for Dan's family.

> *"At age three, she started desensitization therapy, which we did for a year and a half and then for almost a year with a psychologist. She has sensory issues and is quite stubborn. When we did the therapy techniques we were told to do, she vomited or gagged at almost every meal. They told us it might take years for her to improve, but they never helped us with the vomiting and power struggles. We finally just gave up. Now she gags when we ask her to try a new food. She's into dance, and I'm terrified this will all lead to an eating disorder. The way she is around food is so messed up."* — Cori, mother of seven-year-old Louise

Many parents express both relief and guilt when they realize therapies they had hoped would help may have been counterproductive. By discussing harmful therapies, my wish is not to make parents feel bad for following an expert's recommendations, but to empower parents to choose the best course of action for their families. (See the section "Let Go of Guilt" in Chapter 9, page 270). The good news is that children are resilient, and I have seen remarkable improvements when parents have followed the child's lead with feeding.

Keira's parents followed their intuition and pulled Keira out of therapy that they knew wasn't right for her. Keira began feeding therapy at age two for "sensory aversions." The therapist held the spoon near Keira's mouth until she relented and took a bite, offering no eye contact or interaction unless she ate. If she took a bite, he would lavish her with attention, praise, toys, and stickers—all classic behavior-modification techniques. Keira's parents were advised to do the same at home. Keira's mom found it profoundly sad to watch her cry and gag down a bite of food, desperate for interaction. It *felt* wrong, and it took a few sessions for Keira's mom to get up the courage to take Keira out of treatment—but she did.

> **Interventions that withhold the parent's attention and nurturing to get the child to eat are particularly harmful to the traumatized or poorly attached child, or the child who is new to your family. If it feels wrong, or you are disturbed or doubtful of an interaction, trust your gut.**

Shortfalls of a Therapeutic Approach

While some therapies are blatantly harmful, even some of the more standard approaches can impede your child's progress with eating. Allow me to share some of my observations and concerns with a therapeutic approach.

Therapies may slow down progress when:
- The child is not allowed to participate in, but is the focus of, family meals
- Therapy recommendations worsen power struggles
- The goal is to "fix" the child
- One-size-fits all thinking is used
- Little support is offered when therapy is not going well or when the child "fails" therapy

The Focus on the Child

In most therapeutic approaches, the child is not allowed to simply participate in a pleasant mealtime atmosphere, but is the center of attention. All the talk about food, the game playing, and the cheerleading makes what the child is or isn't eating the focus of every encounter with food and often of family life in general. The parent and child get the message that the child is not capable with eating, which introduces doubt and anxiety into the feeding relationship, frequently leading to counterproductive feeding practices. The child hears, "You can't be trusted with eating."

For the sensitive or traumatized child, this focus and pressure robs him of the opportunity to learn by watching, feel capable and trusted, and *move himself along*. This focus on the child and his eating can lead to battles over control. Which brings me to the next concern.

Therapy Strategies can Worsen Power Struggles

The "therapy meals" described above provide endless opportunities for conflict. The child who is locked in the power struggle may be relentless in fighting therapy tactics. Lindsay, mother of Axel, lamented, "*It felt so forced, and it ruined meals. We were supposed to have spit bowls, or he was supposed to blow food into the trash ... He fought every last bit of it.*" Therapeutic strategies that increase conflict and power struggles are likely to make matters worse, not better.

McGlothlin tells of a little boy with a long history of feeding problems and therapies. "Even coming to therapy is pressure for kids who are traumatized, really stubborn, or stuck in a power struggle," she says. "This boy resisted everything, and therapy was not helping. He ended up needing nutrition through a feeding tube, using homemade-blended formula, which helped Mom feel empowered. We stopped all therapy, and once his nutritional needs were met, it helped Mom trust him and support his learning to eat. Within three weeks with no pressure, he started showing interest and asking for foods, and even ate a slice of pizza. Every kid is unique."

You Can't Just Fix the Child

After working with many families, I have great concern when the goal is "fixing" the child without supporting the feeding relationship. More than one parent has confided, "*I didn't feel like part of the process. We brought Max to feeding therapy twice a week for months, but we got no real support or instruction about what to do the rest of the time.*"

If it sounds too good to be true, it probably is. If a therapist claims he will produce "results in weeks," "never" suggests a feeding tube, or has a technique that "always takes care of the problem," beware. **Those who use the terms "never" and "always" may not be open to following the child's lead, and setting up this kind of expectation is risky for the child and harmful to parents who are understandably terrified and struggling.**

It's Not One-Size-Fits-All

Every child is unique, and what helps one child might not work for another. One child may need relative quiet or the secure feeling of a strap on the booster chair, which may lead to tantrums in another child. One child prefers foods at room temperature, while another enjoys hot sauce or ketchup on almost everything.

For example, while Mary responded to encouragement and tried to chew with her "big-girl teeth," her half-brother Marcus had extreme trust issues and would scream for "*hours on end,*" as Sue recalls. "*Any suggestion that he eat something else, or if I even put veggies on his plate, meant an instant tantrum and the meal was over. We tried to do 'lion teeth' with him, but he just said 'no' for months. Finally, as he learned to trust us, miraculously one day he watched and tried chewing with his molars, or 'lion teeth,' on his own.*" With the help of a behavioral psychologist working on general areas like making transitions, addressing behaviors, and building trust, things were improving.

> "The most important thing is that your therapist makes decisions based on what is happening with each child in the context of the family, versus what some book or protocol tells them to do. Your therapist or doctor needs to listen to you and work with you, always following your child's lead." — SLP Jenny McGlothlin

Often, when children don't do well with a particular therapist or approach, it is because of the one-size-fits-all trap. An independent or strong-willed child will fight behavioral modification, even desensitization-therapy meals that are supposed to be low pressure. Did the child "fail therapy," or did the therapy fail the family?

When You've "Failed" Feeding Therapy

When parents and children "fail" at therapy meals or do not reach goals established by therapists or insurance companies to justify services, they feel worse about themselves. Parents may be accused of not trying hard enough or not "doing it right." The therapeutic model of trying to *get* the child to comply with tasks, even as minor as passing a dish or playing with a noodle, may fail to take into account the power struggles, temperament, and development of the child. It certainly sets the family up to fail with the child who is seeking conflict, for whatever reason.

In my experience, when families "fail," they give up and just want to stop fighting. Because parents don't know what else they can do, they resort to feeding Timmy his four accepted foods, separate from the rest of the family, sometimes for years. The family doesn't go out to eat, the child can't attend camp, and parents and children fret over birthday parties and school lunches.

Happily, the Trust Model is an alternative to fighting or giving up. And if you've found the therapist or team that is helping your child with his eating, the Trust Model—that is, feeding well at home—can only help. The Trust Model is so powerful because it taps into the child's natural motivation to mature and grow with eating.

Not Doing Formal Therapy Is Not the Same as Doing Nothing

"If it gets in the way of relationship building and trust, it is not helpful."
    — Lara, mother of Brian, adopted at age two

Not pursuing formal therapy may be the right choice for your child and family, and is *not* the same as doing nothing. Satter's resources, including books, Webinars, and online articles, illustrate the normal range of child development, child eating, and behaviors from one stage to the next. Increasingly, the Ellyn Satter Institute is addressing special needs to more fully support families.

From the Trust Model perspective, following cues from the child, the parent optimizes feeding and trusts the child to do her job with eating and progress at her own pace. With the Trust Model, it is the child supported by her parents in the home, who will do best with feeding. The child will follow through with her own desensitization within the context of pleasant, supportive family meals. She will have the opportunity to see, smell, touch, taste, lick, spit out, chew, strengthen muscles, and enjoy increased variety. In essence, *she will move herself up the hierarchy.*

Lara, mother of biological children and two adopted children with FASD, describes how she came to the realization that formal feeding therapies were not the best fit for her family. When her adopted son Brian was four years old, the OT working on his general motor and coordination issues also tried to address his extreme selective eating and sensory issues. *"The OT didn't seem to know what she was doing with feeding. Basically she was giving him a lot of candy. After a few months with no progress, she wrote him off—and gave up working on his eating."*

Another OT asked the family to do therapy meals and try to actively get Brian to work on desensitization. *"We didn't do what that OT recommended with therapy meals. It was one more thing that interrupted our time together as a family. If it took away from our relationship building, we didn't do it."* Lara had never heard of the Trust Model before we talked, but by focusing on trust and connection and avoiding increased conflict, she was able to trust the process intuitively.

"There would be no quick fixes with Brian," she says, and focused on providing family meals, structure, and connecting through cooking. With this understanding and approach

to the feeding relationship, many families who choose not to pursue feeding therapies, even for children with sensory issues and delays, can help their child progress with eating and learn to feel good about food. (Brian is now 13 years old and is enjoying a wider range of foods, including homemade salsa, which Lara never dreamed he would eat.)

**You know your child best. If something doesn't sound
or feel right, move on. Educate yourself.**

A Few More Resources

The Mealtime Notions Website, which explains Marsha Dunn Klein's "Get Permission" approach, stresses following the child's lead and has a desensitization program. Excellent resources on this site include videos and articles such as "Redefine Try It" and DVDs about homemade blended tube feeds.

Food Chaining: The Proven 6-Step Plan to Stop Picky Eating, Solve Feeding Problems, and Expand Your Child's Diet [15] by Cheri Fraker, et al. may be helpful. Essentially, you take foods your child accepts and make minute changes to increase texture and variety, such as adding tiny amounts of cooked and mashed apples to a tolerated applesauce. Or, if a child seems to like salty or crunchy foods, try to find similar foods—a different brand of waffle or chicken nugget. If your child drinks only one flavor of PediaSure, try a different flavor or add very small amounts of another flavor.

If you have an older child who is agreeable or more analytical in nature, the *Food Chaining* book may be a good fit as it involves the child rating different foods. One mother shared that her son, who had Asperger's (considered part of the autism spectrum and no longer a distinct diagnosis in the anticipated 2013 DSM V manual), was helped by the logical process of rating foods.

Food Chaining also provides a number of other useful tips, and stresses avoiding pressure. "Anxiety and stress will reduce your child's appetite. Anxiety and stress are your greatest enemies in this process." This should sound familiar. I also like the term "food chaining" to help parents imagine what foods to introduce during meals and snacks. (As with other therapeutic approaches, food chaining can still make the child's eating the focus of meals.)

Within the framework of a healthy feeding relationship, there are tips out there that can help your family. I have found something useful in every resource I have read, and incorporated it into my work. But the important takeaway is: *if it pressures, it's not helpful.*

Kim, mother of two grade-school aged children adopted from Russia, explains her non-intervention approach with her child who had a history of unsupportive feeding and had sensory issues: "*It took awhile to adjust to new textures and tastes. Susan would take a hamburger apart and had trouble with lunchroom smells and textures. I even had school lunch with her a few times, sent her lunch with her, and tried not to make a big deal out of it. With time it got better.*"

Another mom, Lucy, explains how knowing the options, choosing a plan, and knowing the next steps made all the difference. At 15 months, Jack, the youngest of four children, had some developmental delays typical of boys with XYY syndrome (an extra Y chromosome). Lucy called, anxious about his feeding and looking for more information before she pursued the referral to the feeding clinic suggested by her son's physical therapist.

Jack was about six months behind with his eating skills, with low muscle tone and core strength, but was able to sit in a supportive high chair and enjoy meals. Lucy's main worry was that he vomited easily, which upset Lucy's husband. Lucy explained all this to her old-school pediatrician, who was not worried. Jack had no problems with breathing, infections, or other red-flag symptoms, indicating there probably was no serious oral-motor or swallowing problem. The fact that the pediatrician found nothing of concern was reassuring.

Jack was otherwise thriving, growing steadily, and was happy at the table. He was undisturbed by his vomiting, intensely wanted to feed himself (Lucy says he's a "stubborn" little guy), and ate an adequate variety to meet his basic needs. His mother worked hard to have pleasant meals for Jack and his siblings.

A handful of times each week, Jack would vomit a small amount, then return to his meal. Lucy and I talked over some possibilities, and she felt a watch-and-wait approach was reasonable. I encouraged her to try to be calm and matter-of-fact when Jack vomited, and to follow his lead. I cautioned that pushing or forcing, or getting into power struggles over food, would probably slow things down.

If things backtracked or didn't progress, she would re-evaluate in a few months. Lucy shares, *"It felt good knowing that I was choosing not to intervene, knowing what my options were, and knowing that I had a plan to help his eating. Equally important was knowing what NOT to do. Not to freak out, pressure, force, play games, or reward him to try to get him to eat."* Six months later, Lucy was happy to report that his vomiting was almost completely resolved, and his eating was progressing nicely, *"but on his own timetable."*

After a workshop at an early childhood center, one of the parent-education specialists approached me to share her story. Her daughter, born prematurely some 40 years ago, had a feeding tube for a month and experienced delayed growth and development. As she transitioned to eating solids, Mom worried about how she would learn to eat, as she was so far behind her brothers at that age. Other than her delays, the pediatrician found no concerns. He calmed this mother's fears: "Don't worry. Pull her up to the table with you and her brothers, and she'll figure it out because she'll want to do what they do." This doctor and mother trusted she would learn, and in this case, with good support, that is exactly what happened.

Rachel, mother of a child with a chronic severe illness, low weight, and severe digestive problems, explains how she is applying the Trust Model at home after stopping formal therapies: *"My son is two-and-a-half and won't eat anything soft other than pureed prunes, which he loves, thankfully, because that's how he takes his meds. Anything else 'wet-looking' he won't even try…YET. It took almost nine months to try a hamburger bun. Now he loves it, and loves telling the story about the first time he tried it. I still offer all kinds of foods and look forward in another who-knows-how-many months to him beaming when he finally decides to try yogurt or cottage cheese or applesauce. Until then I'll keep enjoying them myself, keep serving them at meals and snacks, and pretend I'm not paying attention."*

Better than Praise or Stickers: Internal Motivation

Children want to grow up to be like their parents. They want to learn to be capable adults, and they have an innate, or internal, drive to do that. They try on your shoes, put on your makeup, want to drive a car, and pick themselves up over and over again when they are learning to walk. Eating is no different. Even with challenges, children want to learn to grow up and eat the foods the family eats. This drive to grow up and be capable, called "internal motivation," comes from within the child, and it is a powerful force. It is your best ally in helping your child become a competent eater.

> When the motivation exists in a natural setting—one in which the child has a desire to succeed rather than senses he is being pushed or feels he has to comply or lose face to make progress—it can work wonders. You can't replace internal motivation with therapy, praise, or stickers. For many children, external rewards and pressure undermine and hinder the true, deep motivation to grow up and be capable.

Allow me to illustrate. The independent or suspicious child who is coerced or pushed to try a bite of pepperoni will refuse, but when she is at a party and sees a friend enjoying pesto, without pressure she pushes herself along to try and perhaps even enjoy it. Speech therapist McGlothlin agrees. "I talk to my families a lot about wanting their child to be 'internally motivated' to eat, rather than them having to 'externally motivate' the child."

One family was in their first week of no-pressure family meals after they gave up trying to "get" their four-year-old son Nathan, who had sensory issues, to try new foods. The dad says, *"Nathan observes everything and understands now that he is not expected to eat anything he doesn't want. He remarks on foods, 'Hey, watermelon!' He's eaten some different waffles, which is great. I sense that he wishes there were more foods on the table he could eat."* I often hear this from parents. It is this motivation from the child that, if supported with options and no pressure, will help children like Nathan branch out.

The Power of Internal Motivation: Sara's Story

Many children who are developmentally delayed also participate in therapies to advance other skills. While this may be necessary and helpful, remember that the most powerful motivation comes from within the child, and the role of the parents is to provide opportunity.

Pam, whose story was described in the section "The Pressure of Reimbursement: Is it Influencing Your Child's Diagnosis?" on page 56, adopted Sara from China at age 11 months. At age five, Sara was seeing an occupational therapist for anxiety and sensory integration issues. After Sara had refused for months to take off her shoes and walk through a pan of dry rice during therapy, Pam recalls one afternoon at the park watching Sara and a friend play together in the sand. When the friend pulled off her shoes and ran happily to the slide, Pam doubted that Sara would follow. She watched with wonder as Sara pulled off her shoes and socks, gingerly at first, but then ran through the sand and played happily—barefoot.

This was a task they had been working on in sessions without progress, and here she was doing fine. It was the same with showering: after months of trying to get Sara comfortable in a shower, she followed a friend into the communal shower after a swim at the local Y. Perhaps the work in the therapeutic setting made these breakthroughs possible, but just as likely, the key was Pam's diligence in giving Sara enjoyable opportunities to be challenged and move herself along.

Pam feels that it was critical both to accept her daughter's strengths and determine where she might need a little extra support. For example, the OT's help with transitions, Pam says, was key to establishing a routine that made family meals easier.

Pam says, *"As a society, we think everyone should be doing everything at the same time. Maybe my daughter wasn't swimming at age three, but at age five, she was out on that soccer field. When I can relax and realize that this is where we are right now, this is the support she needs right now, and it might be different in six months, that is when things seem to go better. It's baby steps."*

Progress at Their Own Pace

Whatever you chose as the path for your family, remember that while you are supporting your child and feeding well, it takes about two years for a typically developing child to learn to eat. It may take even more time to rehabilitate a difficult feeding relationship as your child draws on internal motivation and progresses with eating.

The pace of progress varies widely. Some children I've worked with, even "feeding-clinic failures," tried and liked new foods within weeks. Frequently, I see major improvements six to 12 months after initiating the Trust Model.

Here are five success stories illustrating how long things can take to improve:

- Mary's eating, as described above, was greatly improved in about seven months.
- Marcus's frequent screaming tantrums and resistance to even the slightest pressure meant it took a little longer, but after about a year, he had better behavior and increased his variety of accepted foods.
- Brian, with his extreme sensory issues and FASD, needed more than a decade of support.

- Another mother says it took about four years, but her daughter's sensory issues are much better; she now enjoys more variety than many of her peers.
- Oscar, who at 10 had "failed" feeding therapies and relied on only a handful of foods, tried two new foods within a few weeks of supportive and pressure-free family meals.

This process can take what may feel like "impossible patience" from you. If you try to push or hasten the process, you are more likely to slow it down than help.

If your child is learning to eat and there are oral-motor or swallowing challenges, he will need close supervision. Mothers have observed that for children who tend to stuff food or have a history of aspiration, feeding is intensive at the beginning. You may need to give very small, manageable pieces a few at a time or perhaps supervise with thickened liquids. This is where your ST should help guide you. Beverly shares, *"'Family meals' meant I was sitting facing him and monitoring him closely for his own safety. Now, a year later, he is doing much better and I can eat too, but I still keep a close eye on him."* You may not be eating "with" your child initially, but you are setting the stage and feeding in a supportive and safe way.

Putting It All Together

The Trust Model of feeding is most successful for families dealing with oral-motor and sensory issues when parents trust the child to develop her innate eating skills to the best of her capabilities. Even the severely delayed child can make remarkable progress when she is nurtured and supported with several guiding principles in mind.

Guiding Principles

- Follow your child's lead. If your child is receptive, you can play a game, such as the "big-girl teeth" game that helped Mary learn to chew properly.
- If you are getting pushback, it may be because your child feels pressured. If your child is fighting you, look for other options.
- *You* know your child best.
- Compare your child only to himself, not to others his age.
- Over and over, serve the foods you want to eat as a family.
- Establish a predictable routine. Transitions help, like saying, "We will have dinner in five minutes," or rituals like washing hands or asking the child to help put dishes on the table, etc. This can be particularly helpful for an anxious child.

Seek Help When Needed

- Find trusted therapists and avoid therapies that do not build relationships.
- When you are evaluating intervention options, look for a program or therapist

that understands the crucial role the family plays in feeding and has a plan to support you at home.

- If you are in therapy that is working for your family, it is important to have a healthy feeding relationship with pleasant meals and snacks at home. *Love Me, Feed Me*, Ellyn Satter's *Child of Mine* and *Secrets of Feeding a Healthy Family*, or resources from Mealtime Notions can help.

- Be sure your child has adequate baseline nutrition if you are making major changes in feeding. You may need to work with a pediatric RD through the transition. To increase variety and support nutrition, ask for a list of specific ideas for food groups and preparations that match your child's skills. Advance texture and variety as appropriate.

- Ask your social worker or therapist to help with transitions and managing behavior.

- Ask the ST to help your child learn to spit food out (if she can't); otherwise, be sure your child has a paper napkin so she can always spit out food.

Let Them Play

- Expect a mess and allow uncoerced exploration of food. Allow the older child the opportunity to play with her food, within reason, if she hasn't had the opportunity before.

- Have kids help with food preparation as appropriate.

- Incorporate play with and around food if it feels natural. Build a gingerbread house or paint with pudding, but be careful not to pressure during these opportunities. If you are pushing a kid to paint with a Popsicle, he will sense it.

Regardless of the challenges, temperament, or behavioral realities a child may present with, following the Division of Responsibility (DOR) at home is a critical way to reduce anxiety and power struggles and set the stage for the child to mature with her eating. You cannot immediately anticipate your child's unique needs, but following your child's cues without pressure, within the framework of reliable and rewarding meals and structure, will help.

As you prepare to dive into the chapters about specific worries and Transitioning to Trust, remember, ***children with special needs are worthy of our trust.***

Chapter 4

Selective Eating, "Underweight" Worries, and Ending the Power Struggles

"I literally would throw myself on the floor with clown-like antics after every bite my daughter would eat. It was exhausting, but I was terrified she wasn't eating enough."
— Olivia, mother to Janelle, age two years

"Our years of trying to pack in calorie-dense foods had little effect. From what I could tell, she ate less. It resulted in food battles. The day I finally gave all of that up was the day we started to move toward non-stressful mealtimes. Now at three-and-a-half, she eats a decent variety of foods, and is still not quite on the charts, but is clearly normal, healthy, and thriving." — Beth, mother of Annabelle, age three-and-a-half

American mothering these days seems to be awash with anxiety. Many mothers have tiny bottles of hand sanitizer on their key chains, feel guilty if they don't make their own organic baby food, and wrap shopping carts in layers of cloth to protect from germs. Are American mothers so unfit for their task that they have to rely on a bathtub sensor that alarms if the water is too hot? In a conversation about our fearful age of mothering, someone explained, "The ideal consumer is a scared mom."

In my observations, fathers experience less anxiety with parenting. Out of the hundreds of calls I've answered over the years, fewer than five have come from fathers. When I do workshops—even with stay-at-home dad's groups—most questions from men start with, "My wife wanted me to ask you about…" It seems that fathers largely escape the extreme self-analysis and criticism that mothers suffer from on the parenting front. Certainly, with feeding, women have traditionally carried more body image and food baggage than men. While exploring this anxiety imbalance might be diverting, ladies, let's give ourselves a break. If Dad is involved and calm, might there be something we can learn? I know I envy my husband's less anxious approach to parenting and life in general, and it is a calming presence for our family that gives me a valuable perspective as we deal with parenting challenges.

Feeding is no exception. Anxiety about size and nutrition abounds, with special apps for smartphones that add up every bite baby takes, or sticker charts to keep track of how many fruits and vegetable our children eat any given day. How did mothers from a generation ago manage without all these gadgets? My guess is they weren't as worried as today's mothers seem to be. Mothering seems to have evolved from an era of, "Don't worry about anything," to the extreme default of "Worry about everything!"—whether it's a speech delay, selective eating, or how much protein a child is eating. Somewhere between the two extremes is the right balance.

One mother lamented, *"Parents today are really pressured: 'Make sure your child is getting enough of all the nutrients.' One book I read said that children (age four to eight) should eat eight to 10 servings of vegetables a day, a serving size being ½ cup—my child doesn't eat that much food in a day, let alone of vegetables!"*

Bringing home the small or malnourished child, or one who is extremely selective, can be downright scary. Because I see so much overlap around selective eating, small size, or slow growth in my clients' families, and *because the underlying fear is the same,* I am addressing these issues together. The two main worries that drive parents to pressure a child to eat more or different foods are over size and/or nutrition. When a child is much smaller than average, the worry and pressure is often centered on both size and nutrition.

The worry that the child isn't eating enough food, or enough of certain kinds of foods, fuels the counterproductive feeding practices of pressuring, begging, or bribing. Within the broad topics of selective eating and small size, the stumbling blocks parents face as they transition to the Trust Model of feeding are also similar.

What You Will Learn

This chapter begins with a review of general growth information, explains why "failure to thrive" is such a problematic term, briefly touches on slow growth, and offers a more thorough discussion of selective eating. We will look at why parents get stuck in power struggles, include a description of counterproductive feeding strategies, and examine why they don't work.

Finally, I will walk you through what the transition to the Trust Model with the small, selective, or problem eater looks like—all while lessening the power struggles and strengthening your relationship with your child.

The information in this section is relevant to *all* children, whether weight is within the "normal" or "failure-to-thrive" range, your toddler is having some standard finicky eating, or you have a "tween" who has "failed" feeding therapy. If you have a selective eater, read Chapter 3, Pieces of the Puzzle, since there can be oral-motor and development reasons behind why some children are trickier to feed in the first place.

In addition, the information in this chapter is general information and is not meant to provide specific advice. This text is not meant or intended to replace careful

observation, evaluation, diagnosis, or ongoing medical or nutritional care for a child, and should not be used in place of such careful observation, evaluation, diagnosis, or ongoing care. The reader assumes all risk of taking any action or making any decision based on the information contained in this book.

Underlying Worries

Why do parents pressure? From a conventional approach, it seems intuitive that if you could *get the child to eat more*, by any means necessary, she will eat more and grow better. It's calories in, calories out, right? Many parents have heard as much. Desperate parents who truly fear their child will need a feeding tube, or *will die*, do as they are told: they hold an infant's head in place to force in a precious ounce, or they fall into the pressure tactics described in more detail below.

"The amount of stress and despair this was causing in our household cannot be underestimated. Feeding your child is primal; it is a fundamental responsibility of parents to provide food, and when your child won't eat, it is devastating."
— Carrie, mother of Cassie, age three

Reasons Parents Pressure
- Parents are scared:
  - "If I don't get my child to be an adventurous eater, he will be picky forever."
  - "He has to eat five servings of vegetables a day."
  - "He has to eat protein at every meal."
  - "The doctor said he would need a feeding tube if he didn't eat more."
- The added scrutiny associated with fostering and adopting may lead to a fear, on some level, that the child could be taken away.
- Pressure tactics seem to work in the short-term—to get those two bites in, for example.
- Parents are told to pressure:
  - "Do whatever you have to, just get food into that kid!"
  - "Serve green beans and rice for every meal until he eats it."
  - "I've never heard of a kid who would starve himself, just keep trying."
  - "Let's see how far we can push her."

What About Growth?

If you remember from Chapter 1, misunderstanding and mislabeling growth is a major factor in feeding problems. The critical piece is to follow each child and plot growth over time. Ideally, having two points two months apart will show the overall trend. A child growing at below the third percentile must be followed with Z-scores or percent change, *as the standard growth charts, based on calculations, are not accurate at the extremes of growth.* Your pediatrician should be able to do this.

"Her doctor had never heard of Z-scores. I did review Z-scores after calculating them online like you suggested, and her numbers definitely were improving with the weight gain, so it was helpful for me. Plotting weight-for-length was interesting too. She's pretty proportional, and close to the "normal" range, especially for her current height."
— Bethany, mother of Amari, adopted in late infancy from Ethiopia and now two years old

Z-scores are a way of calculating and comparing growth at the extremes—above 97th percentile and below third percentile. As a mathematical expression of the bell curve, it is how far a child is away from the mean, or roughly average. For example, at the third percentile, the child is two standard deviations below the mean, so the Z-score would be -2.[1] If your doctor isn't aware of Z-scores, you can calculate them on your own. The Z-score is more sensitive and thus a way to follow change more accurately, so improvements may be seen in the Z-scores when it is not evident on a standard growth chart. See https://web.emmes.com/study/ped/resources/htwtcalc.htm for a calculation tool. (Accessed 2012.)

Recall that human growth is based on the bell curve, and there will always be part of the population that grows at the extremes. A little less than five percent of the healthy population will plot below the fifth percentile. Steady growth, even at the extremes, is often healthy growth.[2]

That, however, is not how most clinicians think about growth. Traditionally, "failure to thrive" (FTT) is diagnosed when a child's weight-for-age falls below the fifth percentile, though many will diagnose if it is at or below the 10th percentile or if there is a decrease of more than two percentile lines. Importantly, there is no real-world agreement on the cutoff, whether it's the third, fifth, or 10th percentile, and even varies by country. In addition, in a review article that defined FTT, the authors acknowledged that about 25 percent of healthy children will cross percentiles downward in the first few years of life.[3]

The "Failure to Thrive" (FTT) Label

While these weight categories are arbitrary and questionable at best, the term "failure to thrive" has major implications, and clinicians need to proceed with caution. ***Parents, if your child is healthy but small, you must have a basic understanding so you can protect her from inaccurate labels and feeding interventions.***

Kara tells the story of her son Griffin, who has always been small and has food allergies and some feeding difficulties. For two years, Griffin saw a pediatrician who "diagnosed" failure to thrive and warned, threatened, and prodded Kara to get her son to eat more. *"It was unbelievably stressful. I felt like a total failure. If Griffin dared to poop before a weigh-in, I was annoyed. That meant he would weigh less. How ridiculous is that? We switched to a pediatric allergist, who said that our son was not FTT and was growing steadily at about the fifth percentile. I urge any parent dealing with an FTT diagnosis to get a second opinion. All that worry because the first doctor mislabeled our son. Dealing with serious food allergies meant we already had plenty of anxiety. We so did not need this additional piece of constantly fighting to get more food into him."*

I've seen even stoic fathers brought to tears over this "diagnosis." Few words are as painful to hear as "failure to thrive." Remember, children can be small *and* healthy. Not all children growing at the third percentile are healthy, but some are, and we must first *do no harm.*

The label is not inconsequential, because it leads to worry, which leads the parent to pressure, resulting in pushback from the child, thus creating the very outcome they are trying to avoid—a child who eats and grows less successfully. Remember the worry cycle from the introduction, on page 3?

> If your child is losing weight or is not stable with her growth and intake, don't wait two months between check-ins. Children with growth concerns should be closely followed by a doctor and an RD.

The following can indicate worrisome growth:
- Crossing percentiles. This does need to be investigated, but should not on its own be a criteria for diagnosis. More rapid and abrupt shifts of growth are more alarming.
- Low energy and listlessness. There is far more concern if the child is listless than if the child is happy, energetic, thriving, and eats a decent variety of foods with little conflict. Consider the child's overall health and wellness.
- Medical explanations. Coexisting conditions such as iron deficiency anemia, high lead levels, or abnormal thyroid function can contribute to low growth.
- Medications. Certain medications may contribute to the problem, such as ADHD meds, which may suppress appetite.
- Depression and anxiety in the child.
- Counterproductive feeding practices that contribute to the child eating and growing poorly.

Steady growth, even if it is low, is reassuring if the child is otherwise well. Maintain or establish a healthy feeding relationship, address concerns if there is faltering growth, and remember that trying to push a child to eat more is almost certain to backfire.

"She's not on the charts, but her curve was always going in the right direction. She created her own little curve below the chart."
— Sue, mother of Mary, adopted from Kazakhstan at age 13 months

The Malnourished Child Who Experiences Catch-Up Growth

Supporting the malnourished or growth-delayed child with excellent feeding and nutrition is important. Children who experience catch-up growth can grow at 20 times the average rate. Parents tell me about children who outgrow clothes in a matter of weeks.

Growth depends primarily on two factors: quality of care and quality of nutrition. The quality of the caretaking interactions and food intake are independent predictors of growth. That means that if care improves—even if calories and nutrition stay the same—growth often improves, and for some, if nutrition improves and care stays the same, growth improves as well.

> There are increasing resources dedicated to improving nutrition and care around the world for children in institutional settings, such as the SPOON Foundation (www.spoonfoundation.org), so every child has a chance to grow and develop to his or her full potential.

The older the growth-delayed child is when catch-up growth begins, the higher the chance is that he will not reach his full genetic height potential. A three- or four-year-old child may not catch up as robustly as a one-year-old, but it is impossible to predict for each individual child.

Children who experience catch-up growth have special nutrition demands, such as rapidly depleting iron stores, which predisposes them to iron deficiency, with or without anemia (see medical issues addendum).

The Growth-Delayed Child Who Does Not Experience Catch-Up Growth

It's more common to hear about the malnourished child who joins a family where food is abundant and is expected to hoard, stuff food, eat large amounts, and grow rapidly. While many children do this, not all do. Some will continue to be smaller than average but grow steadily at a lower percentile.

"I was prepared for a child who hoarded food, as that issue came up in all of my reading. I was a bit taken aback when I realized my daughter did not really want to eat and was not motivated by food." — Kara, mother of Antonia, age three

Some small children don't experience catch-up growth and may fail to gain weight even at a slow and steady pace. Occasionally, a child has a true growth hormone deficiency, which is more common in small-for-gestational-age (SGA) babies who had growth restriction in-utero, and in children exposed to alcohol. An evaluation is warranted in a child who, despite being well cared for, has a history of poor nutrition and growth delay and is not growing as expected. An endocrinology workup may be in order, other medical factors should be ruled out, and perhaps even the option of growth hormone treatment can be entertained.

> **What if my child doesn't hoard?** For reasons we don't fully understand, some children who experience food deprivation become food-preoccupied for a time and may "overeat" until they learn to tune in to internal factors, while some children who experience malnutrition and deprivation have little interest in food. When I posed the question to Dr. Dana Johnson, founder of the Minnesota International Adoption Clinic, he surmised, "…it may be due to oral-motor or sensory processing problems or to oral aversions that have developed secondary to poor or abusive early feeding practices. We don't know for sure." Follow your child's lead. Parenting, and life in general, is often about managing expectations.

Take-home points on growth:
- Use two growth points two months apart to see the trend. (Remember, if there is concern about growth, work closely with your child's doctor and don't wait two months between check-ins to be sure your child is not losing ground with weight or nutrition.)
- Use Z-scores to follow growth when your child is at the extremes on the growth chart (less than third percentile and greater than 97th), as you may detect improvement before the pattern is evident on a standard growth chart (see Z-scores discussion and resources on page 78).
- If your child was born premature or dates are unknown with a low birth weight (LBW), use the premature or LBW growth charts and a standard growth chart for the first year.
- Consider plotting growth on the World Health Organization (WHO) Z-score chart.[4] Go to The Center for Adoption Medicine Website (www.adoptmed.org) and click on "Growth Charts." (You may first have to click on "Topics.") You may still need to calculate or use Z-score graphs at the extremes.
- Be sure to plot weight-for-height, not only weight-for-age and height for age.
- Steady growth is a healthy growth pattern.
- If the FTT diagnosis is considered, get a second opinion. Do not accept an FTT diagnosis based on low, steady growth alone.
- Insist on a workup if there is a significant or concerning downward crossing of percentiles and/or the FTT label is being used.
- Avoid pressure. Children who are pressured to eat more tend to eat less and don't grow to their potential.

While the term "failure to thrive" strikes fear and guilt into a parent's heart, the other, almost paralyzing, fear is the prospect of a feeding tube. Next we will evaluate how the fear of a feeding tube also distorts feeding, and how clinicians often try to motivate parents with that fear—with harmful consequences.

Feeding Tubes

No one wants a child to depend on a feeding tube for nutrition, and very few children do. Unfortunately, health care providers may use the threat or fear of a feeding tube in an attempt to motivate parents to "get" the child to gain weight. Knowing what you know about how pressure backfires, you can imagine how this plays out. One dad was told at every visit for almost two years, "If she doesn't gain weight by the next visit, she'll get a feeding tube!" After talking with another dad who had fallen into a very dysfunctional feeding relationship with his infant by forcing food, he finally admitted, *"I worry that if I don't figure this out, she'll need a feeding tube."*

Practitioners' use of the fear of the feeding tube, rather than motivating healthy feeding and supporting the child, often fuels desperate measures from parents, worsening initial feeding challenges.

Feeding Tubes Can Be Your Friend

Despite the dread inspired by the thought of a feeding tube, when used appropriately it can support a healthy feeding relationship. Beverly's little boy was born with a rare chromosomal disorder. He was aspirating (getting fluids and foods into his lungs when swallowing) due to malformations of his feeding and breathing tubes. His early months were traumatic, with surgeries, time on a ventilator, weight loss and, finally, at six months, the placement of a feeding tube directly into his stomach.

Beverly, as many other mothers do, expressed surprised relief when the feeding tube was placed. *"I finally knew Danny was gaining weight. I knew he was getting what he needed. It was scary to deal with the tubes, but ultimately it was helpful."* The agony over trying to get him to eat when he struggled to breathe was over. His breathing difficulties and healing requirements meant he absolutely needed good nutrition, and the only way to get that reliably was through a tube. He seemed to sleep better, was more consolable, gained weight, and even got chubby cheeks.

Initially Danny's progress was slow, but getting through that first year with only one hospitalization was a major feat. At 18 months, Danny was more like a nine-month-old in terms of his development. He could sit up, was beginning to crawl, was enjoying purees from the spoon, and sitting in on family meals.

A feeding tube can be an important ally in helping your child learn to eat. Remember the story from the last chapter where the feeding tube allowed everyone to calm down and helped the parents to stop pressuring? The result was a fairly rapid interest on the boy's part to experiment with new foods. The tube can be placed to support the child's nutrition and brain development while rehabilitating the feeding relationship.

Feeding tubes that support nutrition in vulnerable children are placed directly through an opening or "button" into the stomach (also known as gastrostomy, G-Tube, or PEG), where a small tube then delivers nutrition directly into the stomach and sometimes into the small intestine (J-tube). It is a relatively quick and common procedure, and the tube itself should be painless for the child when used. This is different from the very short-term solution of the thin tube that goes through the nose into the stomach or small intestine that is sometimes used with a limited illness or for premature babies as they gain strength and weight.

"Using the tube feeding as a way of *preserving*, restoring, and supporting the *pleasure of normal feeding*, rather than as an alternative to feeding, is the key."
— Ellyn Satter, *Child of Mine*

Many children who are labeled "failure to thrive" have experienced pressure around feeding. One mother took it to heart when the ICU doctor said, "If he doesn't get enough formula by mouth, he'll have to get it through a tube." On discharge from the neonatal intensive care unit, she was told absolute minimum amounts her son was to take in every day. Mom was afraid her son would die if he didn't eat enough, which led to anxious and forceful feedings. Clearly, this was counterproductive feeding that grew from a terrible storm of desperate parents, a lack of support, and poor advice from trusted professionals. This kind of vague and unhelpful advice invites counterproductive feeding and can lead to serious enough feeding disturbances that a child may become nutritionally compromised. Ironically, the threat of the feeding tube may be self-fulfilling.

Supporting Your Child on Tube Feedings

In typically developing children, the initial introductions to solid foods are ideally about learning about food and the experience, not about "getting food in." A feeding tube can free you from worrying about volume so you can focus on a pleasant learning experience for your child. Some guidelines for supporting your child with a feeding tube include:

- If your child isn't getting enough nutrition orally to thrive and gain or maintain weight appropriately, a feeding tube can help.
- Tube feedings can be incorporated into pleasant mealtimes. Perhaps start with food by mouth as he is able, until he loses interest or the feeding is no longer pleasant, then meet his nutritional needs with the tube. Your RD can guide you.
- Make best use of the feeding tube—schedules, amounts, and what you put in the tube—to support nutrition. I have seen families left guessing and lost while managing tube feeds. Ask for an experienced pediatric registered dietitian (RD) to help manage tube feeding, particularly when you are weaning off tube feeds

and trying to balance your child's nutritional needs with allowing her to develop an appetite.

- Try not to be too hasty about wanting the tube out—anxiety and pressure often slow the process.
- Under the guidance of a pediatric RD, consider making homemade blended tube feeds to introduce your child to your family foods and tastes he might get with burping. His GI system will also benefit from the nutrients found in a variety of whole foods.
- Visit Marsha Dunn Klein's Mealtime Notions Website for excellent online resources for feeding tube help.

Beverly was helping Danny learn to eat while supporting his nutrition through the feeding tube. He continued to improve his core strength and hand coordination, and he slowly began feeding himself adapted table foods when he was able. As his skills progressed, he was slowly weaned off his supplemental tube feeds until he no longer needed them. Danny's parents and pulmonologist decided to keep the tube until cold and flu season was past, and by Danny's second birthday, the tube was out. Danny was not eating all the foods his mother prepared, but he ate a good enough variety to support his needs, and he was curious and happy at the table.

Feeding Tube, or Not?

If your child is seriously faltering with her oral intake, growth, and nutrition needs, perhaps due to a cardiac condition, severe oral-motor or sensory issues, dysfunctional feeding, or a combination of reasons, this transition to the Trust Model is likely to fail. Because children often take in less for a while when starting with the Division of Responsibility, a child who does not have nutritional reserves may not be able to transition without the critical support a feeding tube can provide.

It is almost impossible to have mandatory minimum goals for volume and/or calories and transition to the Trust Model at the same time. Some parents, in consultation with their medical and nutrition teams, decide to place a feeding tube to insure adequate nutrition while simultaneously working on developmental skills, physical therapies, dealing with medical issues, and rehabilitating the feeding relationship. These are difficult decisions.

Other times, health care providers and parents may resist the feeding tube and instead continue with desperate and dysfunctional feeding patterns, like in Allison's situation. Allison, mother of a five-year-old, shared that while extreme behavioral therapy "saved" her daughter from a feeding tube at age 18 months, her current eating is characterized by severe anxiety, frequent vomiting, and continued worsening weight and nutrition concerns. The years of pressure and therapy have not resulted in anything close to normal eating for her daughter. Allison wonders now if placing the feeding tube when she was a toddler may have allowed them the peace of mind to rehabilitate her relationship with food. They avoided a feeding tube, but at what cost?

If you are being "threatened" with a feeding tube, it is critical to think through the ramifications of your decisions and feel confident that you have the best team possible advising you through this process.

"I've let myself imagine the thing I was most scared about—that is, a feeding tube. I am finally at rock bottom. I actually think a feeding tube would be better than this."
— Amanda, mother of a three-year-old who is not gaining weight and is caught in a dysfunctional feeding pattern

Now that we have addressed the range of size worries, from small size to thinking about feeding tubes, let's move on from the background information to counterproductive feeding practices and how to turn them around.

Counterproductive Feeding With Selective Eating and Low-Weight Concerns

Families get into trouble with feeding when they cross the lines of the Division of Responsibility (DOR)—when parents allow the child to do their jobs of deciding what, when, and where to eat, and/or the parent tries to take over the child's jobs of deciding if and how much to eat.

Power struggles result, and eating is most often worse, not better, when parents:
- Allow the child to dictate the menu, hoping she will eat *something*.
- Offer other foods or allow the child to get something else after food is on the table.
- Limit foods to what the child readily accepts, which tend to be simple carbohydrates or easy-to-like foods like chicken nuggets.
- Feed the child his accepted foods separately from the family so he is never exposed to the foods he is expected to learn to like.
- Forget about the "when" piece and lose structure, allowing the child to eat all day, which doesn't allow the child to have an appetite at meals and snacks. Many parents are encouraged to push the child to eat all day. I remember one particular call where the mom was clearly out of breath. She explained, *"Oh, I'm fine. I'm just chasing Matthew around the house with his sausage from breakfast."*
- Try to take over the child's job of deciding how much, which results in **pressure**.

What "Pressure" Looks Like

"We took Dora to feeding therapy for her picky eating. The therapist told us to be super-enthusiastic with feeding. It's so frustrating. She seems to progress a little in therapy, but at home she is eating less, and now is pretty much only eating pureed pears and crackers. We praise and beg and reward when she eats, but it's not helping."
— Franny, mother to Dora, age four years

The Most Common Pressure Culprits I See:

- **Bribes:** "You can have dessert if you eat two bites of chicken."
- **Pressure:** "You have to eat two bites of everything on your plate," or "You have to take a "no-thank-you bite."
- **Negotiating:** "Okay, two bites of this, then one bite of that. No? Three small bites of this one then…"
- **Catering with cooking:** "I made you rice, look! You don't want rice? Want some buttered noodles instead?"
- **Guilt:** "You are so lucky you got adopted; think of all the children who don't have this wonderful food," or "It shows Mommy we love her when we eat the food she makes."
- **Begging:** "Please, just take at least one bite. Please, please, please."
- **Forcing:** Physically placing or forcing food into a child's mouth or holding a child's head or hands while feeding.

"'Just make them eat.'—that one gets me every time!"
— Sherry, mother of a five-year-old selective eater

Pressure Backfires Most of the Time

- Pressuring is a lot of effort, causes a lot of turmoil, and research shows it doesn't work.
  - Children pressured to eat more tend to eat less, and don't grow to their potential.
  - Pressure leads to stress, which kills appetite.
  - Stress makes it harder for a child to tune in to cues from their bodies about hunger and fullness.
  - Pressure and stress lead children to seek out and rely on safe and comfortable foods.
- Children pressured to eat more fruits and vegetables tend to eat fewer.

More Subtle Forms of Pressure

In addition to the begging and bribing, pressure can take many forms. Remember that even "positive" tactics like rewards and praise can feel like pressure. Here are a few additional, though less obvious, ways parents pressure.

There are different ways of referring to children who have experienced trauma. Authors Gregory Keck and Regina Kupecky use the term "hurt" child. Others use the terms "traumatized" or "abuse survivor." It implies a more severe history of neglect or abuse, and these children often have increased needs as they learn to trust and attach. Lara, who has adopted two children with fetal alcohol spectrum disorder and fostered several children, recognizes that all adopted and foster children have experienced loss and trauma to some degree.

Praise can also be pressure. "Positive" pressure is still pressure and turns many kids off from new foods. Sticker charts, toys, praise, and high-fives don't help many children learn to like new foods. The "hurt" child in particular will "lose face" if he gives in and eats the darn broccoli.

Distraction: Parents resort to needing kids to "zone out" to eat, usually with TV. Parents describe an almost "dissociative" state, where children only eat if they are not really aware of what is going on. Another example of this is feeding infants only while they are sleeping, simply taking advantage of the suck reflex to get calories in. As the child grows up, "zoned-out" eating has potentially harmful consequences in terms of eating competence and bingeing, which is often characterized by a sense of not being aware of eating.

> ***Is it ever OK to eat in front of the TV?*** Eating in front of the TV and other distractions makes it harder for kids to eat the right amount. It's noise that makes it more difficult for them to listen to their bodies to know if they are hungry or full. Some kids may eat less, and others more, than they would if they were paying attention. As with any change, while you are early in the process, try to be consistent about eating meals and snacks at the table together. Once children seem to get the process and skills are emerging, you can have the occasional snack or meal in front of the TV. See how your child handles it. Maybe it's a snack during a movie on a rainy day or dinner on trays while watching the game. She may eat more or less than she otherwise might have, but since her body is allowed to self-regulate with the Trust Model, her intake should even out, maybe later in the day or the following day.

Rewards, commonly used in many behavioral feeding therapies, may slow the process. Authors Gregory Keck and Regina Kupecky, in *Parenting the Hurt Child*, explain, "The problem occurs when rewards work—when the child becomes the blackmailer, and the stakes get higher and higher."[5]

> An example of a high-stakes reward: After a workshop, a woman approached me to talk about her teenage stepson who ate a limited variety of foods. There were no developmental issues, and he ate a good variety when he was younger. She described the incident: Dad, son, and stepmom are at the table with chicken breast, mashed potatoes, bread, and carrots. Son nibbles on bread and Dad pulls out his wallet and says, "How much to get you to eat just one bite of that chicken?" Son shakes his head. Dad pulls out a $100 bill. Son doesn't blink. Dad pulls out another one. No response. Dad peels off *ten $100 bills* and son still doesn't bite—the chicken or the money.

Sophie's experience with her son's feeding therapy illustrates how rewards might not help. Her son was making some minor improvements in terms of his desensitization therapy (page 58), but still relied only on his top 10 or so foods at home. She described how he was rewarded at therapy with a toy car if he made progress. She knew this wasn't working when he asked one day, *"I wonder what they will give me today if I lick broccoli?"*

Rewards are a power chip. If you reward with praise, stickers, and toys, then the reward is external and provides an opportunity to resist. If the motivation is internal (meaning the child's inborn drive to grow up to eat the foods her family eats), with nothing to fight against, the child will branch out—when she is ready.

Humans have an inherent drive for variety in foods. This is an intrinsic (from within) reward, and that's the best kind. Kids will eventually tire of eating the same thing if we let them.[6]

Food jags: After an overnight with her grandparents, my daughter talked about how she loved "the cheese where you unwrap every piece." When she asked for it, I bought the cheese and let her eat it with snacks. She ate lots for a few weeks when it was on the menu with a lunch or snack, sometimes up to four slices. Very soon, she would only eat one or two, and within six weeks I noticed that the slices I packed in her lunch came back uneaten. Food jags are normal and not just for kids. Many adults say that they eat foods like hummus or a boiled egg with lunch for weeks on end, and then suddenly aren't interested. Incorporate the favored food into regular meals and snacks, allow children to eat as much as they want at those times, and continue to rotate other foods. The key is not to allow a total food jag where all you offer is one or two foods at every meal and snack.

Punishment. I hardly feel like I need to say it, but punishing kids by withholding food, making menus of only rejected foods, or threatening to take away TV, your nurturing, or your interaction to motivate a child to eat will not help.

Sneaking

With the success of the "sneaking" cookbooks recently, many parents are tempted to hide nutrient-dense foods like pureed blueberries or spinach into a brownie mix or smoothie. But even sneaking food can backfire.

Particularly for the child who is working on attachment, is learning to trust you, or has trauma around food, they don't have trust in others. Protect the trust that you are building or have built with your child and don't risk it for a short-term nutritional goal. Don't even do the old trick of sneaking in a spoonful of veggies between those sweet pears for the child learning to eat solids. Kids won't like it, and it will make them wary and more prone to refuse foods.

Samantha, who grew up in her biological family, is a self-described reformed picky eater. As a child, she was often left to fend for herself and her brothers to get meals, was rewarded with food, and was served a fairly limited variety. During a visit to her grandmother, she ate a stew, only to be told afterward that she had eaten bear meat. She became so suspicious of any food served at her grandmother's that she only ate things there that she could recognize, such as crackers, cereal, or individually wrapped items.

Sherry, another mom, told me about baking blueberries into brownies in an effort to improve her selective preschooler's nutrition. She baked furtively at night, taking the blueberry container out to the garage trash to hide the evidence—like cleaning up a crime scene. She was jumpy when she hid the "good" food, because she knew that when her kids found out, there would be a fight and they might not even eat her brownies again, or anything else for that matter. What she was doing felt wrong, but she didn't know any other way to support their eating.

Sherry says, *"The information in magazines, online, and in books that I read (unfortunately, I didn't stumble upon the Division of Responsibility until later) was completely unhelpful. 'Hide veggies in her meatballs,' but she won't eat meatballs, and it is hard to hide veggies in plain noodles with butter on them."*

If you don't want anyone to know you're putting blueberries in the brownies, you may want to reconsider your tactics. Chances are, the kids might not care either way, so if you do choose to add foods or purees to support nutrition, do so in the open so that you aren't getting "caught." You are simply preparing food.

> Many children like frozen treats because of the temperature, consistency, and the fact that they can hold them and control their eating. Homemade frozen pops, like those you can make with the BellyFULL Kit, make use of nutrient-dense ingredients, including gluten- and dairy-free options. You can also experiment with recipes on your own. Your child may enjoy frozen pops with meals and snacks while you are working on the feeding relationship.

If you do choose to sneak, or use shakes and frozen pops to support nutrition, be sure to also expose your children to the actual foods. Let's take blueberries. Go ahead and bake them into a brownie (in broad daylight), but also:
- Bake them into a muffin, or buy a blueberry muffin if you don't bake.
- Make some of your pancakes with blueberries.
- Try offering frozen blueberries in a bowl if your child has the oral-motor skills to handle it safely. Little kids might especially like frozen fruits or veggies straight from the bag.
- Serve frozen or freeze-dried blueberries to a child who likes crunchy textures.
- Serve blueberries in yogurt or buy blueberry-flavored yogurt of a brand your child already likes.

- Try blueberry jam.
- Make yogurt or ice cream, or oatmeal "sundaes," and have different bowls of toppings, including blueberries.

Supplement Drinks

One of the first "answers" that many clinicians reach for when a child is smaller than average or is a selective eater is a nutrition supplement drink like PediaSure. Rather than pursue an evaluation of possible causes, including a review of feeding, these parents are told to get PediaSure and then sent on their way.

"We were handed a coupon for PediaSure by my physician when I tried to discuss my child's picky eating. We served it with meals, and my son didn't want or need to eat any other foods, it seemed. Now, a few years later, I have banned PediaSure and am now struggling with an older and pickier eater." — Alice, mother of Mitchel, age six

You may have seen the PediaSure ads, which feed on a parent's anxiety. Remember, "The ideal consumer is a scared mom." In one commercial, a girl sits at the kitchen counter, turning her nose up at fruits and vegetables while the slogan is announced: "Be 110 percent sure!" A food pyramid floats magically above the girl's head, with all the fruits and veggies disappearing, leaving big holes. Add a dash of guilt to that worry, and how could you *not* want to "feed your child's potential?" Luckily, there is PediaSure to fill in the gaps. Mom reaches out, grabs a bottle, and her relief is visible.

Supplements have the potential to hinder healthy feeding because:
- It is easier and faster to write a prescription rather than have to learn about or delve into other factors, which the doctors may not even be aware of.
- It is easier to open a bottle than to plan and prepare meals.
- The supplements are usually very sweet and may be easy to like for a selective child.
- It can seem like a "quick-fix" and might not help parents work on feeding.
- One in three moms will perceive their child as "picky" at some point, with some studies suggesting that children described as "picky" eaters eat the same amount and grow just as well as children who are not.[7] Put another way, many children who don't need the supplements might get them anyway, simply because of parental anxiety over nutrition.

That is not to say that scared or terrified parents are lazy or trying to take the easy way out. Parents with feeding struggles are often desperate and will try anything. If your child truly is limited with her intake, a supplement, used within the healthy feeding relationship and along with structured meals and snacks, can support nutrition. But most often I see families using shakes and supplements in a way that doesn't help the child learn to eat.

Almost all the children I have worked with who relied on shakes for the majority of their intake were challenging to feed for some reason, but were also in feeding relationships with intense pressure and struggles around getting them to take in more. Usually the parent was told to follow the child around with a sippy cup at all times to get as much in as possible. This clearly ignores the idea of structure and allowing the child to get a little bit hungry. If their tummies always have a little bit of PediaSure in them, it robs them of the opportunity to develop an appetite.

Another couple I worked with would make their child sit in the highchair for 45 minutes or more at each sitting, hoping to get in a few more bites, then follow each meal with eight ounces of PediaSure. This child vomited several times a week. Within days of stopping the post-meal PediaSure and offering only four ounces at a time *with* meals, her vomiting had almost completely stopped.

Some children *can* benefit from supplements to help support nutrition while the feeding relationship is supported:

- Consider making your own smoothies or shakes that you can mix with ingredients like cow's milk, soy or almond milk, yogurt, vegetables, fruits, protein powders, or nut butters to boost nutrition. Ask your pediatric RD for recommendations. One mom wrote, *"We wound up making her homemade smoothies with almond milk, instant breakfast mix, baby rice cereal, peanut butter, bananas, and mangos. She loved it."*
- If you rely on drink supplements and are scared to stop them, first incorporate them into the meal and snack routine.
- Be sure that you also include the child in regular meals and snacks that offer a variety of tastes and flavors.
- If your child truly is not getting adequate nutrition, that in itself can affect appetite. Be sure to work with an RD, follow growth, and have support when transitioning to the Trust Model.
- Consider nutrition-boosting favorite foods when planning meals and snacks, like muffins with pureed veggies or other supplements. Work with an RD to identify nutrition needs.

No matter what the tactic is, from force-feeding to following the child around with high-calorie shakes, most attempts to try to get your child to eat more will backfire.

"Our daughter was a tiny baby and didn't breastfeed or move to solids well. She was, and probably always will be, skeptical of new food. So we made the classic 'mistakes.' We were so concerned about how much she was eating that we only served foods she ate a lot of, which of course are now the only foods she eats. We were so freaked out about variety that we tried again and again to get her to try foods, laying on the pressure, lots of fighting. Exhausting and stressful for everybody." — Nora, mother of Suze, age five

Food Insecurity, Hoarding, Pocketing, and Forcing

"Sam had some hoarding issues, but it didn't last long. We let it run its course. We chose not to have food available to the boys all day and night. I didn't think it would reassure them. I fed them regularly and sat and ate with them. They pretty quickly learned to trust they would get fed." — Mia, mother of two boys adopted at age five and seven

"He liked to hold and play with teething biscuits and would chew at them a little, but he would lose interest and keep it clutched in his hands for hours. If we tried to take it from him, he became very angry." — Sue, mother of Marcus, then 18 months

Hoarding food is a common topic with internationally adopted and older foster or adopted children. "Hoarding" refers to stealing, hiding, or keeping food in a hand, pocket, or bag. If we take a moment to think about what the child's prior experience with food might have been, these behaviors are understandable.

When children are not fed reliably, do not get enough food, or have to compete for enough, they feel anxious. They have not been able to count on being fed, and when they do have access to food, they don't understand or trust that it is coming again. It can take weeks and months of reliable feeding for that trust to build and for them to believe that they will be fed. *Hoarding behaviors are about survival.*

Think about when you were on a diet, were told you couldn't eat a certain food, or had to fast for a blood test. I imagine you thought a whole lot more about your forbidden foods, and when you "cheated" on your diet or finished fasting, perhaps you ate a lot more than you would have otherwise. It's the same with kids and food scarcity, but on a much deeper, scarier, and more emotional level.

Kids who have experienced food scarcity frequently:
- Eat quickly.
- Gobble foods or stuff large amounts.
- Steal or hide foods.
- Eat large quantities.
- Become upset if someone eats something off their plate.
- Become upset if you try to take food away or try to get them to slow down.
- Keep food in their mouths for hours, known as "pocketing" (which may be behavioral or a sign of an oral-motor problem, or both).
- Demonstrate an apparent lack of interest in food (see below).

Many resources on adoption and hoarding advise allowing the child to have snacks in his backpack or carry food in a pocket, or even have Tupperware containers of food in the bedroom at night. Anneliese, mother of two boys, one adopted, one biological, recalls that the main feeding advice she got from her social worker was to let her son carry around baggies of carrots all day: *"I just didn't think that was going to help."*

Consider Marcus, who did not want to let go of his biscuit. He certainly can be allowed to hang on to the biscuit for a while, and maybe even have one in a baggie in his pocket. Follow his lead. If he throws a tantrum about having it taken away, allow him to carry it with him. But the parent also has to be absolutely reliable about regularly providing food. You may need to offer food more frequently at first, perhaps every hour or so.

In a different case, three-year-old Arielle, adopted at 11 months, was on calorie restriction and was experiencing intense food anxiety and preoccupation. Mom tried to let her carry food in an attempt to address her anxiety, but Arielle gobbled it up and begged for more. In this scenario, Arielle's actions were not the "hoarding" behaviors seen when a child first arrives from a place of food insecurity, but were actually symptoms of a feeding relationship disruption due to her food restriction (see Chapter 5). Letting her have her own stash of food to carry around didn't work for this family in this situation.

My main concern with the general recommendation of allowing kids with a history of food insecurity to have their own food stash is that it may make parents feel like they are off the hook for providing regular meals and snacks. Also, the child allowed to get food whenever he wants may *still feel responsible for getting his own food.* It is a missed opportunity to deepen the attachment with your child.

Feeding your child directly shows your child that you will take care of her and builds trust. Completing that cycle of need and meeting her needs, over and over again, is the basis for attachment.

One foster mom had a little boy she couldn't keep out of the fridge. He would eat up to the point of making himself sick on occasion. Mom didn't want to lock the fridge, feeling that restricting his food access was the wrong strategy. Instead, she assigned one of the refrigerator drawers to him. She stocked it with food he liked and told him that the drawer would always be full, and while he could not take food at random, this drawer was his. He checked the drawer often, with Mom's reassurance that it was his food, and he could help chose from it for meals and snack times. Mom made certain it was never empty, and gradually he forgot about it, mostly because Mom reassured him with regularly scheduled meals and snacks.

Another preschool boy adopted from Eastern Europe loved cereal. He would frantically gobble as much as he could and cry if he was limited. His parents finally realized that when he saw an empty cereal box, he thought there would be no more cereal, ever. They were able to reassure him, and for a while had to overstock the pantry with his favorite cereals. At breakfast, he was allowed to eat as much as he wanted, but simple reassurances and a trip to look at the pantry helped him to realize he would get enough. Pretty soon he was eating about the same as his brother and was no longer anxious at meals.

While you can allow access to food or a biscuit to clutch if it works for your child, I caution parents not to use constant access to food as an "easy out" from the task of reliable feeding. The best way to lessen hoarding behaviors is to lessen anxiety about food.

Your child may benefit from frequent reassurances such as, "There will always be enough food." You may even need to show her the pantry during the day, perhaps even as you end a meal, and say, "See, there is always enough food here."

> **More than anything, the thing that will lessen food anxiety
> is to be reliable about feeding—and to not limit the child.**

Pocketing

Pocketing, or keeping food in the mouth for prolonged periods, can also be seen in children who hoard, particularly with older children from institutional settings. There may be a combination of reasons, including oral-motor delay due to poor early feeding. A child may lack even basic knowledge of how to chew and move food around in his mouth and have a history of so little stimulation that he literally doesn't know the food is in there.

Amy tells how her three-year-old adopted foster daughter, Kassa, pocketed and how it resolved. *"Kassa hoarded food briefly and pocketed, keeping it in her mouth for hours. I really believe it was following the Trust Model of feeding that let her trust she would get fed and helped her stop the pocketing. Feeding her reliably also seemed to help her attach to us fairly quickly, when it was clear she had not attached to her previous caregivers."*

Amari's Pocketing

Bethany, an experienced foster and adoptive mother, emailed me in crisis. Two-year-old Amari, adopted at 14 months from Ethiopia, was rapidly getting worse. *"In the last week, Amari hardly drank 1½ cups of milk/day and only takes about three bites at meals. I can force feed her more, but she gags constantly. Now that she's vomiting, the weight gain has stopped and I can't keep force-feeding her. I just can't."* Amari had been seen by her speech therapist, who felt her pocketing and gagging was not due to an oral-motor problem. Although it was scary, I encouraged Bethany to stop pressuring and putting food in Amari's mouth. Often, kids pocket or gag when they are force-fed. *"If the weight starts slipping off, they'll recommend a feeding tube. That wouldn't be fun, but it can't go on like this,"* Bethany replied. I emailed Bethany the manuscript for this book, and we had a few brief calls. With the pressure off, within a weekend, Amari was no longer vomiting and her pocketing had decreased. Bethany was starting to see other encouraging signs, like Amari asking for lunch, and even on one occasion eating an entire piece of pizza.

Kim, mother of two older children adopted from Russia with sensory and oral-motor delays, was also reliable about feeding and family meals. *"The pocketing just seemed to go away, and wasn't even an issue within a year."*

Sometimes, however, pocketing is behavioral, a way of just saving or keeping food there so adults don't put more food into the mouth. Jacob, the son of a family I worked with, was labeled "failure to thrive" and experienced years of extreme feeding difficulties and "failed" feeding therapies. Multiple doctors found no explanation for his lack of appetite and slow growth. Jacob screamed at the sight of his highchair, which was in front of the TV, where he spent hours each day as his mother tried to get in even a few more bites.

He had recently been evaluated by his speech therapist, who felt that his pocketing was not due to an oral-motor issue. Our intake analysis, which includes the what, when, where, and how much the child eats from what is offered and, importantly, the social context, offered insight. Mom wrote: *"I put the cracker in his mouth and walked away from the highchair. I came back 20 minutes later and he still hadn't swallowed the cracker. He knew if he didn't swallow it that I wouldn't put anything else into his mouth."* (See the Feeding and Intake Journal Appendix.)

When kids get into gagging and vomiting, it can become almost reflexive. Amari was likely pocketing her food (See "Amari's Pocketing" on previous page) because if she tried to swallow it she would vomit, but Bethany initially felt that Amari was being naughty by pocketing. Once she understood it as something frightening that Amari couldn't control, she was able to stop pressuring and have more compassion. When Amari trusted that no one would put food in her mouth, her gagging and vomiting quickly improved.

When Kids Don't Feel Good About Food: Rediscovering the Joy

Remember Jacob, with his pocketing and feeding difficulties? Mom was encouraged when Jacob started to actually enjoy and seek out plain cucumbers and spinach—the first time he willingly ate *anything*. The family happily reported the progress to the GI (gastrointestinal) doctor who had been following Jacob's growth, looking for a possible GI explanation. The doctor scolded, "Don't bother with those foods; not enough calories. Douse them in ranch dressing and then give them to him."

Jacob was showing a glimmer of pushing himself along with eating. For the first time, he was expressing an interest and showing pleasure with eating. I don't think it's a coincidence that he sought out foods he had never been pushed or encouraged to eat. By denying and spoiling those first steps to a healthy relationship with food, his GI doctor was doing more harm than good.

> When it comes to feeding, when the *quality* of the eating experience improves for the child, the quantity and variety can then improve, but at the child's pace.

Maren, mother of Katia, shares a similar story. *"…with my very small but ultimately healthy daughter, who was picky from the start, her GI doctor kept pushing Carnation Instant Breakfast, which I couldn't understand as it seemed to be mostly sugar and she never drank it anyway. He told us to avoid things like plain fruit. We were supposed to put syrup or cream on everything sweet and oil and butter on everything else. For a couple of years I added oil to almost everything. But she loved (and still loves) plain fruit, and I refused to mess with that, even though her doctor disapproved."*

Some things to remember while helping your child discover the joy of eating:
- Don't fall into the trap of offering and pushing only high-fat or high-calorie foods.
- Do not "douse" everything in ranch dressing or butter to increase calories, but instead offer and serve some foods with high-fat and high-calorie sauces and some without.
- Remember, feeling comfortable and safe and having a good attitude about food needs to be in place before a child can tune in to hunger and increase intake on his own.
- Offer the foods you want to eat as a family, including high- and low-fat foods.

While Jacob and Katia were able to begin to discover the joy of eating on their own, for some children, eating has been so traumatic, painful, or full of conflict that they are not able to push themselves along. In that case, it may take more concrete steps.

Preparing for the Transition to Trust

"Since mealtimes have such deep meanings about relationships and love and giving and receiving, it's worth all the effort it takes to avoid turning mealtimes into bargaining sessions or battlegrounds." [8] — Mister Rogers, Mister Roger's Neighborhood

We've reviewed how many families have had bad experiences with different tactics and therapies that punished and rewarded. They may have "failed" intensive feeding clinic therapies and feel there is nothing they can do but give up and serve chicken nuggets and mac-n-cheese in front of the TV, or rely on PediaSure. Families may feel hopeless and traumatized and, for the sake of getting along, they give up.

You might feel that your only choices are:
- Fighting to get your child to eat, or
- Throwing your hands in the air in defeat and doing nothing.

But there is another option—the Trust Model for healing the feeding relationship and trusting that your child *can* improve with her eating.

Small and selective children are still worthy of trust.

"When I first held Alicia in my arms, she was a month old and weighed four pounds. I worked hard to help her stay awake for feedings. She didn't suck well. By 10 weeks, the judge who initially approved the adoption accused me of switching babies because she looked so

different! This wasn't the tiny, emaciated baby. She had rounded out so much. I didn't have access to a scale, so I didn't know how much she had gained, but I knew she was thriving."

— Connie, mother to Alicia, adopted from Peru. Connie's son came home a few years later, also severely malnourished. Both children are happy, healthy, and thriving at college.

Rehabilitating the Eating Experience: Starting Over

Children who have experienced trauma around food need a calm environment for eating so they can begin to feel calm and positive around food.[9] Recalling my analogy at the end of Chapter 2, where I compare nurturing a child's eating with planting bulbs and waiting for the flowers, feeling safe and comfortable around food is like the sun. The warm, energy-giving sun, that good attitude around food, is necessary to bring forth the first green shoots and healthy, vibrant flowers.

If you are tense at the table and your child is too, or if your little one panics at the sight of the highchair, she will not eat well. Anxiety, fear, and conflict are appetite killers. If Susie is crying and engaged in a battle over how many bites of carrot she has to eat to earn her Oreo, her energy is focused on *you and the battle*. If your child is in fight-or-flight response mode, she can't begin to imagine tasting the food in front of her. Susie simply has too much going on in her body to tune in to internal cues: the storm clouds of conflict and stress have blocked the sun, and her skills with eating cannot emerge and thrive. Some children may eat more, and some less, than is healthy for them when this happens.

If your child is anxious, the answer is not to distract with TV or let the child tune out with a video, but to re-set the feeding relationship. One place to start is where you feed. Your child may have a conditioned anxiety response to the setting around feeding, so that even when you take the pressure away, she may still feel anxious for a time.

In addition to no longer pressuring or forcing, signaling a change in the feeding relationship by changing the physical setting might help:
- Change the view that your child has been seeing, move her place, change the painting on the wall, or change the curtains.
- Change who sits next to her. For one family I worked with, Dad was engaged in a battle over table manners, so they found that moving him to a seat *not* directly across from his nine-year-old daughter was helpful.
- If your child is able, transition from the highchair to another chair. If he is ready, get rid of the tray on the highchair and pull him up to the table.
- Get some new drinking cups or throw out the plate that your child has been staring at while gagging.

What not to do:

- Avoid serving foods directly from the original container. Some children will refuse to eat a food simply if the wrapping or label changes.

- Don't always use the same cup, plate, or mat. Children on the autism spectrum, or children with rigid thinking, often seen with fetal alcohol exposure, can get so caught up in the visual presentation that they will *only* eat from the purple place-mat or the cartoon plate. Try to avoid this issue from the beginning by changing up dishes and cutlery.

- Avoid scraping your child's face with a spoon to clean dribbling foods, wiping her hands, or otherwise interfering with her while she is eating. Important: You can wipe her hands with permission if she seems distracted or unhappy about messy hands. Try not to do it if it doesn't seem to bother her.

- Have a damp washcloth available if she doesn't like messy fingers, and she can be taught to wipe them herself.

"But my child can't feel hunger and fullness cues. She's never shown me that she's hungry." This is what the mother of nine-month-old Olivia, a healthy older infant with difficulty transitioning to solids, said while we watched her crawl and play. Olivia soon became less interested in her toys and made her way to mom. She stopped socializing and inspecting me—the new person in her home—whimpered once, and played quietly with a ball in her lap. She looked far more serious than the smiling baby who greeted me at the door. Minutes later, she made another small whimper. Mom picked her up and she nursed, though they had to go into another room to avoid distraction. Olivia did have hunger signals; they were just very subtle. In addition, a review of her feeding showed that Olivia was fed every 20 minutes or so over an hour in the morning, with more cluster feeding in the afternoons—on Mom's, not Olivia's, schedule. Mom wondered, *"Maybe if I'm feeding her so often, she doesn't get a chance to really feel hungry?"*

When I hear parents say, "My child can't feel hunger because of his digestive problems" or another reason, here are a few considerations:

- He may not have the opportunity to develop an appetite if he is constantly grazing, encouraged to have small amounts of food, or given PediaSure to get calories in.

- His cues may be subtle: a change in demeanor, a change in activity level or skin color, looking for closeness, etc.

- If he's in a difficult feeding relationship that is characterized by intense conflict and stress, he may be too stressed to feel his hunger signals.

The Division of Responsibility and healing the feeding relationship allows the child to greatly reduce anxiety so he can begin to tune in to those cues of hunger and fullness. Stopping grazing also allows the opportunity to develop an appetite.

A pleasant atmosphere also means that the table is not the place to discuss adult or gloomy issues such as:

- Possible home foreclosure.
- Whether you have to put Fluffy to sleep.
- How nobody appreciates you and all you do (of course they don't)!

- The problems in your marriage (and there will be problems; remember, studies show that marital satisfaction is at its lowest with small children).
- Your son's behavior report at school.

You get the idea. The table is for connecting with your child and your family. Save the drama for another time.

> If you've been using TV to get food in, alas, you will need to turn the TV off. Perhaps allow TV with some meals or snacks, or eat family style for 15 minutes before turning on the TV. Find what works for your family. Often, by backing off the pressure, children are less dependent on distractions to eat. You may need to do this slowly over days to weeks, perhaps with one meal or snack a day, if your child has truly poor nutrition to start. You should be working with an RD if nutrition is compromised to that degree.

Saying Grace or Taking a Centering Breath Before Meals

Saying grace or taking a centering breath is another concrete way of signaling to the family that things are different now, a way of calling truce if you've been battling at the table over who is eating what or how much. With my adult clients, I also couple the centering breath with explicit permission to eat: to eat what tastes good, what appeals, and enough of it to feel satisfied.

Rebecca, early in her transition with her formerly restricted little girl, also took this opportunity to give permission to Adina, *"You can eat as much as you want from what is on the table."*

Taking a moment to pause from the craziness of a hectic day, getting the meal on the table, or rushing in from work helps on many levels. Alexis, newly transitioning her family to the Trust Model, noticed that she had also been eating much faster herself: *"I'm going 100 miles an hour to get the food on the table, and then I match my daughter's fast pace and I never slow down."* Taking a moment to pause and catch her breath has helped her slow down, pay attention to her own eating, and enjoy herself at the table.

As often as you can remember, say a little "grace" or take a moment before a meal to slow down, take a deep breath or two, and connect and transition to mealtime. This might mean a brief "bon appétit, you may eat!" or a more traditional blessing, or perhaps you take a moment to thank the farmer, the cook, and all the participants for showing up. When children lead this "thank-you time," it can be an opportunity to learn some surprising things about what they are thinking about and what they value most.

This breath, pause, grace, prayer, or whatever it is for your family helps calm and center before meals. It also:

- Includes the foster and adopted child in family ritual and helps welcome and cement the child's place in the family.

- Passes on family traditions, like saying Grandpa's funny grace.
- Starts the meal with focus and quiet before passing plates and serving little ones who can't serve themselves.
- Can transition into conversation, such as, "What was the best part of your day?" or "How was gym?" or "Who did you sit with at lunch?"
- Helps you and your children tune in to hunger and fullness cues.
- Helps connect you with yourself and your family, and holding hands is nice, too.
- Makes the mealtime feel special. Maybe even light a candle or two, and let the children blow the candle out to signal the end of the meal.
- Shares values, religious practices, and/or gratitude and appreciation for the cook, the farmers, and others involved.
- Can slow the pace for everyone.

Other Things to Consider as You Prepare to Transition to Trust

Acknowledge Your Feelings

"Once I mentally accepted that my son simply may never like vegetables and he could still be a productive member of society, it sort of released a weight I didn't even know existed." — Sue, mother to Marcus, adopted age 13 months

"The most frustrating thing for me has always been when I go out of my way to make something for my daughter that she has asked for or that she has eaten in the past—and then she refuses to eat it."
— Michelle, mother of Katie, adopted at 14 months from Russia, now three years old

Your children will know that you are upset and frustrated. Ashley Rhodes–Courter writes in her memoir, *Three Little Words,* about an episode where her adoptive mother Gay prepared all her favorites: "*'I'm not hungry.' I stared Gay down. A little thrill went through me as I saw her twitch. I knew she was thinking about how to respond to my rejection of her menu.*"

Children are master manipulators, and I mean that in the nicest way possible. It's their job. They can and will push your buttons, repeatedly. They can often sense your desperation around eating, and that is a power chip. It is normal to feel angry, disappointed, and even resentful when parenting, but if that is how you feel most of the time, you may need more support.

"No one wants to feel angry with their child or dread every meal. Particularly when I knew deep down that his own feelings were something he could not control."
— Peggy, foster mother to Scott, age four years

Cooking, planning, and buying food is a lot of work. Many parents enjoy food preparation and show love for their families through cooking. Moms often tell me they feel rejected and defeated when a child turns his nose up at a lovingly prepared dish. Find a way to get over it. Fume (in private), talk to your partner, or consult with a professional about your feelings.

Sixteen-year-old Yiseth, a self-described picky eater who is new to the Trust Model with her family, says, *"It's not a personal rejection of love if a kid doesn't want to eat something their mom made for them. Maybe it's the pressure, maybe the food, but it's not coming back at the love. It's not about the love. I love my parents to death."*

Realize that you are a good parent because you prepared a variety of foods, you are eating with your child, and you are doing *your* jobs. If you let your mood depend on whether your child eats something you made, or less or more than you wanted, you will make yourself crazy—as well as everyone around you. When you sit down to eat, your job is done, and now it's up to them.

Acknowledging or even identifying what you are feeling when you are overwhelmed, maybe even anxious or depressed, is hard. Sitting down to think about and understand where you are, and where your child is, as you undertake this process will be critical to learning to observe and be responsive to your child. Journaling is one tool that is helpful for you to prepare.

Write it Down

As you get ready for that leap of faith, buy a notebook or journal or use a few pieces of paper tucked in a kitchen drawer. One of the most powerful tools in this process is the journal, or diary of change. The point is: *Write it down!*

Before you begin your new feeding strategies, write down where you are now. What is your day like? Does it start with a child screaming for a bottle or stealing snacks from playmates while ignoring all else? How does it make you feel? How much time and energy are you devoting to what goes into your child's mouth? Get it on paper. As you go through this process, I can promise you that it may be hard to remember where you came from, so the journal has been invaluable for allowing my clients to see clear progress when they may feel like things are going nowhere. Particularly when you don't have someone like me on the other end of the phone reminding you of how far you have come, the journal is a valuable resource.

Avoid Labels

It is important not to label children as "picky," "under-eater," or "too small." This is particularly true with the hurt or traumatized child, described by Keck and Kupecky in *Parenting the Hurt Child* as "hypervigilant."[10] Be careful even not to let them overhear you talking about your concerns with others.

You can't win if you label your child with eating. He thinks, "Huh, I'm the picky one, I'm not supposed to learn to like new foods." From the child's point of view, he is not made to feel capable, but deficient. In addition, children sniff out and learn where your buttons are, so if they hear a lot of talk and concern about their eating, they learn, "I don't eat, and it makes Mom and Dad crazy!"

Wouldn't it be nicer to give the message to an older child, "You'll try new foods when you're ready," or "You don't have to eat anything you don't want to," and then stop talking about it? In fact, the less you say about what or how much your children are eating, the less they will have to prove, disprove, and fight you over it.

Ignore What and How Much Your Child Is (or Isn't) Eating

You may have to fake this at first, but ignore what and how much your child is eating. Don't comment or praise. Most parents I work with on this issue say they spend 95 percent of mealtimes talking about how much and what the selective eater is eating: negotiating, encouraging, and bribing. That has to stop. The child must be allowed to *participate* at meals, not be the focus. Over and over again I have heard from clients that when the focus was off the child, perhaps when Mom tells Dad about her day or they talk to a sibling, *that* was when the "picky eater" would sneak a piece of broccoli onto his plate.

Similarly, when you pick your child up from school or daycare, avoid the temptation to rummage through his lunch box and greet him with, "Did you eat all your sandwich?" If it's the first thing you ask about, you have sent a very powerful message that his eating is what matters most—which is a power chip—and that he can't be trusted to handle it on his own. Be intentional about avoiding this habit. Pretend you are not concerned about it; you can look in his lunch box later when he is not in the room. Ask about art or if he played in the puddles during recess—ask about anything but food.

Many daycare centers also will report about intake at pick-up time. Colby, a client whose son Frank was an extremely selective three-year-old, had to ask the childcare staff not to give her the pick-up report in front of Frank. She also asked the staff not to encourage or scold Frank about his eating. (More on "Dealing With Meddlers" on page 255.) Colby had a meeting with the daycare staff to explain her new approach, and since Frank wasn't gaining weight well and she worried about his overall nutrition, the staff agreed to email her about what he ate at the end of the day instead. Having this information helped her plan her after-school snacks and meals.

Critical to the Transition: Neutralizing the Power Struggles

Many of the feeding problems I work with arise or are worsened because families are locked in a battle for control—the power struggle that can turn dinner into what one parent calls *"45 minutes of hostage negotiations."* One of the key pieces of advice in *Parenting With Love and Logic,* by parenting experts Dr. Foster Cline and Jim Fay, is to "avoid control battles whenever you can."[11] When you are engaged in battle over those two bites of chicken or how many beans he needs to eat to earn dessert, your child's attention is focused on you and on the struggle, not on his own cues of hunger and fullness.

"I really had to learn how to lay off. It's really hard to resist. My biggest hurdle at the table is not getting sucked into the power struggle. All day long, Mommy sets the boundaries. To feel like it's not a parenting failure to let him tell me 'no,' and to know I don't have to have consequences for that—was a huge struggle."

— Riya, mother to Jackson, adopted domestically at 18 months

There is a reason why it feels hard not to fight over food. Kids often want to engage you in the power struggle. Whether it is a traumatized child yearning for control, a securely attached child now working on separation, or a child with sensory issues who doesn't like how a food feels yet, it is their job to manipulate (and I mean that in the kindest, most respectful way). Not allowing them to suck you into the power struggle will get easier with time. As Michelle, three-year-old Katie's mom, recommends, "Be patient, and don't take it personally."

Stick to Your Jobs and Let Your Child Do His

It's worth the time to flesh out the concept of neutralizing battles because it is absolutely essential for the transition to Trust to succeed. The short answer to how to avoid the power struggle is to institute or maintain the Division of Responsibility (DOR). The previous review shows that most parents get stuck or fight with the child because they are trying to do the child's job by trying to get them to eat more, less, or different foods, or because they allow the child to do their job, such as dictating the menu.

See if you can tell where the jobs have been confused:

Scenario 1: Mom Marion makes a lovely dinner with salad, fruit, bread, and stew. While she was cooking, she asked her son Ryder what he would like. He asked for his favorite, plain pasta. When she was serving up their plates, he cried that he wanted rice instead. Marion argued that he asked for pasta.

Answer: Mom has done part of her job—the when and where—and she is to be commended for getting everyone to the table and planning a variety of foods. But alas, she let her son decide the what—pasta. Predictably, he changed his mind, and they are still arguing. Also, Mom pre-plated the meal. Remember that allowing the child to have more control by serving family style is a key neutralizing strategy.

Scenario 2: Dad George gets takeout Chinese with plain rice and a few entrée options. He also opens a jar of applesauce and serves milk. His nine-year-old son Joshua gets up and helps himself to crackers.

Answer: George also is allowing his son to decide the what. Joshua normally likes rice and applesauce, and one entrée was a mild chicken dish that he has enjoyed in the past. He had options on the table he could have eaten.

Scenario 3: Snack time was over 15 minutes ago, but four-year-old Susie gets a granola bar. Mom Deborah and Susie argue over the bar.

Answer: Susie is deciding the what and the when by getting it on her own. Deborah can ask Susie to save the granola bar for afternoon snack, or to eat with lunch.

Scenario 4: Six-year-old Tom wants dessert, but he has to eat two bites of chicken nuggets and two bites of corn before he can get it. He is trying to negotiate down to one bite of chicken and is whining.

Answer: This is the bargaining and negotiating that happens because parents are trying to control how much and what Tom eats. Once the food is on the table, Tom should decide what and how much he eats from what is provided.

If you stick with your jobs and let Junior do his, you will avoid most battles. This may sound too simple to be true, but it is a recurring theme: When parents stop trying to do the child's job and start allowing the child to do theirs, the battles stop—and the mood and atmosphere improve, often quickly. It doesn't mean that the intake or variety improves right away; in fact, they often worsen initially, as you will read below. But the battles stop, and that is the first step.

Serve family style: My clients tell me that in addition to the DOR, the single most useful piece of advice to neutralize the battles is serving food family style. Put all the bowls out on the table, let children (who are able) serve themselves, and help little ones as needed. Many families start meals with an all-out fight. If you put a pre-plated meal in front of a selective eater, and he doesn't even want to see green beans, he may instantly fight or gag. Avoid this battle. The game is over if you start a meal with intense emotions.

What Else Can You Do to Help Your Selective Eater?

Meals and Structure:
- Have family meals, remembering that children need to see, smell, pass a food, and see others enjoy it as part of the learning process.
- Serve meals and snacks every three to four hours for older children and every two to three hours for younger ones. The structure is key to helping a child have an appetite.
- Experiment with different settings like restaurants, samples at the grocery or warehouse store, or outings where food is available, but not the main activity. One mom shared on my blog, "*She watched a young child request seconds, thirds,*

and fourths of pasta and pesto. She would not try it that day, but soon after her curiosity got the better of her and she ate some. Pasta with pesto became a staple for years, and is still a favorite food."

Serving Tools:

- Spoons and other utensils can add frustration and get in the way of how much your child eats. Do not push using utensils.
- If your child is interested in utensils, be sure they are appropriate. Get specifics on the right utensils, cups, etc. from your therapist, or use trial and error to find the right ones. A spoon with a thick rubber handle and a deeper bowl may help.
- For a child with a motor delay, you may need to help load the fork or spoon and hand it to her, or even feed an older child—with permission, meaning the child leans forward and/or willingly opens his mouth to accept the spoon.
- Put paper napkins at each place setting so she can spit food out. The young toddler may just lean forward and spit food onto the tray, as is age appropriate. A four-year-old with normal development should be taught to discreetly spit food into a napkin.

Remember Bethany's daughter Amari from page 94–95, who was pocketing and vomiting? Turns out Bethany had a family rule of no spitting out food. When Amari's only option was to swallow the food, this increased her anxiety and worsened her gagging and vomiting. I advised that Amari had to be able to spit out food. If a child has a history of gagging, pocketing, or vomiting, they must know they have an alternative to swallowing. Also, a child who is allowed to spit out a food is more willing to put food in her mouth in the first place. If a child pockets, ignore it whenever possible. If there is a safety concern, calmly offer the option, "You can spit it out (while handing over a napkin) or swallow it (offer a glass of water), but it's not safe to go on the trampoline with food in your mouth." You can develop a shorthand signal like, "Let's do a quick Cheek Check" if you need to. Stay calm.

What to Serve:

- Enjoy fruits and vegetables yourself. Studies show this is the best predictor of a child learning to like fruits and veggies.[12]

- Texture is often more of a stumbling block than flavor. If you are moving slowly with texture, don't forget to introduce a variety of flavors.
- Serve something your child usually eats at every meal.
- Include dips, sauces, toppings, and sprinkles. Ellory explained her approach with her selective three-year-old daughter. *"One day I put out several small bowls of rice (she was unfamiliar with rice and would not eat it), and let her put different*

toppings on each bowl. She loved the rice with soy sauce, and that's how we added a new food."

- Serve a child-sized portion of dessert with the meal.
- Occasionally serve sweets or other favorite meals with snack and let them eat as much as they want.

NOTE: The last two points on dealing with sweets and treats usually elicit the most doubt and the "yeah, right" response from parents. It is more thoroughly discussed in the "Sweets and Treats" section of Chapter 8, What About the What, on page 230. Pause and read that section now if you are in the "yeah, right" camp.

Menu Planning: Consider Versus Cater

Something that is critical for a child to feel safe when coming to the table is that she sees at least one thing that is familiar so she can satisfy her hunger. That might be bread, rice, pasta, naan, tortillas or some other accepted food. That reassurance that she won't go hungry helps her feel more confident about trying new foods.

If having family meals is new to you, start with the regular foods you are eating now, place the serving bowls in the middle of the table, and eat together. Do this until you get the hang of the schedules and not pressuring. When you feel like you want to branch out, you can keep the familiar food such as mac-n-cheese and add something new like apple-sauce, or make your favorite white chicken chili knowing Sam won't try it (but he won't ever try it of he doesn't see it), and make something you know he likes, like cornbread, to go with it. If the kids also like things like microwaved frozen peas,that can be an option. Visit the Ellyn Satter Institute at www.ellynsatterinstitute.org for wonderful resources on getting into the family meal habit.

> If you are concerned that your child doesn't have the nutritional reserve to begin this process, as her eating may get worse during the transition, make sure you are working with a dietitian and under the supervision of a physician. Some indication that she might not have the reserve is if you rely heavily on supplement drinks for nutrition, or if she is falling off the growth curve, is not experiencing catch-up growth, or has identified nutrient deficiencies like iron.

If you have an entrenched problem with a child who only eats four things, initially, *every meal and snack must include one of these four things during the transition.* Remember to add on; don't take away. Planning what to put on the table is one of the trickiest dilemmas for families who have given up and are used to serving Sam only his accepted foods at a separate time and meal. The following has helped many clients plan meals and snacks:

- Make a list of your child's favored or almost-always accepted foods.

- On a separate sheet of paper or 3X5 card, make a list of foods your child *usually* eats. Include at the bottom of this sheet or card a list of foods he *has eaten* in the past.
- Observe or ask if your child prefers salty, sweet, crunchy, or smooth tastes and textures.
- List any accepted condiments.

If you are fostering or adopting an older child, you can ask your child to help you make the list initially so that you can stock some favored and accepted foods. Here is a sample from one of my intake questionnaires for Kelly, a selective eater:

- **Favored foods:** crackers (Ritz, Club), pretzels, plain pasta, rice, French toast fingers, McDonalds plain hamburger, chicken nuggets, vanilla tube yogurt, maple instant oatmeal made with water
- **Accepted foods:** canned mandarin oranges, seedless red grapes cut in half, vanilla yogurt from a cup, Wheat Thins, plain peas
- **Refused:** fresh fruit or vegetables and anything with mixed textures
- **Prefers:** sweet, salty, and smooth
- **Condiments:** ketchup and ranch dressing

Condiments can be your friend. Parents often express a reluctance to serve sauces and dips, worrying the child won't learn to eat foods plain. Think of ketchup and dips like "training wheels." You probably won't have a teenager pouring ketchup on rice or corn on the cob— that is, unless you are fostering or adopting a teenager who comes to you doing that. The bottom line is that condiments help children learn to like new foods.[13,14]

- The familiar flavor of condiments can be the bridge or link to a new food. If a child likes chicken with ketchup, she may enjoy another meat if it is served with the familiar ketchup.
- For foods like meats, which are tough to chew for small children or kids with oral-motor issues, dips and sauces can add moisture and make them easier to manage.
- One study showed that vegetables cooked with a little sugar helped kids like them more, and another study with grapefruit juice showed that kids who had a little sugar with the juice on the first introduction afterward liked the plain juice more readily than children who had not initially received a sweetened version. So the myth of the sugar and condiments limiting variety is just that—a myth. Ketchup, or even sugar for that matter, helps increase variety.[13,14]
- Have a variety of options, from ketchup to ranch dressing, to homemade honey-ginger dressings to hot sauce.

Put the lists of favored and sometimes-accepted foods on the side of the fridge or in a drawer where you, the parent, can see them. Also make a list to remind yourself of what you like to eat and want to eat again. Many parents tire of eating "kid" foods year after year and are happy to rediscover their own joy in cooking and meals.

Wasting food: *"This feels so wasteful when I make things I know he won't eat."*
Go into this knowing you will waste more food—for a while. Kids need permission to take food onto their plates and not eat it. It's part of that process of learning to eat. A child who is allowed to *not* eat something is more willing to try something new. If your "picky eater" orders pulled pork, avoid the temptation to say, "You know you won't eat that; why don't you get something you can eat, like chicken fingers…" Instead, think, "Well, I'm glad he's open to the idea of pulled pork; if he doesn't eat it this time, he can eat the cornbread and baked potato and I can take the pork for lunch tomorrow." In general, to lessen waste, you can ask your son to serve himself a small portion initially and take more if he wants it.

Try redefining "waste" like one of my blog readers does: *"I struggle with guilt about throwing food out, since I grew up with 'clean your plate' and had to retrain myself to know when I'm actually full. One thing that helps me is to define 'eating food I don't want/need' as wasting. It helps me realize that feeding scraps to the dog or cat is better than eating food I don't want. If a kid tries a bite or two of a new veggie and the rest gets thrown out, is it really 'waste' if it provided an introduction to a food that she might later like?"*

When planning dinner, lunch, or a snack, put out foods *you* want to eat, or food you want your other children to learn to like, as siblings are often unintentionally limited to the accepted menu of the most selective child. Initially, add one or two foods from the favored foods list to the offerings. It might feel silly to have the rotisserie chicken Mom brought home with some microwaved frozen peas and mashed potatoes sitting next to a bowl of plain rice or pretzels, but this is the bridge to helping your child learn to like new foods. If selective eaters come to the table and see *something* they can eat and know they won't be pressured to eat other foods, they can begin to relax, look around, watch, smell, pass and poke, and eventually try new foods.

Sample Menu for Kelly's Family
- **Breakfast:** French toast fingers, yogurt from a cup, and cut-up bananas (allow the child to do the cutting, if willing and able). If *you* are eating scrambled eggs, put them on a serving plate and serve yourself, but make a bit extra.
- **Morning snack:** Pretzels, canned mandarin oranges, and 2% milk (or whole-fat milk if your child likes it and supporting nutrition with increased fat options is a goal).
- **Lunch:** Whole-wheat Club Crackers, whipped cream cheese with a spreader so the child can have fun applying the cheese, turkey lunch meat, and grapes. If he is old enough, he can eat the grapes whole or cut them himself with an appropriate knife.

You may want to eat pita bread and turkey with avocado, so slice some avocado and put it on a plate on the table so he sees it and can help himself to it if he wants.

- **Snack:** Cut-up apple with half the slices peeled, cinnamon-sugar shaker on the table, vanilla yogurt from a tube, pretzels.
- **Dinner:** Chicken nuggets, plain rice, rotisserie chicken, microwaved peas, pan-fried onion and peppers with teriyaki sauce, ketchup on the table, vanilla frozen yogurt (or ice cream) for dessert.

More ways to consider children when menu planning and cooking:
- Hold the spice or chopped herbs, and let everyone add their own at the table.
- Serve a favored side dish if you are making an unfamiliar entrée.
- Serve different preparations of favorite foods; for example, whole-wheat versions of favored foods like waffles or crackers may be a good start.

How long you serve favored foods, and for how many meals and snacks a day, will vary depending on the limitations of your child, how long you have been struggling, and your child's baseline nutrition. If your child is a very selective eater with few choices, I recommend having something from his favored list at every meal or snack while you get the hang of structure and learn not to pressure. Once you have been doing this for awhile, you can try one meal or snack per day where you don't have a "favorite," but instead you serve something from the "usual" list, knowing that in a few hours he will have the chance to eat a favored food again.

Often, the pace at which this progresses depends as much on the anxiety level of the parent as on the skills and interest from the child. Having an RD or a speech therapist familiar with the Trust Model may help.

> With menus unintentionally limited to the preferences of the most selective child, it is often the younger sibling of a child with feeding challenges who initially blossoms. As one dad shared early in the process, *"We put out lentils and chicken and bread and corn. While our daughter ate mostly bread and a little corn, we were surprised when our younger son, Mathew, ate and loved the lentils. I don't think he'd ever had them and he's almost two. This process is making us much more aware of his needs and not limiting his opportunities."*

Many parents have trouble with the menu planning process because they feel so much pressure to get calories, protein and, most challenging, veggies into the child's diet. Parents seem obsessed with veggies, leading to endless bribes and fights. If we look at the *worry*, we see that parents generally want:
- The nutrition, vitamins, and fiber that veggies offer.
- The child to learn to like vegetables.

Here are a few facts that may help you relax and trust this process while working on menu planning:

- Fruits basically have the same nutrient and fiber content as veggies.
- Pressuring, bribing, and begging her to eat veggies will not help her like to eat veggies and will probably make her like them less.[15]

Ashley Rhodes–Courter, author of *Three Little Words,* spent 10 years in foster care before she was adopted and now finds herself dealing with feeding issues with her own foster kids. The following are some of her tips about feeding adopted and foster children, excerpted with permission from the SPOON Foundation Website (www.spoonfoundation.org).

- Understand that you can't win this battle.
- A child will eat what they want, and often balance their own diets in the long term.
- Don't label them as "picky eaters" or let others continually comment on their food intake or put children down for their choices.
- Don't force kids to clean their plates or sit at the table past the normal mealtime. Meals should not feel like a punishment.
- Assume you don't understand all the many conflicts this child may have about food.
- Serve at least one dish per meal that your child will like, but don't get angry if they choose not to eat it.
- Be lenient about sugared cereals—these may be the only kind the child ever knew.
- Have the child pick out foods in the supermarket so he feels he is participating.
- Teach them to cook and bake (everyone loves to have a skill or feel accomplished). Make things around the kitchen fun, and mealtimes a time to share thoughts and jokes, not a source of pressure.

Menu Planning Veggie Tips

- Serve raw versions of the veggies you are cooking with the meal.
- Include dips, ranch or yogurt dressings, ketchup, or other condiments.
- Keep serving veggies, without comment.
- Find different ways to serve veggies. Your child might reject a baby carrot but might eat carrot coins (larger carrots cut into circles).
- Add fat, flavor, and even sugar. Studies show that adding a little sugar helps children overcome the bitter taste of some vegetables.[14] Simmer chopped carrots in a little chicken broth and ½ teaspoon of sugar and a little butter. (Also serve veggies plain.)

Take advantage of convenience foods if it helps: precut veggies or frozen stir-fry mixes.

What Families Go Through as They Transition to Trust

This is a process, with ups and downs, and sometimes progress is slow. When parents have been struggling for so long, it can be hard to see progress. Hopefully you have begun, or will soon start with writing down your "where are we now" in your feeding story.

Documenting Your Journey

Initially the successes will be yours, and these are worthy of noting and celebrating. Celebrate (out of your child's sight) when you:

- Get everyone at the table.
- Start serving family style.
- Serve your child seconds and thirds, even if it makes you anxious.
- Don't have to play food cop anymore!
- Didn't allow yourself to get sucked into a battle.

Throughout this process, use the journal as a prompt to help you observe, be curious, and respond to your child.

Stage One: This Is Scary

With selective eaters and "problem" feeders, some of whom may have "failed" feeding therapies, the predictable response to taking away pressure is that **your child's eating will get worse before it gets better.** The good news is that while his eating may seem worse, families almost always say that they are happier at the table and the fighting over food has stopped. Everyone seems to relax and actually enjoy being there together. That is one of the three goals parents have when they start this work—having enjoyable family meals. This is a big step and is not to be underestimated. Write it down in your journal.

Things Parents Typically See in the Early Transition

- *"He starts with dessert and only eats that plus maybe one or two bites of bread or a favored food."*
- *"He eats less than he used to. How is that possible?"*
- He eats only one or maybe two things from what you put out at any meal or snack.
- His behavior seems to be getting worse.
- You used to be able get him to eat a bite or two of veggies with the dessert bribe, but now he won't eat any.

This stage can last a long time, and as with other transitions, it will pass more quickly if you are truly able to trust your child and adopt the Division of Responsibility. Most families get stuck or struggle because they follow through on parts of the model but have trouble with others, like serving dessert with the meal, for example. Parents either aren't sure of what the DOR means, still cross the lines of the DOR, or they can't yet fully commit.

How to Get Through Stage One

- Pray.
- White-knuckle it—that is, hold onto the chair when every fiber in your being wants to encourage him to eat just one more bite or put that last cracker into his mouth.
- Hold hands with your partner under the table.
- Keep a note on the fridge such as "Trust Jacob" and use it as a mental mantra, or even write out the Division of Responsibility in big letters to remind you of your job and your child's job. (If your child is able to read, you may want to tuck this away.)
- Know that your child may eat less for a while until she learns to tune in. Knowing that it is a necessary part of the process may help you get through it.
- Say the "Serenity With Feeding" prayer (see page 248).
- Tap into any feelings of relief or instinctual confidence in the process.
- Ignore, or pretend to ignore, how much or how little your child is eating.

The **"Rescue Snack"** might help you get through dinner, which is often the most difficult meal because it is usually when the new and "challenging" foods are presented, and people are tired and rushed at the end of the day. Understandably, many parents can't handle the idea of letting a child go to bed hungry. However, if your child senses your weak spot, he may refuse the offered foods, even if there are options you know he can eat, in an effort to hold out for a favored food. If you worry this might happen to you, or it has happened, consider moving dinner up a little earlier, allowing him to choose to leave the table after eating nothing and then plan on a snack before bed if it's at least an hour and a half later. Try saying this: "You don't have to eat anything you don't want to, but this is what's for dinner. Snack is in a couple of hours. Will you sit and keep us company for a few minutes?" Later, the "rescue snack" should be at the table and be an accepted food, but not a favorite like cookies.

Stage Two: Emerging Skills

This sometimes surprises families, as children can push themselves along in a matter of days, but it may also take longer. The first skill to emerge is a better attitude about being at the table. DO NOT underestimate the importance of this. Once the DOR is mostly or all the way in place, you may observe the following behaviors:

- He notices and expresses interest in foods, even if he doesn't put any on his plate or try them.
- He might pass a food and watch you intently as you eat it.
- She might lick a food.

- He might ask for food or wonder when a meal is.
- A child with sensory issues may be more tolerant of foods on the table or near him, now that he is not pressured to eat them.
- He visibly relaxes and fidgets less at meals.
- Patterns emerge in his intake—more at some meals, less at others. These are indications that he is learning to tune in to his body.
- He might eat a "large" meal on occasion or at least a "normal" portion.

"He gradually became more comfortable with baby cereal mixed with milk, and whole milk yogurt mixed with whole milk in a bottle seemed soothing to him. Other than that, it took a long time to introduce each solid to him. Over the course of a year, he has become much more accepting of foods, but it was a long, slow process."
— Gabriella, mother to Mika adopted from Romania at fifteen months

"The 'division of responsibility' and taking the pressure off was a godsend. We are working at removing the pressure, tweaking mealtimes, etc. and we are seeing signs of progress, like her commenting on food smelling good, her moving to eating grilled cheese sandwiches that have a little bit of mozzarella mixed with the other cheese, etc."
— Sally, mother to Anisa, adopted from Ethiopia at nine months, now four years old

There will be good days and bad. Sometimes progress comes quickly, but for other families more slowly. Knowing that it may be two steps forward and one step back, and being prepared for gradual and subtle progress, will help. Your child is probably not going to suddenly and reliably start eating large quantities of a variety of foods.

"I feel so hopeful when Ruby has a bigger meal, and then dashed when she goes back to the usual nibbles for the rest of the day. It's hard to keep the progress in mind, and there has been amazing progress in only one week: saying she's hungry, being happy at the table, one time eating an entire egg, but then there are still those meals that go by and she eats so little."
— Carrie, two weeks into the transition, who describes the process as a roller coaster

Mom Bethany shares Carrie's frustration with the process but found it helpful to think back on their own journey and how far they have come. It is why journaling can be so critical: *"I know compared to where we were a month ago, when she was vomiting several times a day and only getting nutrition from Boost drinks, this is a huge improvement. It's hard not to want it to go, well, faster. It also helps to remember how miserable we were and how none of what we had tried before helped, and where it got us. No sense going back to that."*

Bethany's Journey

Amari, age two, was adopted at age 14 months from Ethiopia and initially did some hoarding. After being home for about a year, her eating changed dramatically, with no identifiable cause. While underlying medical causes were being evaluated, Bethany needed help with their difficult feeding relationship. The following are excerpts from Bethany's notes on the first few months after reading the first draft of *Love Me Feed Me,* with a few brief emails and about an hour total of phone support.

February 10th: A few months ago, she started to get pickier and ate less and less, eventually eating about five bites at each meal and down to two cups of milk a day and gaining nothing. She would pocket and take an hour to finish those bites. In one year home, she grew four inches and gained only nine ounces . . . We saw a nutritionist who told us how to sneak calories into her food. We saw a speech pathologist who determined that the issue was "psych" and barely glanced at her. In the last week, Amari has gotten SO much worse. She hardly drinks 1 1/2 cups of milk/day, drinks nothing else, and takes about three bites at meals. I can force feed her more, but she gags constantly and has developed a tongue thrust so she can't take a full bite. I've gone back to tiny, infant spoons only about half full if I want the food to stay in her mouth. I do still think this is mostly a psych issue, though I wouldn't mind her having a better exam to determine if it is physical. She gets distressed, with this glazed-over look in her eyes (we have parented deeply emotionally disturbed children through treatment foster care before and I have seen this look too many times to not recognize it) after a few bites and completely disassociates. We have tried EVERYTHING. We have ignored the issue, we have put her in a quiet room with no distractions, gotten angry and screamed. We even tried to punish her (I know, bad move, but we just thought... maybe?!?). Now she's puking all her food at least once a day. I am screaming inside. I don't want to do this any more. I am tired. We have had one fight after the other for this girl and I love her deeply, but this is sucking the joy out of parenting. I need to know what to do. We have an appointment to see a psychologist — a month away.

February 12th: We are just allowing her to eat as much as she wants (one or two nibbles) and offering her food more regularly throughout the day. It goes against everything the nutritionist said, but this is not a "normal" situation . . . While I cannot be 100% certain this is a psych issue, I am about 95% sure that it is — or that it has become one. In other words, if she has a physical issue, psychological trauma is still presenting itself through this issue . . . At this point, we have been fighting for this child for nearly two years . . . first to get her home, then to get her to walk, then to get her to talk . . . I am just weary.

Feb 14th: I've read about half the book. We are totally willing to try this, but I am leery about whether or not this will work with our daughter . . .

Feb 18th: The vomiting has stopped completely, in one weekend! Seems to be pocketing less as well. I'm not sure if it's because feeding overall is more relaxed or because she hasn't put something in there that she doesn't like. Now, if only she'd start eating more. I am appreciating less stress around eating, but I still feel so defeated at the end of the meal when she's only had a few bites. It is very tempting to start up with feeding her again to get just a few more calories in, but I know where that leads, so hopefully I can avoid it . . . Eventually she will have to start eating more, though. Three bites, three times a day isn't going get her to grow.

Feb 23rd: I wonder how much she needs to gain weight? For lunch, she ate 1/2 slice of bologna, one oz. of cheese, one tsp. of hummus, and two crackers. Breakfast was 1/3 of a banana a 1/2 cup of oatmeal. I don't think that's enough, but maybe it is?!? It's certainly better than three bites. I have helped her to take a few extra bites at both meals, but she did so happily. So glad I did review Zscores, she's definitely improved with the weight gain, so it was helpful for me. She's close to the "normal" range, especially for her current height.

Feb 26th: Good days and bad, good meals and bad. I am still really struggling with what to do when she cheeks food. I know that the simple answer is to let her spit it out, but it angers me. I know that she can swallow it—she just swallowed other bites. I don't know how to mentally get past that to let her spit it out. I've tried, I swear I have. My husband has the same struggle. For now, we're just having her sit in her highchair until she swallows it. She eventually does, but it can take a LONG time.

March 12th: Amari is doing much better. She only ate about three bites of food for breakfast, but she was asking for food two hours later. I had her wait until lunch and she ate half a cheese stick and about 2/3 of a hot dog plus a few crackers and other things. We're seeing about one full meal per day and she's happily eating more like six bites at most meals — vs. the three she was doing before . . . If she has gained weight (I think she has), we don't want to see GI. I'm afraid all of that will just traumatize her and set us so far back. I'm not seeing her dislike any certain type of food like we were before. She even asked for chicken the other day and took and swallowed two bites without any prompting from me . . . sometimes Amari refuses to try a bite of something that I know she will like. I have asked her to lick these things and then she always wants a bite after that. So far it doesn't seem to upset her, but I don't want that to turn into a battle, ever. I feel like I am better able to gauge and respond to her reactions.

Six weeks after the initial contact, Amari had gained 10 ounces, more than in the entire previous year.

April 3rd: And... just like that, she eats normally for 3/5 meals. Amari still likes to cheek things and it still drives me crazy, but it no longer seems to cause any kind of back slide for the next meal when she decides to do that. I would honestly say that MOST days she eats 2 decent meals. They're small, but so is she. She will never be big. Her Zscore is going up and she's even almost on the regular charts. I call that a HUGE win.

Handling Common Obstacles During the Transition

Your child will challenge the new system of the DOR. It's his job, and he is figuring out the new rules and deciding if you really mean it this time. He will eat worse, less, and push every button he can. Hang in there. Here are common questions I hear over and over from my clients:

- *"Every time I put food on the table, he immediately says, 'Yuck, that looks gross.' It's so discouraging. I try to tell him, he loved it last week, but it doesn't matter."* That is typical of small children. You reply: "You don't have to eat it, but please say, 'no thank you.'" Then move on.

- *"Everyone says to introduce a food at least 10 times before he will like it. Our feeding therapist has us keep track, and with a big smile, remind Jeremy that he has to try it TEN TIMES! So far, he refuses, and then I keep serving the same food 10 meals in a row. I'm sick of it."* I would be too. The idea is to have a checklist and cross off each try—which he would agree to after your rational explanation—and he would decide he liked some and not others, right? You know by now that's not how it works. Ten times would be nice: A selective child, one with a difficult feeding past, oral-motor issues, or sensory concerns, may take dozens or even *hundreds* of neutral exposures before liking a new food.

  Even the "adventurous" child might take years to learn to like salad or tuna fish. Serving it 10 times in a row is not realistic. That's not how families eat, and it puts the focus on the food and not on enjoyable meals. Serve tuna or salad when you want to eat them. Serve the foods *you* want to eat, over and over again. Consider his tastes when menu planning, but don't cater. Then wait. As my colleague Pam Estes, RD, says, "They don't, they don't, they don't, then suddenly they do!" I often get calls from clients six months to a year after our initial one or two sessions, with cheerful news of recent breakthroughs. Hang in there.

- *"We noticed a few times with family-style meals, when a bowl was almost empty, and I'd say, 'I'm going to finish the peas if no one minds,' he would suddenly want to try the peas, or would be willing to put them on his plate. Can we trick him into trying more by doing this more often?"* What you're seeing is the result of scarcity. That is, when something is limited (think of "ONLY ONE LEFT!" kinds of advertising), it piques our interest. I get this question from all kinds of families who have noticed this scarcity effect, and I've seen it at my table as well. It's human, it's normal, it applies to food, and it's tempting to exploit. The fact that you asked the question means that you are thinking the right way. You are examining your own motives, and it feels wrong because you need to "trick" him. If you do use this technique, chances are he'll figure it out, and it will slow the process down. You can see what happens and be curious about his reactions, but don't do it intentionally too often. Also, if your child has experienced food scarcity or insecurity in the past, trying this tactic may increase his anxiety and not help him with his eating. Proceed with caution.

- *"We feel really stuck. We are at the table now, which is great, and we put out all the food, always with one of his favorites; however, he still gets up mid-meal and gets what he wants. Last night it was chips. I don't want a tantrum in the middle of dinner so I let him do it."* First off, you are sensing this is going against the DOR by allowing him to go and get food because you are feeling conflicted and anxious about the interaction. He is trying to take over the "what" to serve, even though you have done a great job of offering him choices he can handle and likes. This annoys you because you can feel that it is a power play. Pay attention to those feelings. When you get annoyed, or think, "What do I do now?" check back in with the DOR. He is testing your rules, and alas, he is winning. He is finding out that your fear of a tantrum means he can do whatever he wants.

Now you have choices:

1. You can choose to avoid the tantrum because you can't handle it right now and are happy enough that everyone is at table; it's pleasant and you are serving family style. This is a viable option. Be kind to yourself, decide what you will take on, and perhaps leave it for another day. If you feel overwhelmed, you may need to make these choices, but recognize that his progress may be slowed if he is still allowed to dictate what he is served.

2. Do what is "right," but it will be painful for a few days. He may protest when you ask him to put back the chips. When he doesn't put them back and you give him a warning, he will pout but try to eat them. When you take them away from him, he may have that tantrum. But ultimately, he is testing and wants to know that you are in charge and that you are in control. That makes him feel safe. He will pitch a fit and might even miss dinner, but you can allow a snack of accepted foods before bed. He might try it again a few more times, but if you stay firm, he is likely to go along with it and behave better at the table in the long run. Remember, feeding is parenting, and if he learns he can flout your rules over chips, what else will he try to get away with? (See stage-specific feeding for a brief discussion about discipline, page 204). If you are dealing with severe behaviors, attachment difficulties, or a child with FASD or other issues, talk to your therapist about ideas to redirect and meet his needs while maintaining the DOR.

- *"We are so frustrated with how slow this is going. He hasn't tried more than a few new foods for weeks."* As Marsha Dunn Klein of Mealtime Notions says, "change your definition of try." Children learn to like new foods through experience. First, they need to see you eat and enjoy a food. If he is eating only nuggets, and then you eat "grown-up" foods after he goes to bed, his initial learning isn't happening. It's like expecting a child to learn to swim but not letting him near the water.

 After watching you eat something, he might pass the bowl and let it sit next to his plate. He might look at it when no one is watching him. He might even poke it with the serving spoon. He will smell it. Maybe after he's seen it for a while, he might put some on his plate for a closer look. He might dip a favored cracker into it or lick some off his finger. A few weeks or months later, he might dip his fork in it and lick his fork, or pop it into his mouth, chew it, and spit it out again.

It might be months or even years before he chews and swallows a challenging food. Focus on keeping the table pleasant, offering a variety of foods, and don't give up.

- *"He wants to play with his food, and he's four. I wouldn't let my biological kids do that."* You probably did let your other kids play with food, but they had the chance when they were closer to eight or 15 months old. Playing with food is often a sign of emerging comfort with food. If it's exploration and fun, and he might never have had the chance to smear applesauce on a tray or bite a noodle into a fish shape, let it slide. Playing with food is part of learning how to eat. You can explain to your older children that they also got to play with food, or let them join in for a while. If the "play" is disruptive or has crossed a line to making a mess just to get you angry, you will know. Trust your intuition.

- *"My son is crazy for sweets, and I feel like our family keeps sabotaging our efforts. Grandma dropped by with a cupcake the size of his head right before lunch. Give it to him, or tell Gran to keep it?"* Managing unexpected and unasked-for foods will get easier. You can let him eat it now if it's a rare occasion, although it doesn't sound like that is the case. You can teach your son to say, "Thank you," then give him a choice, "Do you want to save it for snack time, or dessert with dinner tonight?" You are not saying "no," and you are giving him some control. He will tantrum at first to see if he can get you to cave in. Grandma might throw a fit too. Try to stay firm and calm. You can also decide to serve the whole cupcake as a "treat snack" with milk and a banana (See section on "Sweets and Treats," page 230) or half or even a quarter for his dessert portion with dinner, and the next half for the next day. You can also talk to family and tell them you appreciate their kindness, and suggest they bring some stickers instead or a few less treats per week. Work with extended family to come up with other ways that they can bond or have special time with your son.

- *"What if he doesn't want to eat anything for snack or dinner?"* That's okay. He might be testing your resolve, or maybe he is not hungry. Remind him a few times that there will be another snack in a little while, but the kitchen will be closed until then. Don't use these reminders as a threat to try to get him to eat, as in, "Are you sure you don't want to eat now? There will be no more food until dinner; you just think about that!" Consider a "rescue snack" (see page 112). If you need to, you can serve the next meal a little earlier, but that will be your idea, not his. You can say, "You don't have to eat, but we'd love your company. You're an important part of this family. You can leave in a few minutes." When my clients do this and don't pressure the child to eat, they usually report that within a few minutes, the child is eating something and is pleasantly partaking in the meal.

- *"My son eats a variety of foods at his daycare and for Grandma, but not at home. I feel like we are always fighting over what and how much he eats."* Of course he is "better" for other adults. You may be the safe adult or the one to be tested. I hear this all the time from many of the families I work with—adoptive or not. If your child is new to you, he is working on trust and testing, but after he is securely attached, he will still need to separate. He will need to become his own person within the safety of your family. He does this by opposing you. While he has to oppose you, you have to get the fight and the power struggle off the menu to allow him to even think of eating a better variety at home. Fake it at first if you have to, but stop caring whether he eats his broccoli tonight. Having a pleasant table and good attitude about food are much more important.

- *"He tried mashed potatoes the other night and was asking us to praise him. We used to, so it feels weird not to praise. I think he senses it too."* If he does try something new, don't react. Look away and talk to your partner or another family member. Pretend you don't see it. It sends the message that trying new foods is normal and expected, and he is capable. Many clients tell me they see the child sneaking that broccoli when no one is looking. If he does ask for praise, try something like, "Oh, I'm glad you liked the mashed potatoes; Mommy loves them with a little butter. Were you line leader at school today?"

- *"Our son is a slow eater, and doesn't eat much of his packed lunch. I'm so worried about how much he is eating, I dread opening his lunch box when I pick him up and seeing his sandwich still sitting there. He complains about everything I pack, even if it's something he likes."* If he's staying on track with his growth, there may not be much to worry about, though it's awful to think of our little ones not eating. When you first pick him up, don't ask him what he ate or rifle through his lunch box. (Parents do this all the time.) Pretend it doesn't matter. Give him the message that he can manage his eating, even if he is still learning. Maybe a phase of being less hungry at lunch, or distracted, has now turned into something more: a power struggle, a way for him to engage and test limits? He has a power chip—your worry about his hunger and nutrition. Here are a few ideas to turn things around. With an adequate offering at breakfast and a planned snack, he will probably be just fine. If he's drinking milk with lunch (flavored may help), he'll get several ounces of protein and a little fat. When he gets picked up at school, don't give him what's left from lunch, that makes too much focus on lunch, feels punitive, and becomes a battle point. Plan instead on serving a balanced and substantial sit down snack with a few choices: crackers with cream cheese, or cheddar with pear, oatmeal cookie with banana or apple slices. Let him eat as much as he is hungry for. (See my short YouTube video about snacks.) Pack foods for lunch that are easy to unpack and eat. While involving him with lunch planning is fine, moms tell me that even when they involve their children with shopping, cooking, and growing food, that is no promise the child will eat. Further, when kids are involved, this can invite battles, as in, "You chose those crackers, now eat them!" Think outside the box. If sandwiches don't get eaten, try sending a thermos with microwaved corn, or edamame (shelled or not) or left-over stir-fry with rice. How about a handful of crackers and cheese, with rolled up turkey and a little container of Miracle Whip. You can add a "treat," like a mini-Snickers, fruit leather, or a Go-Gurt if you want. Sometimes foods are eaten, sometimes not. As for the food waste, it stinks. You might want to cut down on how much you pack for now until the issue is improving, or accept, as I tell my clients, more food waste now, and less later.

I'm sure your child will invent other obstacles and roadblocks to challenge you, but my hope is that as you learn and begin to incorporate these principles, you will feel confident addressing what comes up day to day. Don't worry, there's much more in this book to help you transition to this new way of feeding—particularly Chapter 9—and it will get easier with time.

The Paradox of "Underweight" to "Overweight"

When families bring home a small or undernourished child or a preemie, there is pressure to get the child to grow. Parents are encouraged to concentrate formula or breast milk, add oils and fats to foods, and get calories in by any means necessary. As we've explored in this chapter, many children who are pressured to eat don't grow to their potential.

Other children, for whatever reason, whether they are more compliant, like food more, have less discomfort with fullness, or are more interested in pleasing adults, are taught to overeat.

Hydee Becker, RD, saw this trend while working in a clinic and seeing young children with rapidly accelerating weight. *"These were often preemies who had been tube fed, and then the parents were sent home with instructions to concentrate and add fats and oils to everything. The parents worked really hard to get these kids to gain weight. They pushed and did all the tricks they could. It seems like someone forgot to tell them they didn't have to keep doing that. These children had never been trusted to eat based on what their bodies were telling them, and some learned to eat more than they needed."*

When I spoke with a NICU nurse in charge of follow-up care, she too described increased rates of high weight in former preemies. It seems these children were either put off eating or learned to eat more than they needed. In almost all cases, the early fear and focus on weight, as well as the fact that these kids weren't trusted and were fed based on external cues, meant they were not fed in a way that supported self-regulation. It is notable that preemies were referred to as "feeders and growers" when I did my pediatrics rotations—clearly what mattered was weight.

Hopefully, whether your child is smaller than average, bigger than average, or some-where in between, you are beginning to see the wisdom in helping her eat based on internal cues. She is much more likely to grow up to have the body that is right for her and be healthy and happy.

It must be very confusing for a child who has experienced early starvation or catch-up growth to be encouraged, pushed, and praised for being a "good" eater, to be sud-denly told, "No, you have to eat *less*," when his weight gain accelerates. This is one of the scenarios we will explore in the next chapter about overweight worries and food preoccupation.

Chapter 5
Food Preoccupation and Concerns About Weight Gain

"She has begun to show anger toward me. She isn't interested in anything but food. Will I get fed again? Will Mommy be upset that I'm angry that I can't eat more? Will Mommy be impatient with me? Will she try to distract me with another stupid toy? Why does my brother have a banana?"
— Rebecca, mother of Adina, age 2½, adopted from Ethiopia at age 8 months

"This feels so good. You're telling me I can treat her like everyone else, which is all I ever wanted to do!" — Rebecca, six weeks later

The issue of how we deal with unhealthy weight gain, "overweight," and "obesity" is particularly interesting to me because it is where I see our current cultural "war on obesity" and the advice to parents that *causes* harm—and that is simply unacceptable.

Parents receive harmful feeding advice from the very experts they turn to, those who are unaware of the research and don't understand that restricting children is harmful and can destroy the feeding relationship, making trust and attachment more difficult. Trying to get a child to eat less most predictably leads to a child who is preoccupied with food, eats more when she has the opportunity, and may weigh more than nature intended. *First do no harm.*

In this chapter, I will examine the issues of food preoccupation—both with and without unhealthy weight gain—because the underlying common fear is that the child is or will be "too fat." That fear leads to the feeding mistake of trying to get the child to eat less or different kinds of foods, with predictable results. As the approach to turning both situations around is essentially the same, I will address these issues together, as I did with selective eating and low-weight worries in the last chapter.

What You Will Learn
We will briefly explore the terms "overweight," "obese," and "food obsession" or "preoccupation" and why the time of catch-up growth is particularly risky for unnecessary and harmful intervention. Once there is an understanding about the worries that lead to feeding errors, we can begin to apply the principles of the Trust Model and turn things around. In addition, we will consider the child with a history of food insecurity (not having adequate food enough of the time) and growth delay, and how restricting a child with this history is particularly harmful.

I use the term "food insecurity" for two reasons. First, it is the correct term to describe the state of not having reliable access to enough food, and second, *food* and *security* go hand in hand. It's about more than just calories; it's ultimately about feeling safe, trust, and not worrying about survival.

Address the Worry: What Is "Overweight" or "Obese?"

If you are familiar with Chapter 1 and the "Misunderstanding Growth" section, you will already know that the words "overweight" and "obese" might need some clarification. When I use "overweight" or "obese" in quotations, I am referring to the arbitrary cutoffs and labels on the standard body mass index (BMI) and growth charts. The child growing above the 85th percentile is considered "overweight," while the child growing at or above the 90th percentile is labeled as "obese."[1]

Are these category labels really meaningful? Consider:

- In other countries, the cutoff points for "normal," "overweight," and "obese" are different.[2] Does it make sense that a child at the 90th percentile in America is "obese," but if he travels to England, that same child would not be "obese," but merely "overweight?" He didn't lose any weight on the trans-Atlantic flight; they just use different cutoff points. This is another clue that these labels are not necessarily clinically meaningful for an individual child.
- A decade or so ago, the child growing at the 90th percentile was considered "at risk" of becoming overweight, and as with adults, the cutoff points and classifications were lowered. Overnight, almost 30 million American adults who went to bed with "normal" weight woke up "overweight," with no change in their actual health status.
- In a young child, five pounds can span the label of "normal" to "obese," and 1/8 of an inch can change the "diagnosis."[3] While the clinical significance of a few pounds is questionable, the significance of the label is not.

Labeling children has not been shown to improve health and is more likely to make the child less healthy. Regardless of actual weight, children labeled "overweight" or "obese" feel worse about themselves in every way,[4] exercise less, and are more prone to practice disordered eating, diet, and *gain* weight.[5] Parents who are told their child is overweight also tend to resort to trying to get the child to eat less, with more dieting and, ultimately, weight gain. In this case, "knowing" is not necessarily a good thing.[6]

Children are often labeled or "diagnosed" based on a single BMI measure, in spite of the fact that both the Center for Disease Control and Prevention (CDC) and National

Institutes of Health (NIH) assert that "BMI is not a diagnostic tool." For example, a child may have a high BMI for age and sex, but to determine if "excess fat" is a concern, a health care provider would need to perform further assessments. These assessments might include "skinfold thickness measurements, evaluations of diet, physical activity, family history, and other appropriate health screenings."[7] In most doctors' offices, however, BMI alone is used to label and "diagnose."

The original BMI calculation was developed by Adolphe Quatelet, a Belgian mathematician (and not a physician), in the mid-1800s to describe population trends in the physical characteristics of military recruits and attempt to relate it to statistics and the bell curve. The calculation wasn't labeled as "body mass index" until the late 20th century.

Remember that a child growing consistently—even at a high percentile—is, by definition of the bell curve, larger than the majority of her peers. But to label her as "overweight" when she is probably at a perfectly healthy weight *for her* is wrong, and implies a health risk that may not be there. Most of the clients I work with who are referred for "overweight" or "obesity" fall in this group, at least when the alarm bells are first sounded. Almost always, the child is a larger-than-average but healthy child, enjoying good nutrition, with a lot of effort on the part of the parent. Then a worry, either from the parent or from a health care provider who plots out BMI and labels the child as "overweight" or "obese," sets off the cycle of worry, restriction, and food preoccupation and weight gain.

From birth to age two, growth should also be plotted on a weight-for-height chart, not just weight for age and height for age. After age two, BMI can be followed, but a weight-for-height chart is usually adequate. BMI charts tend to visually exaggerate even small changes.

Admittedly, following growth charts can be difficult. Remember that your child should have at least two measurements about two months apart to follow a trend. If your child is experiencing catch-up growth, that complicates matters further.

Obesity and poverty are clearly linked[8] and may partly explain why children in foster care tend to have higher rates of "overweight" and "obesity." We know that food insecurity affects how people eat and is related to higher weight. Understanding that feeding well and reliable access to enough food helps: studies show that children who participate in school lunch and breakfast programs have more stable and healthy weight.[9]

Ethnic Differences in Body Shape

This comes up fairly frequently, particularly with international adoption, but also in foster care and domestic adoption. Different ethnic groups tend to have certain typical physical characteristics. For example, there is evidence that Navajos tend to have a more dense build,[10] and data on Hispanic American children suggests similar differences in build and BMI.[11,12] Certain Central and South American groups tend to have a more dense body type with relatively more muscle mass.

The "mean," or average, for these kids may be closer to the 85th percentile on the standard U.S. growth chart, which means that roughly half of the children with these body types will be above the 85th percentile and half will be below. The bell curve moves in essence, to a higher weight range. Many more kids who are healthy, but bigger than the average on the standard growth chart, will potentially be mislabeled as "overweight."

Connie, mother of Ric, adopted at birth from Guatemala and now age 17, was frustrated at the lack of understanding about her son's body shape. *"When he turned eight, he gained weight and grew into his square, Mayan body. He was around the 85th percentile, and the doctor got really nasty about it. For two years he kept talking about it and wanting Ric to go on a diet."* During those two years, Ric stayed stable around the 85th percentile and was active in multiple sports, and he ate a variety of wholesome foods. His body was simply more dense, but the pediatrician misinterpreted and labeled that as "overweight."

Similarly, Tia, age 10 and also from Guatemala, had always grown steadily on the high end of the growth curve. A few years ago, a doctor said she was "almost obese" and recommended "portion control." Mom Tara says, *"We started cutting back her intake and harping on portion control, and it's all gone downhill from there. Now she really is gaining more weight."*

> Different ethnic groups are built differently, with some tending to have a more dense build and higher average BMIs, and others with a more lean build. Be aware that growth charts from some countries are often based on decades-old data that may actually reflect poor nutrition and national growth delay. Regardless, there is no guesswork or worrying about which chart to use—whether its the World Health Organization's or the standard U.S. chart—if you *follow your own child's growth.* If he is following a percentile that is fairly stable, even if it is below or above average, and he is otherwise healthy, his growth is probably normal and healthy for him. If your child is growing significantly above the 97th percentile, your doctor will need to follow Z-scores, or percent change (see page 78).

Catch-Up Growth

When a child has experienced inadequate nutrition, growth is often stunted. To preserve fuel for the vital organs such as the heart and brain, the body uses a complex hormonal process in which growth hormones shut down and the child has a marked slowdown in growth or, as is often the case, stops growing altogether. Weight falls off the curve first, then height and, in severe cases, head circumference.

The starving or food-insecure child places survival ahead of growth.

Fannah, adopted from Ethiopia shortly before her fourth birthday, experienced malnutrition and catch-up growth. Fannah's mom, Elsa, contacted me after listening to a Webinar I presented on weight and food. Fannah's growth history was indeed impressive. Fannah had spent the first few weeks of life with her birth mother. When she arrived at the orphanage, she was severely undernourished and had scarcely regained her birth weight at three months. Her weight increased in the orphanage, but continued to lag behind; when she came home with Elsa, she was in the 5th percentile.

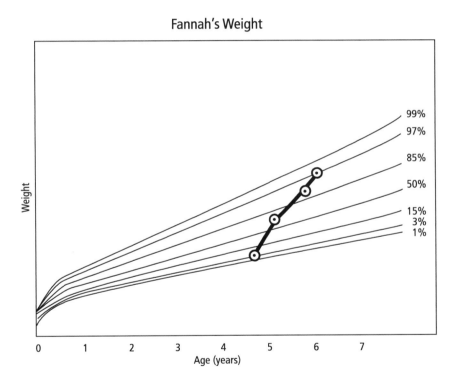

Fannah's Weight

Fannah was adjusting well to family life, joining in with family meals, and eating everything she could. She accepted almost all foods, ate quickly, and added weight and height at an astonishing rate. Children who are malnourished can grow at 20 times the normal rate of a child the same age.

At first, family and physicians were delighted, but by her third visit, eight months after coming home, Fannah was officially in the "obese" range at the 90th percentile. Her concerned pediatrician began asking about how much juice and sweetened beverages she was drinking. (Incidentally, the answer was none.) The doctor warned she would become "obese" as an adult and suffer from diabetes. Although Fannah was already slowing down on her own in terms of how fast she was eating and seemed to eat less than when she first arrived, the doctor recommended changing to skim milk, limiting treats, and serving a limited amount of calories to decrease her portions and slow her weight gain.

Luckily, Elsa looked for more information. When we chatted, I shared some resources and talked about trusting Fannah with the process. A review of her growth data showed that her weight acceleration was slowing and her height was continuing to accelerate, something that became apparent only when the more sensitive Z-scores were calculated. Fannah was probably still experiencing catch-up growth, and to try to cut her intake during that time may have affected her adult height and resulted in predictable food preoccupation.

As Fannah's mom said so wisely, *"Right now we're focusing more on her heart needs than on her weight."*

The beauty of their situation is that by taking care of her heart needs and continuing to support her eating, Fannah will be more apt to grow up with a stable and healthy weight. As you can see by her follow-up growth points, her weight acceleration stopped and her growth is moving toward the mean, as children at the extremes often do. Fannah is showing that she is capable of self-regulation.

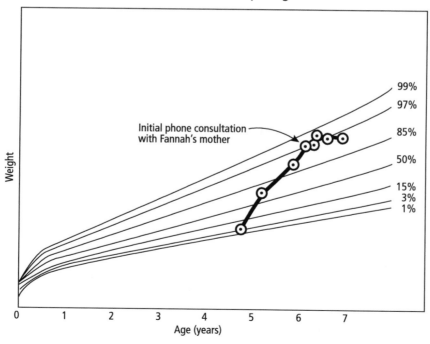

Fannah's Follow-Up Weights

It is rare, but sometimes a child is actually older than parents are initially told. Fannah, for example, was about a year older than what Elsa believed her to be for the first two years. Dental exams and X-rays to determine bone age may reveal that a child is older than previously thought. This can have implications for following growth, and is another reason to compare a child only to herself and to follow the growth pattern. It is a possibility to consider.

Dr. Dana Johnson, of the International Adoption Clinic at the University of Minnesota and a lead researcher on growth in internationally adopted children, says that catch-up growth usually takes about a year, but may be longer in the severely growth-delayed child. Many children will not reach average heights, even with catch-up growth.

"We don't really know a timeframe in terms of growth, and the time it takes for hormone systems to recover," he notes. "For example, the changes we see in the daily variation of cortisol last for much longer than the catch-up growth period. It can go on for years. It may not readjust quickly. There is so much we are still learning. But it's important not to worry about overeating in the first year."

Since the hormones that influence growth are affected possibly for years after malnutrition and growth delay, it is reasonable to expect it to take some time for eating and growth to regulate.

Getting Caught in the War on Childhood Obesity

I am hearing from more and more parents of children who have experienced malnutrition, then re-feeding and catch-up growth. How amazing and resilient these children are, and yet, just as they begin to thrive, a new worry is introduced. The national panic over childhood obesity intersecting with this issue is particularly troublesome. These little survivors are getting caught up in the war on obesity in many ways.

Calorie Restriction Studies

Studies on adults who have cut calories to lose weight show that when a body is deprived of nutrition, there are hormonal, metabolic, and even muscle fiber changes to conserve energy.[13,14] Bodies become more efficient and metabolism slows, so it takes less calories to maintain weight and even more restriction to continue to lose weight. These changes drive the body and mind to seek out more food that is energy dense, and the body stores energy (fat) more efficiently. The body perceives, "I am starving; I am going to conserve energy and do everything I can to get back to my pre-starvation weight." *The New York Times* reported on early research showing these changes can last as long as six years.[15] This information has helped clients to have patience with the process when their children have experienced malnutrition. It takes time.

Take Rebecca's example. Adina had been home from Ethiopia for 18 months when her mom reached out for help. Adina had experienced neglect and growth delay due to a lack of nutrition and nurturing in her early months. She spent a short time in an orphanage where, with adequate calories and care, she experienced some catch-up growth in height and weight. Upon arrival in the U.S., she was declared "overfed" and at an "unhealthy weight" (at a weight-for-height measure of about the 80th percentile) and was therefore restricted in the amount and timing of her formula.

Rebecca was in tears on the phone. *"I've had her on a diet basically since day one. I've spent thousands on attachment specialists, but I know she can't trust me until I can feed her. She begs for food all day, but the pediatrician reprimands me because she thinks I'm not trying hard enough, and scares me about her health. This all feels so wrong."*

Rather than trust Adina to learn to tune in to her hunger and fullness cues, from day one she was fed on a schedule and with certain amounts. Adina finished every bottle and cried for more—a story I have heard repeatedly. These children are not trusted to decide how much to eat, and are limited, which heightens their anxiety and interest in food. They then tend to eat quickly, stuff in large amounts of food when they begin to self-feed, and seem to confirm the fear that they have an uncontrollable hunger.

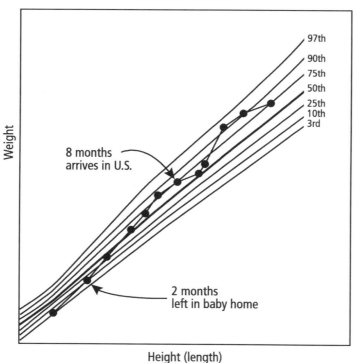

Adina's Growth

What Adina's pediatrician didn't know was this: Restricting a child with a history of food insecurity will heighten her anxiety, hamper attachment, and almost guarantee she will overeat when given the chance. A diet is incredibly harmful to a child who has experienced hunger on a level that most of us can't begin to imagine.

Should "Obese" Children Be Placed In Foster Care?

A topic that attracts a lot of media attention is whether or not extremely obese children should be placed in foster care. As usual, it is complex. Consider:

- Foster care is a radical and untested solution. It should always be a last resort.
- Effective "treatment" of "obesity" is rare.
- Rates of "obesity" in children in foster care are higher than the national average.[16]
- Three years into the foster system in Los Angeles, more children were "overweight" and "obese" than when they entered the system.[17] This is hardly a "cure."
- The message to the child is, "You are fat and that is the only thing wrong, so we will return you to your home when you lose weight…"

A child's extreme weight gain presents an opportunity to ask, "What is going on in this child's life that she is no longer able to grow in a healthy way?" After a complete medical evaluation; an intake analysis, including timing and behavior at meals; and witnessed or videotaped meals and snacks, there should be a complete child and family developmental assessment to determine the source of the child's high body weight. Is it genetics, errors in feeding, stress, chaos in the home, neglect, lack of access to food, abuse around food such as withholding or punishing, or a combination of the above? If there is indeed a problem, parents must be given appropriate support, including food assistance, and have a chance to correct any feeding and parenting errors. If they can't or won't, then foster care may be a last resort. As Ellyn Satter writes, "… the reason for placement is not the child's weight but the fact that the child is being physically or emotionally neglected or endangered."[18]

Food Insecurity

Food insecurity is common in children who are adopted or in foster care. Children who did not get fed enough, were fed without appropriate support, or who lived in an institutional setting, a chaotic home, or foster care situation are food "insecure." That means they could not count on getting enough food. They could not count on when they would be fed.

Imagine you are a child, utterly dependent on adults to care for and feed you, and they can't or don't. This leaves scars that are physical and emotional as well as physiological (growth hormones and metabolism), that take time to heal.

Weight

When a doctor immediately presses the panic button about weight, or does so only a few months in, it is anything but helpful. Expecting a child to come to a new family, perhaps a new country, and be able to self-regulate (in the "normal" weight range), and eat a variety of foods—all within months—is not reasonable.

Cut the kids some slack. Trust that they will figure it out. It may take many months or a few years, not weeks, and your child may never be slender, but she can be healthy and happy. But I can almost guarantee that a food obsession that is *not* addressed in the child will likely lead to a lifetime struggle with food and weight.

What Is Food Preoccupation, or "Obsession?"

"I don't even worry about her weight much, but her food obsession scares me to death. I struggled with an eating disorder, and I feel like the only thing she thinks about is when and how much she will eat." — Alexis, mother of Greta, age 2½

A child's preoccupation with food is a major worry and can be outright terrifying if the parent has a history of or is actively struggling with an eating disorder, his or her own weight, or worry about the child's weight. Usually a parent knows when the child's interest in food is excessive, because dealing with it takes intense energy and effort, it makes the parent upset, and it causes a lot of frustration.

> The word parents use most often is food "obsession." I prefer the term "food preoccupation" so as not to confuse the heightened interest, awareness, and anxiety over food with the more clinical "obsessive-compulsive" behaviors. In addition, the word "obsession" has a more negative and blaming tone toward the child, while "preoccupation" invites empathy and understanding.

You will note that the interest and energy around food preoccupation takes away from time for other activities, to the detriment of the child's social or emotional development. The following are signs that your child may be preoccupied with food to an unhealthy extent:

- The child eats very rapidly and gobbles and stuffs food.
- You have to make an effort to get the child away from the meal or highchair by using games, TV, and other distractions.
- You bribe the child with a favored food to get him to leave a meal.
- The child is frantic, clingy during meal prep, or around any food.
- At playgrounds/parties, the child is more interested in eating than playing. She eats, whines, or cries to eat the whole time.
- The child exhibits high emotion around meals, whining and crying while waiting.

- You feel that you are a "food cop," not a parent, going to elaborate lengths such as these to not go near or mention food.
  - Other children are fed at different times.
  - You are not allowed to mention food.
  - You plan outings and vacations based on your child's food issues and where you can best manage them.

The occasional pestering for sweets or for food while you are cooking is normal. These behaviors may also be normal if your child is still settling in and has experienced food insecurity. The difference becomes apparent with consideration to the severity, length of time, and extent of interference of the behaviors with other aspects of being a kid.

Hoarding behaviors usually resolve over the first year or so with supportive feeding, while food preoccupation tends to be more chronic and a result of restrictive or unsupportive feeding.

My toddler has a huge belly. People comment on how fat he looks. If your child has newly arrived home and malnutrition is a possibility, the round belly on a small frame may be a sign of severe malnutrition or abdominal distension, so ask you child's doctor. However, many healthy children can look "fat" or "pregnant." Even children who are smaller than average can have that round belly. This is not fat. Children have relatively underdeveloped abdominal muscles, which can push out. If your child also struggles with low muscle tone in general, this can look even more pronounced. Use leggings if pants are hard to fit with a larger belly size, and find baggy tops that don't cling. Defend yourself and your child from the comments of others. Know that most children will outgrow this by grade school, although for some it takes longer. My friend Elizabeth laughs at her gymnastics photos from when she was eight, with muscular arms and legs and her round little belly. I also recommend lots of belly kisses, blowing raspberries, and laughter—which is great for strengthening abdominal muscles.

Restriction and Diets

Why Health Care Providers Recommend Restriction

Like the rest of us, many clinicians simply aren't aware of the research. They cling to simplistic ideas like, "It's just calories in, calories out," and the belief that cutting a few calories here and there adds up, like a math equation, to a certain number of pounds lost. But the issue is far more complex.

The vast majority of primary-care physicians get little training in nutrition and certainly none in feeding dynamics or responsive feeding, despite stacks of published research. I did not know this data, and will admit to being ill informed when I was in clinical practice. I had to learn for myself, seek extra training, and even undo a lot of misinformation. So I do not accuse my colleagues of bad intentions; I know in fact they are dedicated, caring, compassionate professionals who really want what is best for children, but they are unaware, and this has serious consequences.

> If you are a health care provider, ask yourself how it feels to practice in the current standard approach. Does it work? Do you dread talking to families about weight? Are you confident that what you are doing is helping and not harming? These were the questions that helped me approach this issue with an open mind. I was not satisfied with my outcomes with the standard approach, which both my patients and myself seemed to intensely dislike. I can honestly say that when working in the Trust Model, I deal with issues of health and weight with confidence and enjoy the process because it works, is affirming, and is health promoting, rather than hopeless and shaming.

Clinicians, like the rest of us, tend to focus on *what* children are eating and ignore *how* children are fed. They assume the child who is accelerating with weight is simply drinking too much sugar-sweetened beverages or eating too much fat or too many calories. Their approach most often will be one of cutting calories or trying to get the BMI below the 85th percentile, even if a higher number may be healthy for your child. One pediatric registered dietitian (RD) shared that the goal at the weight-loss center she worked at was for *all* their child clients to reach the 50th percentile.

> One mother reached out to me after the RD she saw at a university-based pediatric weight loss clinic recommended diet soda and Crystal Lite as "preferred beverages" for her two-year-old. This felt wrong to her, and despite following the calorie and "red-light-food" limits for six months, her daughter was becoming more food "obsessed" and her weight was accelerating.

A Diet By Any Other Name is Still a Diet

Most of us know that diets don't work, and while most clinicians are more savvy and no longer recommend an outright "diet" for children, they will still talk about letting "weight catch up with height," "portion control," "green-light, red-light," and other kinder and gentler descriptions. (Many clinicians still do recommend outright diets with strict calorie limits.) The bottom line is that if you are trying to get your child to eat less so she will weigh less, it's restriction, it's a diet, and it will *increase* her interest in food and probably increase her weight as well.

A study in California followed children for several years.[19] The ones that gained more weight over time ate no more calories, no more junk foods, and were not breast or bottle-fed any differently. Two factors that predicted problematic weight gain were:
- Parental worry about weight in the toddler and preschooler years.
- Difficult feeding relationships in the toddler and preschooler years.

In an attempt to get the child to eat less, parents restrict by using the following tactics:
- Using a highchair tray longer than necessary to keep food out of reach.
- Pre-portioning foods and giving the plate to the child.
- Making the child wait 20 minutes before she can have more.
- Pushing low-calorie, "green-light" foods.
- Not allowing favorite high-calorie or high-fat foods (red-light foods).
- Trying to fill the child up on water before eating.
- "Running out" of favored foods.

Why Parents Restrict

Research shows that when parents worry their child will be obese, they restrict more often from the start.[20,21] In addition, parents who themselves struggle with weight tend to restrict.[22,23] It makes sense. The parents have been told that *they* eat too much, and parents desperately want to do better for their children, so they try to get the child to eat less. Ironically, those parents who worry about weight and try to make kids thinner may contribute to the very outcome they fear most. Restriction tends to lead to higher weight.[24,25,26,27]

Fear of obesity is what led Greta's parents to alter how they fed her. When I talked with her adoptive mom, Alexis, it turned out that Greta's birth mom struggled with high weight, and Alexis and her husband, Mike, were worried that Greta would be very fat. They didn't feel that Greta could be trusted, so from day one, after Greta finished off her specific number of ounces, that was it—she was never allowed her to have more. They gave her what they were told was an "appropriate" amount. By the time Greta started solids, her interest, enjoyment, and the quantities she ate were impressive, and extended family commented—and we know how unhelpful that is. Alexis and Mike cut back her portions and would try distraction to get her to eat less. However, it seemed that the harder they worked to get Greta to eat less, the more obsessed with food she became.

What Happens when Parents Restrict: A Case Study

Greta's Food Preoccupation

When I first heard from Alexis and Mike about Greta, they had been working hard to limit her since she was about nine months old (though prior to that they had limited the amounts of formula they gave her). At 2½, Greta was "food obsessed." Everyone was miserable, and the fear that Greta would always struggle with food, and probably with her weight, was terrifying for Alexis. She described her stress around feeding as "ten out of ten." As time went on, it got worse, and Alexis and Mike had to work harder to keep food away from Greta. Greta would whine and cry and cling and fuss as her parents tried to get meals ready. She would skip playing if she sensed the possibility of food and whined and cried most of the day for more food.

Greta's Growth

Growth charts often tell the story of how feeding is going. Before Alexis and Mike started with restricting, Greta had stable growth, mostly around the 25th percentile. As their struggles increased and Greta became more demanding, her weight increased. Her real weight acceleration started when she was about 15 months old, which is a typical pattern. Though serious efforts to restrict started at nine months, the pre-mobile and pre-verbal child is easier to control in terms of limiting intake. (Note: early in the transition, weight acceleration may continue, but then evens out. Some will see a decline in BMI, while others will stay high and steady for some time. The key is stopping the acceleration.)

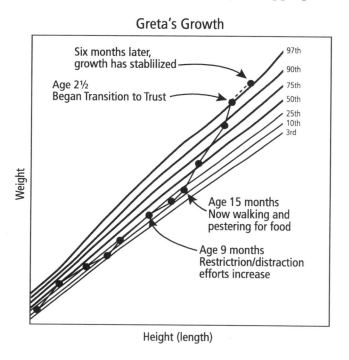

When the toddler becomes more mobile, the tantrums and "pester power" wear down even the most vigilant parent. That is often when weight accelerates. The anxious toddler is able to hold out and often get more food than she needs. I remember one client caving in to cookie demands after six hours of the child's whining. *What children learn is that they can outlast the parent.*

Greta's growth chart was a surprise to Alexis and Mike. They weren't worried about her current weight, but now Greta was in the 90th percentile and would be labeled as "obese" at the next doctor visit. Their intuition that something was seriously wrong was showing up in Greta's growth.

Greta's Intake Analysis

This is the point where most people would expect to see Happy Meal after Happy Meal, lots of fruit juice or soda, and higher calorie and fat intake than the expected range—and that does happen. However, it may surprise you to learn that what I see on our comprehensive intake analyses, time and again, are families serving what would be considered exemplary choices and whole foods, parents who cook, and families who eat together—often in spite of epic battles. (In my practice I tend to see parents in the higher socioeconomic range.)

While Greta's analysis did show a slightly higher intake for calories and fat than the recommended range, about half the intake analyses I see for kids with food preoccupation or high weight have intakes within the recommended ranges for calories and fat, or even below it, as in the case of Adina.

Greta's Macro analysis		
BMI 90th%	Actual Intake	Recommended Range
fat (% total calories)	30%	30-40%
protein (grams)	71.4	> 15
calories	1511	1100–1500
veggies (cups)	2.4	1
fruit (cups)	2.3	1

Adina's Macro analysis		
BMI 75th%	Actual Intake	Recommended Range
fat (% total calories)	38	30-40%
protein (grams)	42.9	>16
calories	1188	1300–1500
veggies (cups)	0.8	1
fruit (cups)	2.1	1

As a group, "overweight" and "obese" children eat the same types and amounts of food as their lean counterparts. [28,29,30,31,32] Study after study has confirmed this, with authors often expressing surprise at their own findings, whether the results reveal that lean and fat children are drinking the same amount of soda[33] or that children who drink whole milk have a lower BMI.[29] My experience with intake analyses confirms this. Most of the children I see for "overweight" and "obesity," as well as food preoccupation and accelerating weight, actually eat within the "normal" range for calories and fat. Body weight is far more complex than "calories in, calories out;" genetics, metabolism, feeding and dieting history, hormones, stress, and more play a role. Read on if you are intrigued or doubtful.

Opportunities Emerge

Even without the full nutrition analysis from our pediatric registered dietitian, the intake often shows key areas to support feeding. Greta's and Adina's feeding and intake journals on the following pages show common opportunities that show up:

- Inadequate snacks are one of the biggest culprits. See the circled snacks in Greta's and Adina's feeding and intake journals: dried pears or just Rice Chex. What do these snacks have in common? They are not balanced, with inadequate energy, no fat, and little protein. Parents have been told that snacks shouldn't "spoil" the appetite and should be low-fat, ideally some fresh fruit or veggies. While it's great to include fresh fruits and veggies, they are generally not an adequate snack on their own. Adina was legitimately hungry much of the time.
- Foods offered are too low in fat. In an attempt to control weight, parents are advised to serve skim milk and low-fat cheese and avoid fat, but 30 to 40 percent of calories for the young toddler should come from fat.
- Too much time passes between eating—up to six hours. By this time, the child is really hungry, probably pretty grouchy, and more prone to overeat. Often, parents try to skip snacks if a child is busy, again in an attempt to limit calories.

> Lack of variety often explains nutrition gaps or excesses. For example, the intake of one family's daughter showed she ate very high amounts of saturated fat. This was clear before even reading the final analysis, because almost every snack included cheese. The parents felt stuck with what to offer because their daughter liked cheese, it was easy, and they thought it was healthy. It *is* healthy, but offering cheese several times a day meant that variety was lost. Snack ideas that included high, medium, and low-fat options helped balance things out, without limiting or cutting out cheese or switching to a fat-free version.

From the intake analysis and growth information, as well as fleshing out the picture with Greta's parents through written questionnaires and phone calls, a sense of the feeding relationship became clear. Opportunities emerged to support Greta's parents as they moved away from trying to *get Greta to eat less* to trying to support healthy eating. And so began their transition to the Trust Model.

What if you can't afford a full analysis? Many insurers no longer cover dietetics services for "obesity." In our area, parents pay out-of-pocket for an RD evaluation, which can range from $150 to more than $300 for the initial analysis. While an intake analysis by an RD can be very helpful, most of what I recommend and work on with clients around structure, variety, and the Division of Responsibility (DOR) doesn't change based on the analysis results. You don't need an RD to look at intervals between meals and snacks or get an idea about variety when it's written down. (In addition, many RDs will do the analysis and offer restricting advice if they are not working in the Trust Model.)

FEEDING AND INTAKE JOURNAL

Name: _Greta_

Meal/Snack	Time of day	Food(s) and/or beverage(s) offered	Amount(s) consumed	Notes
(pre-breakfast)	6:30	8 oz 1% milk in a bottle	8 oz	Wanted more (she drinks in bed w/us while reading books)
brkfst	7:40	2 slices toast with peanut butter	2 slices 1 Tbsp PB, whole apple	Made 1 sl toast. Cried for more toast before finishing first slice (begged for more apple, toast); 1 apple eats fast, doesn't take time to chew well
snack	10:30	dried pear snack	1 bag	Begged for more
lunch	12:00	chicken broccoli sweet potato avocado	2 1/2 oz 1/2 cup 1/2	Eats quickly at all meals, asked for more and had another 1/2–1 oz chicken and 3 pcs broccoli. She is upset when we tell her lunch is over. Use distraction, favorite toys to get her to leave the meal
snack	3:30	home-made choc. pudding/yogurt popsicle	1	
dinner	6:15	1 serving Trader Joe's Shepherd's Pie 1/2 cup grape tomatoes steamed kale plum avocado	1 1/2 cups 1/2 cup 1/4 cup 1 1/4	Wanted more of everything. Watched Disney movie during dinner which helps slow her down. Always eats every single thing. Never leaves any food on her plate. We don't put food on the table bc if she sees it she cries. We have to hide all evidence of food in the kitchen or she whines for it
snack	7:15	1% milk	1 cup	

Name: _Adina_

FEEDING AND INTAKE JOURNAL

Meal/Snack	Time of day	Food(s) and/or beverage(s) offered	Amount(s) consumed	Notes
brkfst	9:00–9:45	almond milk with vitamins	2 oz	Cries and whines for bottle on waking. Frantic until gets it. Bottles are on lap. Meals in kitchen in highchair. Screams while I get breakfast ready.
		rice thins	3	
		almond butter	1 Tbsp	Use toys and TV to get her out of highchair.
		hard boiled egg	1	Let her finish her apple wandering around to get her
		apple	1/2 medium	down. Whines for food and clings to me most of morning.
		blueberries	1/4 cup	
snack	12:00	sunflower seeds	1/4 cup	She loves them, is always asking for them
lunch	1:00	tortilla chips	about 15	Tantrums as I get her to leave the table. Feed other
		hummus	3 Tsp (?)	children first so she isn't screeching and begging for
		applesauce	1/2 cup	their food. Most of afternoon sits on my lap sucking
		strawberries	7	her thumb. Occasionally asks for "snack." Doesn't play with other kids.
snack	4:30–5	rice chex	1 cup	Snack while walking around
dinner	6:30–7	gluten-free pasta	1 cup	With the whole family. Dread it. Always begging for
		tomato sauce (jar) ?		more, reaching for others' food.
		meatballs (beef, homemade)	2 avg. sized	My older kids don't like family meals. All I do is manage Adina. I don't even eat.
		carrot sticks	8–10 small	Never slows down even after all this food! I distract again to get her out of chair. Cries for bottle at bedtime, I give her bottle with water.

Many times I do recommend an intake analysis, because more often than not it is incredibly reassuring to parents. For example, parents commonly worry and pressure on protein amounts, but almost every analysis has shown that the child is getting adequate protein, and in some cases, several times the minimum amount. It allows parents to see that their child is actually within the normal range for nutrients, calories, and fat, or that if there is too much fat overall in the diet, it can be addressed by dealing with structure and adding variety, not by trying to cut foods out or limit portions.

Busting Myths About Weight, Health, Portions, and More

You Can Be Fat and Healthy—Really!

"Can my child be healthy if she's above average weight?" This is the fear that lies behind the struggles my clients face with food preoccupation, accelerating weight gain, and weight worries. I hear you. This was my main stumbling block as I learned to believe in this Trust Model of feeding.

This section will seem to defy every cherished belief about weight and health that our culture and most medical practitioners hold true: The idea that every "extra" pound shortens your lifespan—that weight is linearly related with death and sickness. It is not. There are many healthy people at a variety of weights.[34] Yes, some conditions are *correlated* (different than causation) with higher weights (mostly BMI of 35 or 40 and above), but in studies when fitness level and other disease risk factors were taken into account, the level of fatness did not predict disease.[35,36] In addition, more and more research is confirming that health improves (as evidenced by blood pressure, blood sugar, and cholesterol improvements) with more healthy behaviors, even *without* weight loss.[37,38,39] You can be fat and fit. If you are reacting strongly to this statement, you are not alone; I remember literally scoffing the first time I heard this.

This is not a book in which to review stacks of research; nor can I convince you in the next few pages of something it took me years to grasp. My main point is that if you hear yourself saying, "Yes, but she *can't* be healthy and be overweight," I urge you to read and learn more. If you don't believe your child can be healthy if she isn't slim, it will be difficult to trust her through the Trust Model. The following books can help start the process:

- *Rethinking Thin* by Gina Kolata
- *Big Fat Lies: The Truth About Your Weight and Your Health* by Glenn Gaesser, PhD
- *Health at Every Size* by Linda Bacon, PhD
- *Your Child's Weight: Helping Without Harming* by Ellyn Satter, MS, RD, LCSW

> Even if you can't accept that you don't have to be slim to be healthy, research shows that trying to get your child to eat less is likely to backfire and may lead to the very outcome you are trying to avoid.

The following are some of the specific study findings that surprised me as I was learning, and may help you begin to accept that health and weight are not synonymous:

- In children, fitness was more predictive than fatness for fasting insulin response.[40] (Abnormal fasting insulin is an early warning sign for impaired insulin function, which can lead to diabetes.)
- In older Americans, those in the "overweight" category (BMI of 25-30) had the lowest mortality.[41]
- The thinnest older adults have the highest mortality.[42]
- Fat people survive heart attacks more often than their thin counterparts.[43]
- Women who followed low-fat dietary recommendations for seven years were no thinner than women who did not.[44]
- There is a correlation between illness, mortality, and weight at the extremes, beyond a BMI of 40[42] as well as at the lowest ranges of BMI. (For reference, a BMI of 30 and higher is considered "obese" at current cut-offs.)
- A recent meta-analysis showed that the child who maintains stable, even high, BMI into adulthood is less likely to experience health problems such as diabetes and hypertension than the "under" or "normal" weight child who gains as an adult.[45]
- A study banning sodas in schools made no difference in intake or BMI, and also found that the fat and lean children drank the same amount.[33]

It took me two solid years of reading the research, challenging my training and my biases to embrace the Health at Every Size Approach endorsed by Linda Bacon, PhD, author of *Health at Every Size: The Surprising Truth About Your Weight*. As Bacon explains, this approach asserts that ". . . good health can best be realized independent from considerations of size. It supports people—of all sizes—in addressing health directly by adopting healthy behaviors."[46]

> The Health at Every Size approach is not an excuse to "indulge" children or ignore accelerating weight, as some critics may claim. Feeding a child well and supporting healthful behaviors takes effort and planning. The Trust Model and Health at Every Size simply endorse and support health rather than weight as a goal, and a more stable and healthy weight often results.

Remember:
- BMI is not a reliable predictor of health for the individual.[47]
- Regardless of weight, you can improve your health by taking care of yourself.
- You can improve your child's health, and chances of staying healthy, by feeding her a variety of foods within the Trust Model, and providing opportunities for her to be active.

I know this to be true for myself. I weigh around 160 pounds, at the high end of the "normal" BMI range, but according to various experts, about 20 pounds more than "ideal." Had I struggled against this set point (I have weighed within 15 pounds since high school), I know in my heart I would have done as millions of others do and lost the weight, only to regain it plus some, over and over again. With a Health at Every Size approach, I eat well, provide for myself, get enough sleep, exercise because it makes me feel better and it is good for me. I can tuck into a plate of pasta and veggies and enjoy dessert without guilt; I love my healthy body and what it can do. I do none of these things for weight loss or maintenance, and I am healthy and happy.

When a client says, "*Yes, but I don't want her to struggle with her weight like I did.*" I find it helps to ask the parent: "If your child continues to be restricted, food-obsessed, and bingeing when she gets the chance, what do you see for her future relationship with food and her body?" After some discussion, we usually come to the same conclusion: that the child will struggle with her eating as an adult—and be heavier than nature intended her to be.

What Children Weigh Now Does Not Reliably Predict Adult Weight

I cringe when families tell me that restriction and outright diets are recommended based on a child's weight at age two or three years, and even as young as four months! As larger-than-average children grow up over the years, they trend toward slimming[48,49] IF they are supported well with eating and activity. (That is a big IF on purpose.) Child BMI is not reliably predictive of adult BMI. According to the U.S. Preventive Services Task Force, "a substantial proportion of children under 12 or 13, even with BMIs higher than 95th percentile, will not develop adult obesity."[50] (Note: There is increasing predictability as BMI increases, and the older the child.)

The youngest age at which I have seen outright restriction recommended was in four-and-a-half-month-old Mia, an exclusively breastfed baby. The pediatrician told Mom that Mia was "obese," to cut out all nighttime feeds, and to try to hold Mia off her feeding for 30 minutes when she seemed hungry. Mom cried in one room while Dad held Mia, screaming, in another room. Within weeks, mom's milk supply was down to nothing, and this family was on the road to dealing with a child with an increased interest in feeding. When Mom reached out, just after Mia's third birthday, the family was already doing so many things well. Mom enjoyed cooking and family meals and Mia got plenty of activity, but they limited Mia's portions, and Mia didn't like it. We had one visit and a few follow-up calls and emails, mostly to reassure Mom that Mia could be trusted to decide how much to eat. Within a few months of instituting the DOR, Mom reported that Mia was happier and far less preoccupied with eating. In this case, the doctor recommended ignoring Mia's cues and feeding in a way that was not responsive to her needs, which set up their feeding struggles.

For an example of a child trending toward the average over time, consider Tracy's daughter Nora, who was off the charts in the "obese" range for years. When her growth spurt occurred with puberty, she ended up as a teen with a BMI in the "normal" range, below 75th percentile, with no diet or restriction. The term "losing the baby fat" is a reality for many children, with statistics showing that around two-thirds of preschoolers in the "overweight" and "obese" range will not be obese as adults.

Is this REALLY the first generation of children who will have "a shorter life span than their parents?"
This "fact," which gets repeated in almost every article on childhood "obesity," came originally from an opinion piece in *The New England Journal of Medicine*, with no studies to back it up. Because it sounds so scary, it has been picked up and reported as scientific fact in countless resources. I've even seen it reported as, "This is the first generation of children that will die before their parents." It's like a childhood game of telephone, with anxiety-provoking consequences. It is routinely one of the lines that gets used to justify the "war on obesity" and unproven interventions. As Bacon and others point out, during our current "obesity epidemic," we have seen death rates from heart disease and cancer decrease, and some experts and agencies, including the Social Security Administration, think our children will actually live *longer* lives than we do. Here is another reality check: the rate of overweight and obesity in children has remained stable since 1999.[51] Just a friendly reminder to always question what you hear.

It's Not About Portion Control or Smaller Plates

You probably have heard that the problem of "obesity" is all about portions. In fact, portion control education is popular, with many posters showing "correct" portion sizes hanging in school cafeterias. Another popular piece of advice is to eat off smaller plates, presumably to trick you into eating less. Some studies show that in a research setting, larger portions and larger plate size lead to increased intake.

I have some questions that the studies don't answer:

- Do the folks in the study who ate larger portions then eat less throughout the day? In other words, do they self-regulate and eat less for the next meal or day because they ate more at that sitting?
- Are there things about a study setting that make tuning in to internal cues more difficult?
- Was there a subgroup of people who did *not* eat more based on plate size? In other words, was there a group of people who were eating competent and who stopped when they were satisfied?
- Why aren't they studying people who *are* eating competent and self-regulate? I imagine there would be a lot to learn from a study like that.

At least two studies contradict the assumption that portion control or serving food on a small plate is the answer.

- **Portion control:** In one study, adults were told before a meal the amount of pasta that comprised a "half" portion and a "whole" portion. (They were told they were there to rate the taste of a pasta sauce.) The portion-size information *did not change* how much the study participants ate.[52] Importantly, none of the study participants were dieting, so they stopped when they were full; *hunger* predicted not only how much they ate but also how well they liked the sauce. (This explains in part why having structured meals and snacks helps selective eaters. Allowing kids to be a little hungry for meals helps them have an appetite and makes food more appealing. As they say, "Hunger is the best cook.")
- **Plate Size:** In a study looking into plate size, researcher Barbara Rolls, Ph.D, found that her study participants ate the same amount no matter what the size of the plate, which she replicated in three different scenarios.[53] Hunger and how the food tasted determined how much they ate, not the size of the plate.

This is good news. In both studies, we have examples of eating based on internal cues, not relying on external cues like the size of a plate or portion-size recommendations. If you want to eat off smaller plates, that's fine. But using the "small plate" tactic to try to get a child to be smaller or eat less probably won't work. It is far better to raise a child to eat based on internal cues than to rely on external cues.

Weight Stigma and Bullying

If your child is bigger than average, assume he has been teased or bullied. Weight is probably the most common reason that children are teased.[54,55] Even worse, studies show that more than one third of children are teased about weight by members of their own families.[54] But children with a high BMI *can* feel good about themselves, and the key factor is their parents' support.

It isn't easy being fat in America, particularly now with the "war on obesity." Fat people have become an acceptable group to target, facing job discrimination[56] and health care discrimination. Fat bias is documented among a significant proportion of doctors[57] who believe that fat patients are "lazy," "sloppy," and "noncompliant." These doctors may make assumptions about health and lifestyle based on appearance, at times resulting in missed diagnoses or improper care. (See Adina's story on page 317 as an example of weight bias in the medical setting.)

If your child is bigger than average, the desire to protect him by trying to make him thinner is actually part of the problem. Love your child as he is now, unconditionally. Support his health with balanced foods, the DOR, and the opportunity for fun physical activity. Know that trying to make him thinner will probably make him fatter, less healthy, and not as happy. Learn to be open, be a safe person for your child to talk to about weight bullying, and address it at school if it is happening. Examine and challenge some of your own beliefs about weight and health if you need to (see reading list above).

Transitioning to the Trust Model With the Overweight or Food-Preoccupied Child

Because the Trust Model is universal, it works for all body shapes and concerns. The Trust Model is healthy feeding. For the child who has experienced food insecurity, which is common in the fostering and adopting families I work with, the key is to take away the child's worry and nurture and take care of the child in terms of food. *You* provide, plan, and feed so your child can let go of the anxiety, fear, and worry that is making it hard for him to tune in to his internal cues and eat well.

You get to think about and plan food so he doesn't have to.

"This all makes sense. I did a similar exercise in my recovery from bulimia: fill your cupboards, including all the food that was not "good." I remember feeling relieved that I would not run out of food. It helped. It strikes me that our kids need that same reassurance. In the times we've had plenty of food on the table but it looked more bare because of limited serving dishes, or because it's all combined in a casserole or some such, I'm aware that to my daughter, it may feel scarce and scary. Sometimes I put stuff on there, like grapes, to fill up the space." —Emma, mother to Nussa, age three, adopted from Ethiopia

Guiding Principles

Follow the DOR. You decide: *what, when, where*. Your child: *how much* from what you provide. And:
- Accept your child as he is right now.
- Don't focus on your child's weight.
- Focus on behaviors, such as sitting down for breakfast or not grazing.
- Establish and maintain bedtime routines and aim for adequate and regular sleep.
- Provide the opportunity for regular, fun movement.

Ideas for Meals and Snacks
- Serve a small portion of dessert with the meal.
- Two to three times a week, serve a "treat" snack that includes "forbidden foods."
- Eat meals together if you aren't already.
- Serve family style: put all the food out in bowls.
- Be sure you have plenty of food.
- Be *absolutely reliable* about serving regular meals and snacks—every two to three hours for smaller kids, every three to four hours for older kids. **You don't get to forget. You have to remember it so they don't have to worry about it.**
- Make snacks balanced and filling. Yes, offer her more—even if you are worried about weight. When a child can be satisfied in terms of hunger at meals and snacks, she can stop thinking about food until the next time to eat in a few hours.
- Include low, medium, and high-fat choices.

- Don't "accidentally" run out of the fattening, high-calorie, or "red-light" foods.
- Don't lie to your children. Trust is the goal.

"I was told to lie to the kids by our RD. It felt absurd. My kids were smarter than that. They figured out that I only 'ran out' of the stuff they really liked and wasn't supposed to let them have, like rice, pasta, meat..." — Leah, mother of two

> For a thorough discussion of dealing with formerly forbidden foods, see the section "Sweets and Treats" in Chapter 8, What About the What.

Transitioning to Trust: How the Process Usually Unfolds

Before you begin with this process, just as I advised parents of small or selective children, I recommend beginning a journal to document the journey. Again, this journey is not linear, but instead characterized by progress and what appear to be setbacks. Progress sometimes feels slow. Write down where you are now, what your days are like, how much time and energy you put into keeping food from your child, how does it feel to your child, how do you feel? Writing it down will help you through this difficult process. Use the journal as a prompt to help you observe, be curious, and respond to your child.

Once parents institute structure and the DOR with their children, this is how the transition, which can be divided into two general parts, typically unfolds with my clients.

Stage One: "This Is So Scary"

Predictably, at first the child will seem to prove he can't be trusted with eating—that he really has no stopping place. This is when, without proper preparation and support, most parents panic and give up. Many parents I hear from have already "tried" to let the child decide how much and couldn't get through the transition. It was simply too scary.

Amy, mother of Teresa, age four, wrote on my blog, *"We did it for four days, and I couldn't stand it. She ate more than my husband, so we went back to pre-plating her meals."* Another mom wrote, *"Our three-year-old eats so much. Sometimes I have to leave the room since it makes me really anxious. My husband is better at handling all this."*

"We've been shocked with the amounts, like eight bowls of cereal with yogurt for breakfast yesterday." — Mom Alexis, two weeks into the transition with Greta, age two-and-a-half

Of note, just one week later, Greta was already showing signs of recognizing what it felt like to be full, leaving food, and leaving the table without extraordinary measures. *"Today at lunch, she didn't eat much, asked for more of something, then as soon as we gave it to her, she said she was done. Another day, she left the table voluntarily to go play, something she had never done in her two and a half years.*" Writing these successes down helped Alexis to see that Greta's skills were emerging.

How Do You Get Through Stage One?

The approach almost identical to the list in Chapter 4, because you are trusting that this will work—it's a leap of faith.

- Pray.
- White-knuckle it—that is, hold onto the chair when every fiber in your being wants to take her plate away.
- Hold hands with your partner under the table.
- Keep a note on the fridge such as "Trust Greta" and use it as a mental mantra, or even write out the DOR in big letters to remind you of your job and your child's job. (If your child is able to read, you may want to tuck this away.)
- Know that your child needs to "overeat" to learn to tune in. Knowing that it is a necessary part of the process will help you get through it.
- Say the Serenity Prayer (page 248).
- Tap into any feelings of relief or instinctual confidence in the process.
- Ignore, or pretend to ignore, how much your child is eating.

> You don't often get told to ignore your child, and I don't really mean *ignore* her, but you do have to try to not notice or react to how much she is eating—so "ignore" is a useful image. During the transition, your child will eat more than what you are comfortable with. Don't count slices of bread or pizza, and don't comment. This is tough. You will want to chime in with, "That's your fourth piece of bread. Honey, aren't you full yet?" It won't help, and it could make her want to eat more. It is a distraction from her internal cues. When you pick her up from a party and her friend's mom says with a frozen smile, "She is such a good eater; she ate six pieces of pizza," try to deflect attention and say, "Oh, I'm glad she enjoyed it, sounds like it was a great party. Thank you." Avoid explaining or apologizing in front of your child. Stay calm and send your daughter the message that you trust her, and she will figure it out.

"In a way, it's easier than I thought. I've spent the last two years trying to not let her eat. I'm worried and I'm scared, but part of me is also relieved. That burden of having to constantly try to get her to eat less is lifted. It is such a relief, I can't even describe it."
— Rebecca, mother of Adina, now age two-and-a-half and in Stage One

"Normal" in the Transition

Knowing what is normal will help you get through it. During the transition, your child is aware that things are different and is trying to figure out the new rules, such as by asking if she can have more chicken, even with chicken already on her plate. This is normal and healthy. She is learning to trust that she is in control of *how much* from what you offer and that she doesn't have to be preoccupied about when she will eat next, because you are being reliable about that. This will all help her learn to tune in to her cues from her body, instead of being ruled by anxiety and that feeling of scarcity.

"I am beyond thrilled to see the changes, and I feel like I'm probably halfway there. Seeing her play with her food, biting a piece of toast and saying, 'it looks like a fish—watch him swim!' There are so many more subtle (but significant) signs that she is finally feeling more secure around food—something I thought I'd never see. We were at a play date the other day, and she saw the food, had 2 crackers, and GOT BACK DOWN TO PLAY! We will keep working on this, and even though it may take a while longer, we are on the right track now." — Rebecca, mother of Adina, four months into the transition to the Trust Model

Stage Two: Emerging Skills
If parents can make it long enough to see even these earliest glimmers of self-regulation emerging, as well as less food obsession, it helps build faith in the process. Stage two is characterized by increasing examples of her emerging skills, but she may still "overeat" and seem food preoccupied much of the time.

"Well, we went for a burger, and lo and behold, she had about half the bun, one bite of meat and said she was done. We were so surprised. I have learned that what she loved one day does not always mean she will like it in the same amount or at all the next— which is a change, because she used to eat anything and everything in large quantities."
— Alexis, mother of Greta, in Stage Two

"A month ago, she ate two whole bagels with cream cheese. Today she had a quarter of a bagel, said she was done, and went to play. This is a totally different child."
— Brittany, mother of two-year-old Sarah, one month into Stage Two

"We have noticed a bit less urgency before meal and snack time."
— Alexis, two weeks into the transition, now in Stage Two with Greta

More signs of emerging skills to look out for (and journal):
- She is less frantic or preoccupied with food.
- His rate of eating is slowing down.
- He is playing with food.
- He is opening up to the idea of sharing foods, as in, "this is for my brothers," or "I had mine, now that is Daddy's." (Even if he goes on to eat the food, acknowledging is step one.)
- She may appear to savor foods more, rather than gulping or stuffing.
- She will leave food on her plate.

- He will leave a meal voluntarily.
- She becomes more choosey about what she will or won't eat.
- He is consuming large meals but also smaller ones, as in, *"He ate a huge amount at dinner, and it was really scary, but I noticed he ate less at breakfast the next day."*
- She engages more with others at meal times, and plays at play dates and parties after checking out the food.
- He is beginning to exhibit patterns, such as more at breakfast or after nap and less midmorning.
- He is getting a little more "naughty" at the table. In some ways this is reassuring. He's not preoccupied with how much he can eat and is testing other limits like any other child.

Freed From Worry, Room to Play

Many parents describe their "food-obsessed" kids as listless, inactive, and uninterested in play. This can be confusing, as many of these children have come from institutional settings, where some motor and developmental delay is expected. However, these children are often so preoccupied with food that they cling to or hover near the parent, with most of their waking hours spent trying to get food: they don't play at the park or on play dates, but instead linger near the food or the parent. They cry and whine for a bottle or snack, ignoring the pile of toys next to them.

I have been pleasantly surprised when more than one family has told me that once the child was less preoccupied with food, spontaneous play and movement increased on its own—even very early into the transition. The child who in June wouldn't leave her mother's side at the beach (because she was constantly begging for food) was running and splashing in the water by the end of summer. These children discover the playground when they are not wandering from one parent to the next, panhandling for snack handouts. It makes sense.

As Adan's mom said, just one week into the transition, *"It's as if his mind is freed of food and now he realizes that he can move... who would have known? His spontaneous movement has improved. We actually cancelled a physical and occupational therapy evaluation after just seeing the few days of improvement."*

Realize that people (kids are people too) differ with their level of interest in food. Some children will always eat faster than their peers or take more pleasure in food than others. (There are studies that suggest this is an inborn trait, with "picky" eaters showing different sucking patterns even as infants.) Clearly, some children get more pleasure from eating, and this is not a problem within the context of a healthy feeding relationship.

Remember also that these are *emerging* skills. She will still pester you about treats and perhaps eat quickly or "overeat" at times. In addition, many of these behaviors are normal for small children, and even the child who is eating competent will occasionally beg for treats and "overeat."

"She was also playing with the applesauce she picked up with the spoon. She was licking it, offering it to her doll across the room, and talking in-between bites quite a bit—as opposed to her usual non-stop putting food in her mouth." — Toni, a mother seeing emerging skills

"We were all still sitting at the table talking when she announced she was DONE and wanted to get down to go and play. I let her down with no comment, of course, but I was jumping up and down inside!!" — Rebecca, mother of Adina, age two-and-a-half

Common Questions and Challenges During the Transition

- *"She eats so fast. Can we tell her to slow down so her body can catch up?"* The fact that I hear this question repeatedly tells me that parents have tried it, and it has predictably backfired. If it worked, they wouldn't ask. Most often, when an anxious child is told to slow down, it triggers anxiety and gobbling. If that is what you observe, be patient. Try to eat calmly and at a normal pace yourself. With time, rapid eating or stuffing most often improves on its own.

- *"Do we sit with her the entire time? She keeps eating and eating after we are finished, so one of us (sometimes both) gets up to start clearing dishes."* Play this by ear. At meals, try to sit for about 30 minutes and keep her company. For snacks, maybe sit with your tea or water and chat or join her with her snack; then life goes on, and if you need to load the dishwasher, you can. You are still near and being companionable. This will also get easier as she gets older. With a severely anxious food-preoccupied child, she may be willing to sit and nibble for hours. *When* you cut off meals is up to you. A general rule of thumb is that 20 minutes or so is adequate for snacks; 30–40 minutes for meals. If you need to get moving sooner, your child will know the difference in terms of your reasoning. She will know with time that it feels different to say, "Dinner is almost over, and we need to get ready for bed," versus, "You've had enough!" Prepare her in advance for the transition, "Dinner is almost over, and after, we can do some coloring." She may eat more and more rapidly with the warning, but that is okay. Over time she will learn to trust that you are not trying to get her to eat less.

- *"Can I train my three-year-old to recognize when he is hungry? My friend talks about 'starving, kind of hungry, hungry, not hungry, full, stuffed,' and even has her kids use a chart sometimes to point to what they are feeling."* I don't think that the food-obsessed child, particularly if he has known food insecurity and has been restricted, can initially feel or interpret cues. It's possible that all he feels is "starving" or "stuffed," and he can't even tell what that means. From my experience, children learn to tune in to those cues and tell what they mean, with:

· Time
· Permission to eat and "overeat"
· Regular meals and snacks that are balanced
· Coming to the table without anxiety or conflict

After careful adherence to the DOR and structured meals and snacks, with my clients' toddlers, it takes about 4–6 weeks, to see abilities emerge with eating—all without charts or a lot of talk about it. In general, experience is more meaningful than trying to explain these tricky concepts. If you have an older child who is more cognitively advanced, these kinds of charts and direct teaching techniques may or may not help.

- *"She is always asking for more, even after eating a huge amount."* She is testing you to see if you really mean it when you say, "You can eat until you are done." I have heard from so many clients that the urge to cut the child off is strong, but that often after giving the child more, she took a bite or two and declared she was full. The important thing is that *she* decides when the meal is over.

- *"I'm really scared to let her have her 'treat snack,' with all she wants of her favorites like cheese or cookies."* When you try that "treat snack" with cheese or other favorites, she will probably eat large amounts at first. Consider serving it with a favorite fruit or vegetable if that helps you feel better. She will be okay with high-fat foods, and she does need access to those formerly "forbidden foods" within the structure of meals and snacks. Start with something you find less scary, such as homemade oatmeal raisin cookies versus chocolate chip cookies. You have to feel comfortable with this process as well, but if you have trouble allowing your child access to sweets and treats, you may need to examine your own eating and attitudes in order to better help your child (Chapter 9).

- *"It is okay to begin to ask her when she slows down at the end of a long meal, 'Is your tummy full?' or 'Is your tummy still hungry?'"* When in doubt, you can try it out, and see how she reacts. You can model, "I am still hungry, so I'm having more beans," or "No, thank you, I don't want more; my tummy is full." One or two mentions are okay, but repeated mentions might be felt as pressure. You can ask if she's full, and if she would like to color or read a book. If you are responsive to her, you will be able to tell if she is pushing back—for example, if she gets frantic and grabs a ton of food when she gets down, then you may want to back off a little.

- *"Shortly after a satisfying meal, even if he ate until he was 'done,' he will say, 'I'm hungry.'"* This is a normal, almost automatic response. Remember, it's been his life to worry about food. Avoid, "You can't be hungry, you just ate!" Reassure him that snack time will be "soon," and redirect to another activity. When these kids are bored, they often default to "I'm hungry."

- *"If we give her a pudding pop or a Rice Krispies treat as dessert with her meal, and she wants more, do we give it to her? Is dessert unlimited as well?"* Dessert with the meal is one child-sized portion. "That's your share, and we'll have (that dessert) again soon. If you're still hungry, you can have more corn, potatoes, or chicken."

- *"Maggie wakes up groggy, and we don't seem to have time for breakfast. I worry that she will feel restricted if we hurry her along."* Breakfast is tough. Sometimes families can start a little earlier, or maybe even think about moving up bedtime. Perhaps plan to have easy-to-eat foods when she is ready, like peanut butter toast or Go-Gurt. This is where your family has to find what works, such as an earlier start or allowing her to finish a milk box in the car. (I am not a fan of young kids eating in the car, as it is a choking risk, but families do it all the time.) If she is eating in the car, make sure it is with foods that are easily chewed and swallowed. Being rushed at breakfast will not spoil all your other efforts. She will get it that she is being fed reliably, and it's not about trying to get her to eat less. Some schools have breakfast programs, which is another great option on days you are running late or as an everyday plan.

- *"He seems to be acting out more now at the table."* Some of my clients are somewhat dismayed at new behavior issues, from throwing utensils to refusing to set the table. See it as a positive. Free from the anxiety and stress around food, he can now connect, play, and interact with others at the table. Part of that means testing *other* boundaries. So, deal with it like you deal with other discipline issues. Use your "time-out" or other consequences—whatever your preferred discipline or teaching strategy is—and tell her that when she's ready to be pleasant, she can come back. If she tantrums over food or the dessert choice, you can say, "I'm sorry you're sad we aren't having rice. We can go to your room, and when you are ready to be pleasant, we would love to have you back at the table." If she needs help calming down, you can do that, and then let her finish the meal. Ask your therapist for support and suggestions if you are working on behavior.

- *"He still seems anxious that he won't get enough."* Use simple reassurances when you think he needs it, such as, "There is always more if you are hungry," and "You can have more chicken when you finish the chicken on your plate." Don't get too caught up in words; it is the actions over time, that help most.

- *"We've been at this for a few days, and he is eating like crazy. We are supposed to go to a party with a buffet, and I don't know how to handle it."* This is a common scenario. While still in the eating-like-gangbusters stage, you find yourself facing a food-based event such as a party with the entire extended family. Parents are tempted to limit children in public, but doing that can confuse and slow the process. Early on in the process, he will probably eat a lot at parties like this and not want to play. He might hang out at the buffet, and family and others may comment. You have choices. You can skip the party if it's just too much to deal with publicly right now. That's okay. (Obviously, if your son is excited about it, reconsider, or don't let him know why you aren't going.) Or you can go and see what happens, being prepared for him to eat a ton. You may or may not want to tell family what you are up to with his feeding in general. My clients have had different experiences with this. The child will often check in, not believing at first that he can really eat as much as he wants (as long as he is not depriving others of food). He may eat a lot and only eat, or he may eat a plate or two and then run off to play. This is more about your comfort and anxiety. One client decided to skip a cousin's party because she didn't want to deal with the comments and explaining around her toddler's eating. Another client went to a party and admitted she felt embarrassed by the amounts her daughter ate, while yet another went to a party and was surprised that her daughter played with her cousins. Manage your expectations and see what happens.

- *"What do we do when he eats several servings, says he's 'done,' gets down, and then when we start cleaning up he says 'more dinner?'"* Short answer: When eating is over, it's over. Remind him before he gets down, with something like, "That was yummy. Lunch is over, and we'll eat again soon." When he comes back asking for food, you can say, "Lunch is over, but we'll eat again soon. Let's play." It is very different from "You've had enough! Go play!" or trying to get him to stop eating to make him thinner by distracting with toys. You are doing your job, which is the when, or structure piece. He is doing his job, which is figuring out the new rules and testing limits.

- *"What if she wants more shrimp, but we love it too, and I want my share? If I say 'no,' will that trigger her anxiety?"* You are important to the family too, so if you want some of her favorite, you can have it. She is going to learn to share and will know the difference between being told, "You can't have more because you've had enough food," versus "You've had your share, and Mommy and Daddy like squash, too. I'm sorry you're sad there isn't more squash. There is more rice if you're still hungry." You can model asking if you can finish something, such as, "Does anyone mind if I finish the salad?" I thought it was a hoot when my then four-year-old used the phrase she learned from her older cousins, "Am I depriving anybody if I finish the shrimp?" Find words that feel natural to you. Sometimes, when a child sees that you are going to finish something, they suddenly become interested and may try a new food. It's good to acknowledge her feelings of disappointment, but as all parents do sacrifice, sometimes she gets more than her "share," and that's okay, too. I trust that you will figure it out. It will get easier with time.

- *"He vomited last week after overeating his favorite food. Come to think of it, we did miss snack that day."* He will "overeat" and, rarely, vomit. It's not common, but it happens. Try to be calm and not overreact if it does. If he is vomiting frequently, be sure there isn't a medical or anatomical reason. If you find no medical reason, look again at structure and the DOR to determine if there is room to improve so that he feels satisfied. I have not seen overeating to the point of vomiting continue to be a problem once the Trust Model is in place.

Further Along in Trust: Looking Back on the Transition

"I honestly no longer even think about Sarah's eating. Her little sister eats more than she does, and she is only in the 50th percentile for weight. Sarah no longer obsesses about food and it is certainly not the focal point of her day. In fact, we were at a birthday party on Sunday, and I had to pull her away from the sandbox to get her to eat just four bites of pizza. A lot of times she refuses to eat dinner, and as frustrated as my husband gets with her, I am secretly glad to see some 'normal' preschooler behavior. Don't get me wrong, she still loves food and often times eats more than the other kids, but it is no longer an issue in our house. I think of you often and I am so grateful for your advice!"
— Brittany, mother of three-year-old Sarah, just more than a year into the Trust Model with her BMI slowly trending down

"We are three years out with this process. I can tell you it was hard for a while. My husband and I had to simply believe it would work. Knowing that everything else we tried failed so miserably helped. We saw small meals sometimes, and pretty big meals at others. He was way off the growth charts, and it's taken years, but slowly he is coming down on the percentiles—but still in the 'overweight' category. I try not to think about his weight much, since I know I can't control it. I'm just grateful he is strong, healthy, and happy. Grateful we turned this around."
— Pia, mother of Antoine, adopted at age 16 months, now age five years

"It was really hard to trust it in the beginning, but now almost always this feels really right and natural. I have to admit, occasionally I watch her eat a huge plate of pasta and think I should stop her, but I know better; she's proven she can be trusted. It's just hard to undo all that training where we think we have to limit portions or control what our kids eat." — Mary, mother to Cindy, age eight years

Transition at Your Own Pace

I used to recommend that all parents make a clean break and go "all the way," and many clients have had success with this approach. However, I am learning to trust my clients to progress at a pace that is in their family's best interest. There's that word "trust" again.

Adopted children, or children in foster care, may also need to be eased into new routines. Samantha is a mom who decided it was too overwhelming for her to make all the changes at once. Initially, Samantha removed the highchair and kept everything else the same. Next she tackled the bottle for her then three-year-old, Rosy, adopted from Guatemala. Previous attempts to go "cold turkey" from the bottle, as recommended by the dietitian, ended in disaster, with a trembling child who was "catatonic" for days. The bottle time was simply moved into meal times, then to the table where Samantha followed Rosy's cues and need for closeness and sat next to her with their arms touching. It won't be long before Rosy will be ready to let her bottle go, but for now, it is incorporated into meal and snack times and isn't interfering with the structure.

What About Exercise?

"Okay, I understand that my son shouldn't diet, then how can I get him to be more active?" — Oliver, father to Jeremy, age 11 years

If you have been paying attention to the general philosophy and language around the Trust Model, you might have noticed something in that last sentence. Did you catch it? The question is, "How can I *get him* to be more active?" If we think of our responsibilities as parents within a trusting framework, a better question to ask is, "How can I support my son so he has the opportunity for physical activity and can learn to move his body in enjoyable ways?"

Allow me to illustrate the notion of "control" versus "trust" as it relates to physical activity. One chilly fall afternoon, my daughter and I were at the swings at a local park. A little girl with a beautiful, toothless grin ran up, hopped on a swing, and started pumping her legs. A lean man strode over and shouted, "That's lazy exercise, Sally! We didn't come here for lazy exercise. Get off the swings and run around." Sally's smile disappeared as she walked slowly away from the swings.

I imagine Sally's dad had good intentions. Perhaps he read the Center for Disease Control and Prevention's recommendations or a handout from their pediatrician recommending children get "60 minutes of vigorous supervised exercise daily." He was doing his job, right? But what did Sally learn that day? Did she learn that exercise is fun or a chore? Did she learn to trust her body or to fight it?

We want to raise children who are happy and healthy, who enjoy moving their bodies and have a good level of fitness. We know that fitness is a better indicator of health than fatness, so how do we help our kids be active without turning into a drill sergeant who might turn our kids off from physical activity altogether?

The Division of Responsibility With Activity

You learned that with feeding, the DOR means your job as a parent is to provide *what, when,* and *where* the child eats, and the child decides *if* and *how much.* With activity, the parent's job is to provide the opportunity for physical activity, the structure, and support—and leave the rest up to the child. The more you push, the more children are likely to resist. Sound familiar?

Also know that when a child is told she is "overweight" or "obese," she is likely to become *less* physically active. As my client Becca told me, *"I look back now at photos of my softball team from when I was a kid, and I looked like everyone else, or pretty darn close. But after that doctor visit where I was given a calorie list and told I was too heavy, I was convinced I was a hippo. I dropped out of softball and stopped pretty much every sport and activity I enjoyed. It's so sad! I don't want that to happen to my daughter."*

Trusting kids with activity, as with food, can be tough. If you have a chubby or "obese" child who loves to play on the swings, the impulse to make her get off and run is understandable. Your child's doctor, or even family members, may have even given you stern lectures. One parent commented on my blog, *"My two-year-old is big and loves to swing, but my mom will only take her to a park where there aren't any. Some days she hops off the swings and runs around, while other days she mostly swings. The important thing is she loves being at the park, and I don't want my mom to spoil that."*

Like Sally's dad, this concerned grandma is trying to control how her granddaughter moves to get her to be thinner. This has a high chance of backfiring. Other often-recommended methods that may backfire include:

- Using a pedometer. (One of my blog readers wrote that if her parents had tried that, she would have sat in the bathroom tapping away at the pedometer to add steps as an act of rebellion.)
- Signing a child up for any class with an obvious name like "Slim Down" or "Trim Kids." Again, the message and primary goal of any activity should be fun, enjoying the challenge of reaching a goal, a social outlet, and building strength and fitness, but not with the expected payout of weight loss.
- Requiring that your child run around or do jumping jacks during commercials.
- Enforcing the use of exercise equipment, like treadmills or stationary bikes, which I have seen for children as young as age three. Most adults find exercise machines boring, and they are less fun for kids.
- Having strict goals and limits, such as these examples from a pediatrician's handout:
  - At least 60 minutes of supervised vigorous physical activity a day
  - Don't allow more than 30 minutes of sedentary time in a row

I don't know many families who achieve either of these goals every day. What if your child is doing homework? Does he need to run laps around the basement every 30 minutes when a timer rings?

How Different Body Types Factor Into Activity

An individual's interest in activity may be determined, in part by genetics or an expression of temperament. We all know the person who "doesn't feel good" unless he gets in his run, or the person who recharges by relaxing with a good book. Studies on newborns, with little bands around their limbs to record movement, have shown wide variation of natural movement from "almost constant" to "very little."[58] The leanest babies seemed to move the most, and interestingly took in the most calories, while their fatter counterparts seemed to move less, but also *ate less*. Some eating characteristics also appear to be inborn. Remember the personality traits when it comes to food, on page 52? Children described as picky eaters tended to have a slower suck pattern as infants.[59]

Have you heard of the terms endomorph, mesomorph, and ectomorph? They were coined in the 1940s to describe body types and were associated with certain temperaments and traits. These three classifications have been fun for me to consider, in a not-so-scientific way.

1. The **ectomorph** is like my father: naturally long and lean, doesn't gain weight easily, has a high metabolism, is active, craves exercise, and prefers brown rice to fries—really.
2. The **endomorph** is like my father's sister: rounder, gains weight more easily, doesn't seem to need rigorous physical exercise as much, and finds that sedentary pursuits are energizing.
3. The **mesomorph** is like me: somewhere in between.

A parent might have a hard time empathizing with or understanding an experience so different from her own. For example, the lean parent, not much motivated by food, may have a harder time feeding a child who needs to eat regularly, particularly if the child is stocky or "overweight." One mom wrote, *"I have always been lean, and I forget to eat pretty regularly. I don't see why I have to feed Gavin every three to four hours. I don't think he needs to eat that often."*

While Connie, another mom, could go without a meal or snack, she realized pretty quickly that her daughter Alicia needed to eat every three to four hours or she would get very cranky and even lightheaded. Although food wasn't a priority for Connie, she was responsive to Alicia's needs, even though they were different from her own. She carried trail mix and other foods at all times.

It has helped me and some of my clients find a way to think about movement, weight, and temperament, particularly if there is a mismatch between parent and child. No type is good or bad, and it's hard to change a mesomorph into an ectomorph; all can be healthy and happy.

What type are you? What about your kids? If you are slight of frame with a high metabolism, and your child is stocky, gains weight more easily, and doesn't love running like you do, are you fighting against biology to try to get him to be a lean runner? Are you truly not bothered when you "forget to eat," while your partner or child turns into a monster if it's been more than four hours since the last meal? People feel hunger differently and metabolize differently. There are people who forget to eat, and others for whom that is inconceivable. Both are okay.

Activity Levels Vary

A child who may ride in the stroller one month might run nonstop during the next visit to the park or sculpture garden. The swing, the sole object of interest at the playground for weeks, may one day be forgotten. It's been fascinating to watch my own case study—my daughter. Her interest in activity seems to go through cycles—very active as a crawler and toddler, a little less so around two and three years, then more active again.

Some days she would sit and play with her crafts and watch a little TV, and other days she would run around the house in fairy wings, start spontaneous games of bowling with cups and materials scavenged from the recycling, jump on our secondhand jogging trampoline, and launch herself onto piles of beanbags.

Supporting Activity

Children need to play and move their bodies to be healthy and happy. Just as with food, the goal of avoiding pressure and providing opportunity is key. Don't push it, and allow your child to find his natural rhythm. Make a point to be active as a family in a fun way, and make fitness about having fun and feeling good. Be positive. Telling children they are fat or need to lose weight is the best way to get them to be less active. Don't talk about weight, including your own.

Be responsive to your child and consider his temperament and interests. Are team sports ideal for a social child, or geo-caching at a state park for the one who loves maps and treasure hunting? Help your child find something he likes to do, and help him find time to do it. Limiting screen time (TV and computer) helps kids move more than following them around like a personal trainer.[60] Keeping the TV out of the bedroom is a great start.

While sports are healthy and fun, be careful not to over-program your kids to the point that you regularly miss out on family dinners. (I told you this stuff isn't easy.)

Organized Activities
- Sign up for a class at the local recreation center or gym, such as karate, dance, or swimming.
- Join a sports team or running club at school.
- Train to participate in a fun run or fundraiser for a good cause. However, "fighting childhood obesity" would not be an appropriate cause for a fun-run for kids, though I am seeing this increasingly.

Being Active as a Family

- Go for winter-lights walks. Bundle up after dark and bring a flashlight. Even if you have to bring little ones in the stroller or wagon for a while, get in the habit of moving together in a fun way, if you can.
- Let your kids see you having fun. Instead of sitting around at the park while they run around with friends, grab that basketball and shoot some hoops.
- Find child-sized rakes, snow shovels, and brooms, so kids can join in and "help."
- Family walks or bike rides may be just the thing for a child who is anxious or having troubles with separation.
- Ride bikes along a historical train path.
- Play in the pool at the local health club or recreation center.
- Go to family night at a local gymnastics center and bounce on the trampoline with your kids.
- Head to an indoor playground instead of or before the movies.
- Plant a garden or sign up for a community plot, if available.
- Consider getting ice skates, snow pants, and boots for yourself. I found that my being cold was the limiting factor for most outdoor play. Local schools and recreation centers often have free ice rinks and skate rentals, too.

Make Time to Be Active

- Have a box in the trunk of the car with a few balls and a Frisbee. Stop at a park on the way home if you have time.
- Ask the person picking your child up from school or daycare to stop by the park for 20 minutes on the way home if they have time.
- Encourage your school to increase play and recess time.
- Walk or bike to school if it's safe and you have time. Many schools are organizing programs to support walking to school.

Low-Cost Fun

- Move furniture out of the way so kids can jump on couch cushions, or try indoor bowling with empty bottles from the recycling bin.
- Play music with a great beat and have a dance party.
- Make a list of scavenger items for a walk that they can either collect or mark off on a list, such as fire hydrant, white house, mailbox, etc.
- Provide cushions and masking tape to make an indoor obstacle course.
- Check out your local recreation center's open gym hours.
- Stock up on outdoor gear, which is an important consideration in northern climates. Hand-me-downs are great, but Goodwill, Once Upon A Child, and Craigslist are also good sources for cheaper gear. Insist on snowpants and waterproof gloves.

Other Great Ideas From Parents

- *"We bought a smaller house in a walkable neighborhood. There is a park, corner store, and we can walk them to school."*
- *"If it's not too many flights, we take the stairs. We race, and it's fun."*
- *"I started workout DVDs at home, and they like to join in, and my daughter loves yoga. Check out* Namaste Kid.*"*
- *"We found a cheap tumbling class, challenge our kids to race, or do silly things to get their energy out. We have a lot of fun."*
- *"We belong to our local community center; the kids can play sports or work out there, too."*
- *"Hula hoop and playing Twister. Then going to the to park to throw sticks off the bridge and being in nature."*
- *"Playground time. Bring snacks and water. It's lots of active, independent play."*
- *"My boys love to play chase around the 'track' (our kitchen/living area). All it takes is a suggestion, and they are off."*

A Word About Catch-up Growth and Adult Obesity

Purposefully, I left this brief discussion until the end of the chapter because I wanted to first lay out the story of food insecurity and malnutrition, followed by catch-up growth or high weight leading to restriction and subsequent food preoccupation. I do not want to unnecessarily add to any worries, but I do want to address the concern that growth-restricted children seem to have a higher risk of developing metabolic problems like diabetes. (If worry distorts feeding, the last thing I want to do is cause worry.)

Epidemiological studies (statistical studies based on large groups of individuals) suggest that children who were growth-delayed, and experienced catch-up growth, may have higher rates of some health issues, possibly related to the early malnutrition and hormonal disruptions. (See the sidebar on self-regulation in Chapter 1, page 14).

- Girls have a higher chance of entering puberty early.
- There are reported to be overall higher rates of "overweight" and "obesity" after adolescence with perhaps an increased risk of metabolic syndrome (high blood pressure, increased abdominal weight, and diabetes) in those who may have experienced early malnutrition and growth delay.

I don't think these studies give the whole story. I would like to see more science related to several issues:

- How many of these children are from ethnic groups with higher mean BMIs, where a BMI of 85th percentile may actually be in the "normal" range?
- What about the feeding relationship? There is a good chance that many of these children were pushed to *eat more* early on because of weight and nutrition worries, they were restricted, or both—pushed to eat initially, perhaps learning to

overeat and ignore internal cues, only to gain weight and then at some point instructed to eat less.

- I would like to know if eating-competent adults who experienced early growth restriction are healthier, like the eating competence research shows in other populations. There is much we simply don't know.

I surmise that most of these children were not supported to learn to eat based on *internal* hunger and fullness cues. Remember that with time, a child can be taught to *ignore* and lose touch with those cues and eat more than is healthy for her. Certainly, even if the risk is there, feeding differently to try to avoid high weight will probably backfire and cause the outcome you are hoping to avoid.

Premature Puberty

Premature puberty is more common in girls adopted internationally. (Rarely, part of the picture could be that the child's age is not accurate. Sophia, for example, was surprised when a bone-growth study and other tests showed that their "four-year-old" from Ethiopia was closer to age seven.) The theory is that a history of growth delay due to malnutrition, and then catch-up growth, triggers hormones that precipitate early puberty.[61]

Aside from the social implications of early development, early puberty can be cause for concern, because it can result in premature closure of growth plates and a lower adult height than the genetic potential. In general, if true puberty is occurring, with breast development and other indications, a discussion and evaluation with a pediatric endocrinologist who has experience with premature puberty is in order. There is the option to treat the child with hormones to delay puberty. Dr. Dana Johnson at the University of Minnesota International Adoption Clinic says, "The trend is toward treating and delaying puberty, if it occurs before eight or eight and a half." This is an incredibly complex decision, without a clear "right" answer. Finding a knowledgeable doctor who will listen to your concerns and questions, as well as reaching out to other adoptive parents who have been there, may help.

Big Kids Are Worthy of Our Trust, Too

There is no way to predict whether your child will grow up lean or larger than average. I hope the information in this chapter has reassured you that big children can grow up to be healthy and happy.

What we can predict is that if you struggle with feeding, your child is food-preoccupied, or her weight is accelerating (after catch-up growth), and you try to *get her to eat less*, she will tend to eat more and struggle with her relationship with food and her body for years to come. You may have known this intuitively, and now you have a roadmap for a better way forward, a path to health and happiness.

Part II:
Making It Work: There's More You Need to Know

Part I addressed the main concerns that I hear about from families, from oral-motor delays and sensory issues, selective eating, and low-weight worries, to food preoccupation and worries about accelerating weight.

In Part II, things are different. In the next several chapters, I will share the challenges that come up when working with clients with all kinds of concerns. This half of the book addresses a variety of topics, including research on how our feelings affect nutrition, how a parent's eating disorder history can make feeding more challenging, calming common nutrition worries, and how to support the feeding relationship when your child is on a special diet.

Chapter 6

The Eating Experience: Feelings, Eating Competence, and Eating Disorders

What You Will Learn

This chapter will explore how feelings and attitudes affect our own eating and how we feed our children. We begin with a more in-depth look at the ultimate goal: Eating Competence. I will review studies pertaining to attitudes, pleasure, taste, and how *relying on our brains* (the head game) is a less reliable guide for our eating than listening and responding to cues from inside our bodies.

We will then examine how emotions and feeding intersect, from bottle-feeding to sweets to aid attachment, to helping children learn to tell the difference between emotions and hunger and fullness cues. We will also look at how the way we talk to kids about food and nutrition matters, and end with a brief discussion about eating disorders and disordered eating.

Eating Competence and the Food Attitude

Eating Competence (EC) refers to a way of understanding healthy adult eating. Eating Competence is not measured in calories, phytochemical composition, avoiding refined sugars, or against any pyramid or plate. Rather, it looks at people's attitudes and habits related to providing themselves with food. In essence, you are *how* you eat.

Research in adults shows that those who score as "eating competent" had better blood sugar measures, had better cholesterol levels, and tended to have a lower body mass index (BMI)—*in spite of higher energy intake.*[1] It's not just calories in and calories out. EC adults in the study also had higher adherence to the Mediterranean diet and higher fruit intake. Earlier studies show that EC folks tend to diet less and have lower and more stable BMI, a more balanced intake, less disordered eating, and better nutrition.[2]

Eating Competence is essentially the Trust Model for grownups. The Trust Model is a way to raise EC adults.

You are important too; take care of yourself like you would care for your child. Plan on feeding yourself a variety of tasty foods at regular intervals. The good news is that because you are already doing this for your child, you can easily join in.

You, too, have inborn capabilities with food when it comes to self-regulation (eating the right amount for your body) and food acceptance. Those capabilities might be buried from years of dieting, a history of an eating disorder, or not taking care of yourself with feeding, but those capabilities are there. You can be trusted. When you stop fighting and support your body, eat based on your hunger and appetite, acknowledge pleasure, and turn your back on shame and deprivation, you are more likely to maintain a stable body weight and enjoy improved nutrition.

Michelle Allison, nutritionist and author, writes on her blog at The Fat Nutritionist, *"Feeding myself from a trust perspective has meant a lot of letting go of external rules and expectations around nutrition, and finding my own guidelines. I've discovered that I have a real, internal desire to do things that are good for my body, and that I don't need a drill sergeant to 'get' me to do anything. I will actually eat vegetables on my own, but I will also call it good enough. My focus is on preserving my long-term relationship with vegetables instead of force-feeding myself in the moment."*

One of the most exciting aspects of working with families around eating is that improvements in the child's eating is often a motivation for parents to look at their own relationships with food.

After Halloween, a comment from a parent on my Facebook page said it all: *"Honestly, watching him manage his stash so well has totally changed how I view candy too, for the better. No more bingeing because it's there. If I want a piece, I choose my favorite and actually enjoy it."*

How We FEEL About Food Does Matter

To me, one of the most exciting themes emerging in the research is that attitude matters, and how we *think* about food matters. EC adults feel good about food and feeding themselves. They plan and cook; they don't waste mental energy worrying about food and calories.

One of the first things I help clients with is rehabilitating how feeding feels, or finding and rediscovering joy. If the family has approached the table with dread and is battle-weary, step one has to be improving the attitude and atmosphere at mealtimes. If your child is already thrashing before she is put in the highchair, or crying or whining before her first bite, the game is over. The mood must improve before feeding and weight concerns can be effectively addressed.[3] I have reviewed how to do this in Chapter 4, including page 97. The following is why it is so important.

How We Think and How We Talk About Food Is Important

How we feel about food is central to good health and nutrition. This sampling of studies illustrates how our thinking and attitudes affect how we eat, and even how nutrients are absorbed.

A few helpful terms:
- **Hunger:** the physical need for food to sustain energy and bodily functions.
- **Satiety or satisfaction:** the feeling of being done, or satisfied after eating or drinking, usually achieved best when hunger *and* appetite have been met.
- **Appetite:** the desire to eat or drink, based on smell, how food looks and tastes, and so much more.

Feeling That We Are Being "Sensible" or Deprived May Make Us Eat More

- Consider a 2011 study called "Mind Over Milkshakes."[4] Study participants were given the same shake and told on the first occasion that it was "sensible" and "no-fat," and on another occasion they were told that it was rich, creamy, fatty, and "indulgent." Guess which one they thought *tasted* better? (It's the same shake.) Answer: the "indulgent" one. No surprises there, but the new finding was that despite identical calories, fat, and nutrients, what the study participants *thought* about the shake affected the body's measured hormone response.

  Thinking "indulgence" meant lower hunger-hormone (ghrelin) levels, and presumably, less hunger. "Sensible" (a.k.a., deprivation), meant that the "hungry-hormone" level did not fall as much. In spite of the same intake, these "sensible" shake drinkers had higher hormone levels associated with *more hunger*.

  When we feel "sensible," or that we have to use "willpower" to get through the day, many of us feel deprived. In the magic that is our mind-body connection, the *feeling* of deprivation may result in higher hunger-hormone levels. A "sensible" mindset equates to hormone levels associated with hunger. How we think about food affects how much we enjoy it and how our bodies respond. The authors concluded, "Mindset meaningfully affects physiological responses to food."

  This study contributes to our understanding of why diets—no, not only diets, but often "sensible" eating and even grudging "moderation"—don't work for most people. Consider the study of teens, where even "healthy" weight maintenance or weight-loss tactics, such as trying to eat more fruits and veggies or using moderation—in other words, they tried to watch what they ate—resulted in heavier teens with more disordered behaviors.[5]

  How can this be, when moderation seems so, well, *moderate*? To most people, "moderation," in terms of food, means eating *less* than they want in terms of quantity or perceived enjoyment, and we are beginning to understand how important that enjoyment is.

"Eat cookies *in moderation*" makes me want more, almost like that food-insecure child. If I tell myself, "Enjoy the cookies, as many as you want, with a glass of milk at the table, and really enjoy them," I'm usually satisfied with one or two. And if they are fresh out of the oven and taste amazing, I might eat three or four and not want any more. Maybe at the next opportunity, I have less of an appetite for the cookies. Ironically, an Eating Competent diet, based on internal cues and *permission*, like the Trust Model, ends up being an intake of moderation, but it is the *result* of competent eating, not the goal. This is tricky stuff.

Pleasure and Taste Affects How the Food Is Used and Absorbed in the Body
- A series of classic and oft-quoted studies review how pleasure and taste affect how nutrients are absorbed. Swedish women were fed a meal of spicy Thai food, and a group of women from Thailand were given the same meal. The Thai women, who presumably enjoyed the flavor more, absorbed far more iron, the studied nutrient. Further, when the meals were pureed, presumably making for a less pleasurable way of taking in the same food, absorption of iron decreased across the board.[6]
- Another study showed that minerals were not absorbed when the participant was stressed, versus when taken in under calm circumstances.[7] Stress, and how appealing a food is (appetite), plays a role in absorption of nutrients.

In Chapter 4, we spent a lot of time reviewing how stress kills appetite. Research backs this up. Think about the last time you were afraid or anxious. Perhaps you don't like flying. Were you hungry on the plane? Before a big presentation at work, or at the city council, were you hungry? Another piece of the puzzle is that adults and youth who restrict or diet tend to eat more in times of stress,[8,9,10] whereas those who don't diet tend to eat less.

**Understanding how stress and emotions play a role
will help you build a healthy feeding relationship.**

When We *Think* About Calories and Fat, We Tend to Make Errors
- Several studies have looked at how our thinking about calories and fat affect food choices. When study participants ate what they thought were "low-fat" or "low-calorie" foods, even if they were the high-fat and high-calorie versions, they reliably ate *more* calories for the rest of the day, presumably to make up for those "lost" calories, also known as the "halo" effect (people think they are being "good"). Studies have shown that even the "organic" label makes people tend to eat more.[11]

In Summary

- Thinking a food is low fat or organic means people tend to eat more the rest of the day to compensate (external cues rather than internal).
- Stress decreases absorption of nutrients and appetite.
- Pleasure and good taste are important to absorbing nutrients.
- The feeling of deprivation, regardless of what is eaten, might make a body feel hungry or less satisfied.

The irony was the last sentence of the "Mind Over Milkshakes" study: "Perhaps if we can begin to approach even the healthiest foods with a mindset of indulgence, we will experience the physiological satisfaction of having our cake and eating it too."

Better yet, why not approach all foods with indulgence and joy, so if we do indulge in a piece of cake and eat in a tuned-in way, we will feel satisfied both cognitively (our thinking brain) and physiologically (our bodies). When we reject the labels of "good," "bad," "healthy," or "unhealthy," we can also feel that a ripe, juicy mango is indulgent.

When we rely on our bodies, not our brains, to guide our eating, we tend to do better.

How Kids Think About Veggies

Maybe part of the reason why kids don't seem to like veggies is that we oversell them, preparing them plain because it is "healthier," talking about how healthy they are, and bribing with dessert. Children learn that veggies must be bad if we are working this hard to convince them or if they have to slog through the veggies to get to the "good stuff." Rather than teaching children to rely on the body's natural drive for variety and pleasure, these veggie tactics introduce the "head game" and it gets in the way. What kids learn to think about veggies matters, and most of our efforts thus far to induce children to eat more veggies haven't worked.

Incorporating nutrition and food groups in our meal planning helps us meet our needs for hunger, fullness, and variety. Then we can get the head game off the table and eat based on guidance from our mouths and bodies, and not rely on mental trickery.

My favorite resource for helping adults with eating competence is Satter's *Secrets of Feeding a Healthy Family*, which one blog reader called a "blueprint" for addressing her own selective eating and self-regulation skills. If you are seriously struggling with food, help is available. The process of learning to trust and provide for yourself can take time. Another resource worth checking out is *Intuitive Eating* by Evelyn Tribole and *Health at Every Size* by Linda Bacon.

Helping Our Kids Have a Healthy Relationship With Food

It is not helpful to label or refer to your child as the "picky one," the "undereater," or the "overeater." How we label and talk about food to our kids also matters. One of the saddest trends I am seeing, which I believe is a direct result of the "war on childhood obesity," is increasingly harmful messaging to children about nutrition in schools, in the home, on TV, and in magazines. It is all around us. Consider a kids' coloring activity, from a summer trip to the farmer's market, that asked: "What is the healthiest option (fewest calories)?" and had the children chose from:

- Fruit salad plain
- Fruit salad with 2 tablespoons of orange juice
- Fruit salad with ½ cup of low-fat yogurt

All too often the choices presented to children are simplistic, and demonize fat, calories, or food in general, and are not presented in ways that are age-appropriate. Untrained staff and teachers give common and harmful "nutrition" messages. Even other children are getting in on the action; my daughter reported one day that two of her kindergarten friends told her 1% milk was bad for her because it had "too much fat."

Shaming children around food is not helpful. Michele Gorman, RD, past president of the Minnesota Dietetics Association, cares deeply about how food messages are communicated, particularly with children. She shares her personal story about shame and nutrition messaging: *"My mother left when I was six. My father, a blue-collar man, raised his children with little help. He worked a lot and made sure we had food in the cupboard. My early recollections of food are simply that it was just part of life. We never heard messages about being too fat or too thin, we were simply told we were loved, and eating at the dinner table was a requirement, even if it was pasta or cereal. Looking back now, I see what an accomplishment that was.*

"I remember clearly learning about the food groups in second grade. Already feeling much like an outsider since all of my schoolmates were raised with a mom, I panicked and intuitively felt that something else was wrong with my family—we didn't eat that way. We had cola, sugar cereals, and not many vegetables. I felt a lot of shame, fear, and somehow responsibility beyond what a seven-year-old should feel. I went home and declared we were ALL going to eat GrapeNuts for breakfast! (I was the only one who did.) Looking back, I wish that I didn't take the burden of worry. I wish there was a compassionate side to that discussion in school about food."

"We are creating a world of anxious adults. Let kids be kids and food be food."
— Michele Gorman, RD

Teaching Nutrition

Should we simply put our heads in the sand? Was it "irresponsible," as one mom accused on my blog, to skip the nutrition lecture with my then-preschooler? Gorman says, "I think it is important that children can understand that our bodies get nutrients from foods to do things such as think, see, play, etc. and to understand nutritional sciences like other biological sciences." But how we do that is critical. There is a great potential to do harm here as well.

What to Do
- Focus on health, not weight.[12]
- Have discussions that are age-appropriate. For example, small children may be able to learn that a banana is a fruit, but don't need to know the word "protein."
- Focus on modifiable behaviors, like eating breakfast or stress reduction, rather than factors kids have little control over, like weight.
- Respect body size diversity.
- Promote self-esteem and healthy body-image.[13,14,15]
- Provide opportunities for fun physical activity.
- Support the Division of Responsibility in feeding in the schools.[16] (See online resources at the Ellyn Satter Institute.)
- Teach about food in a fun, positive way, stressing taste, not nutrition.
- Support family meals as much as possible.
- Address teasing or bullying with school officials if it is happening at school.

What Not to Do
- Condemn cultural food differences, such as stating that eating dinner at eight at night is "bad" or rice or tortillas are "unhealthy."
- Judge children using food and nutrition, such as you are "good" if you do this and "bad" if you don't.
- Incite shame or fear, as in, "If you don't do this (eat from these food groups daily) you can become ill and die." As Gorman says, "It didn't help my family; it only made me worry."
- Pressure children to try new foods. It is not okay to force children to taste and swallow a new food, even if it is locally grown and organic. For example, a farm-to-school presenter I talked with required children try food out of "respect to the farmer."
- Use language like "overweight" or "obesity."
- Use "fat is bad" messaging, such as "fat people eat too much"[12] or fat people eat the "wrong" kinds of foods. (Remember, as a group, fat and lean children eat no differently.)
- Teasing and bullying at home.

Shame and fear do *not* motivate healthy changes. Poor body image, shame, and fear most often lead to an increase in behaviors, like dieting and disordered eating, that contribute to both eating disorders and increased weight.[12,13]

Emotions and Eating

Much is being written about the dangers of "emotional" eating. While it is true that many people use food as a coping mechanism for emotional upsets, people of all shapes and sizes do this. Using eating as one of the sole ways to (not) deal with difficult emotions contributes to disordered eating and some eating disorders, and perhaps weight gain for an individual. However, the advice you may hear, which is to *separate* emotions from eating, is impossible and won't help your children.

> "Kassa's birthday is the day after Christmas, and it was her second full day with us. We had a small party and she mostly slept through it and cried. I know that birthdays are negative emotional times for a lot of kids in care, though she seemed happy about hers **this** year. Because we knew it wasn't an ideal time for her, we decided to have another 'unbirthday' party months later, once she was truly attached and settled in. I defrosted the frozen birthday cake and we had candles, balloons, and a few presents. This let her have a positive memory. This sprang to mind because the cake was a part of it and I'm glad my partner Holly had thought to freeze her Princess Tiana cake after her real birthday when she didn't really want any, because it did let her have that whole birthday experience later." — Amy, mom to Kassa, age three, adopted from foster care

Eating involves emotions, and that's okay. Culturally, we eat together to celebrate holidays or enjoy a wonderful meal on a date. Feeding a child is a loving act, and enhances emotional attachment not only by meeting their physical needs, but also by sharing in food preparation, the ritual of a family meal, and the pleasant aromas and flavors. Think about how a particular dish or even a smell might bring back a flood of wonderful memories of a treasured aunt or a trip abroad.

Eating a warm, delicious homemade chocolate chip cookie *can* make us feel good, and that too is okay. Even eating two or three can make us feel good. Eating a dozen, while not paying attention to how they taste and not being aware while we are doing it, is not a healthy way to enjoy cookies—or deal with emotions.

> **To try to make eating just about hunger, fullness,**
> **and nutrition is unrealistic and joyless.**

Problems can arise if eating is frequently used for emotional reasons, or if eating is one of the only tools a person has to deal with difficult emotions. Eating that is done in secret or elicits guilt, shame, or feeling out of control are signs of more disordered eating habits. The guilt, shame, and secrecy often fuels the emotional eating, another of those cycles, if you will.

While this section is not meant to address "emotional eating" in adults, I will introduce some of the elements where emotions and feeding intersect, and how you can increase the odds that eating will be *part* of a healthy and joyful life for your child.

Feeding and Attachment

Do you recall the earlier Fred Rogers quote about feeding being an early expression of love and trust? The infant or child has needs that include feeling hunger, needing attention, and being wet, cold, or too warm. The attachment cycle is fulfilled by meeting those physical and emotional needs over and over again. Food is simply one of the most reliable and obvious opportunities to help a child feel safe and cared for—and to build trust.

Is Food Love?

You may hear "food is love," but when you think about it, *feeding* is love. Food is sustenance, feeding is nurturing. A scrambled egg on a plate is delicious and fulfills nutritional needs, but scrambled eggs shared over a smile and a chat about weekend plans brings you together. Remember the World Health Organization quote from Chapter 1, in which feeding practices are often more important than the food in terms of a child's growth? That shows us that food is food and feeding is love. Add a pinch or a generous handful of love to every meal.

Sweets or Candy to Aid Attachment

Some specialists recommend regularly and deliberately using sweets like chocolates or caramels to enhance attachment, almost as a metaphor for the sweetness in breast milk. Parents might hold out a chocolate treat and only let the child have it as a reward for making eye contact. I do not recommend this as a general bonding activity, and believe that it should be reserved for more extreme behavior and attachment needs, and with the help of a well-regarded therapist.

For the vast majority of adopted and foster children, I think there are other ways of attaching and showing love than with handouts of sweets. This practice seems to have the potential of making unhealthy emotional eating more possible, and frequent sweets may worsen dental problems that are more common in adopted and foster children. Again, if it is working for your family and you have considered other options, trust that. I mention the practice of using sweets for attachment because I don't believe it should be a first-line approach or necessary in most situations.

**Reliably meeting your child's needs is the most important
aspect of feeding and attachment.**

The Bottle

Using the bottle, or "regressing" when the child has skills beyond bottle-feeding, is also commonly recommended to aid attachment. Certainly, if your child needs the bottle at a later age because of developmental delay or oral-motor issues, using the bottle is in order, and you are responding and feeding your child based on what she can do, not on how old she is.

Simply holding and rocking an older child promotes bonding. If you decide not to bottle-feed, you can still enjoy physical contact that promotes attachment. Don't let the bottle-feeding be the only time or reason for holding, cuddling, or rocking. Dr. Bruce Perry, a trauma specialist, has this to say about physical closeness: "Providing hugs, kisses, and other physical comfort to younger children is very important. A good working principle for this is to provide this for the child when he/she seeks it. When the child walks over and touches you, return in kind. The child will want to be held or rocked—go ahead."[17] Following the child's lead is important. Forcing hugs or bottle-feeding on a child can bring back memories of trauma and make the child feel powerless again.

If you have an older child for whom playing "baby" or eating from the bottle is pleasurable and allows positive physical contact, this can be a helpful bonding experience. Amy recalls how her then-foster, now-adopted daughter Kassa initiated and enjoyed baby play. *"At three, Kassa does do a more-than-average amount of baby play, where I hold and rock her and she says, 'goo goo ga ga.' I give her imaginary bottles and food, especially when stressed, but this is not something I'd ever push on her."*

Thinking about the whole child and context is critical, as is listening to your gut. Amy explains how they considered the bottle question: *". . . we had to get her ready for preschool, and that meant drinking out of a cup with no lid. I was afraid that drinking from a bottle, even in some contexts, would set that back."* In their case, pretending and not using an actual bottle met Kassa's emotional needs while not undermining other family goals.

If you wish to "regress" and use bottle-feeding for an older child who has the skills to eat table foods, having a social worker or other trained professional involved may help. Again, always follow the child's lead. If you are pushing her to bottle-feed, it is not the tactic for you. Also, be careful with using the bottle for older children, as it may distort the feeding relationship. Be sure that you are supporting feeding with regular snacks and meals, giving a variety of foods and flavors, and not getting stuck in counterproductive feeding practices—for example, not allowing the child to dictate that he will eat only if you spoon-feed him at age five, or regress to only feeding baby foods.

"Am I Hungry, or *What?*"

Part of normal development is the process of learning about and differentiating what our bodies are telling us. Is that feeling in the pit of my stomach hunger, nausea, or anxiety? Am I lonely or hungry? Children who are working on attachment issues, children who have lived through trauma, or children who have a poor feeding history might be delayed with this skill as well. Many adults still struggle with this.

The Division of Responsibility (DOR) will help children learn this process, and it's part of why systematically using food or sweets for attachment can be problematic. Children will learn to tell the difference between emotional and physical needs over months to years—and how you feed them and react to their "mistakes" can help or hurt that process.

When you are fighting or locked in a power struggle at meals or around food, it makes differentiating emotion from physical sensations close to impossible. Anxiety kills appetite and even affects how food is absorbed. Having a pleasant atmosphere around food will begin to help kids listen to signals coming from their bodies, and learn, "Am I hungry, am I full, or am I just really upset because I have to eat these three bites I really, really don't want to eat?"

How can you help your child learn to "hear" what her body is telling her?

- Listen to and observe your child.
- Have calm and pleasant meals and snacks.
- Be consistent about providing regular snacks and meals. *You* think about providing the food so your child doesn't have to.
- Limit exposure to TV commercials. The constant barrage of food commercials can make it hard for kids to know if they are hungry or susceptible to suggestion.
- Identify boredom. Many children, particularly with a history of restriction, will say they are hungry when they are actually bored. When this happens, you can say: "Snack time is soon, shall we play some Legos?" Avoid, "You can't be hungry, you're just bored."
- Offer language to begin talking about emotions; find a resource from your social worker or therapist to help with this.
  - "You seem very sad."
  - "You seem angry."
- Model emotional awareness and health.
  - "I'm a little sad; can we sing a song together?"

Dr. Bruce Perry's *Bonding and Attachment in the Maltreated Child* [17] advises helping the child understand that: 1) "All feelings are okay to feel—sad, glad, or mad (more emotions for older children);" 2) "Teach the child healthy ways to act when sad, glad, or mad;" 3) "Begin to explore how other people may feel, and how they show their feelings: 'How do you think Bobby feels when you push him?'" 4) "When you sense that the child is clearly happy, sad, or mad, ask them how they are feeling. Help them begin to put words and labels to these feelings."

Gorman tells a lovely story about helping her then three-year-old son to listen to his body. *"He was crying, seemed really out of balance, and was asking for ice cream."* She asked, "How are you feeling?" When he answered with "I feel sad," she asked him if he would like a hug, and that's when he said he needed a hug. He didn't ask for the ice cream after they had time to hug and connect. Gorman recognized, *"It was his sadness that he was responding to, and not hunger. I believe it helped him to clarify and distinguish the difference between emotions and physical sensations."*

The following are *not* helpful for learning to separate emotions from physical sensations:
- Using food as rewards for good behavior, grades, etc.
- Offering food regularly to soothe upset or pain.
- Pressuring or trying to get kids to eat more or less than they want.
- Praising children for eating or punishing when they don't eat (promotes eating for reasons other than hunger or fullness cues).

Is It Okay to Sometimes "Use" Food?

If you want to celebrate the end of the softball season with a team outing to Dairy Queen, or your child gets a sucker with an annual shot or uses candy to take the occasional foul-tasting prescription medicine, that's probably fine. (Studies suggest that sweet tastes lessen pain.[18]) However, if every time your child scrapes his knee he gets a sucker or a cookie, he is not learning a variety of coping skills to deal with difficult situations. If you've had a rotten day and give your son crackers to help you make it through that run to Target, it's probably okay. If crackers or candy are the *only* thing that gets you through every day, or every transition to daycare, you may need help coming up with other strategies to deal with behavior or anxiety issues.

Self-Soothing and the Need to Suck

Amy's daughter Kassa was three years old when she came to their family through foster care. She sought out self-soothing through oral stimulation, constantly sucking her thumbs and everyday objects, and had a problem with eating nonfood items like hair bands (pica). Using a straw cup or giving the child appropriate items to mouth and chew or suck on may help with this issue.

For Kassa, within a year, most of the oral-stimulation behaviors lessened as they bonded as a family. Amy had little time to prepare for Kassa's arrival. She recalls, *"I had 10 days to prepare for parenting a three-year-old. I read Ellyn Satter's book* Child of Mine, *and didn't read any parenting books. I think that was absolutely the right choice and the key to the huge success we've had."*

Many children from food-insecure living arrangements may arrive and hold food in their mouths or pocket food. (This may or may not be a sign of an oral-motor problem, so if your child is pocketing, an evaluation by a speech therapist may be in order. Find more on pocketing in Chapter 4 on page 92.) In most of the families I've talked to who have experienced this behavior, the common experience was that after a while, it went away on its own. *"After a year or so, it wasn't an issue anymore,"* recalls Kim, the mother of two children adopted as grade-schoolers from Russia.

As with all aspects of feeding, be attuned and responsive to your child's needs while also focusing on relationship building.

Thoughts on Eating Disorders

"I am scared to DEATH of passing on my eating disorder, and your easy intro to family meals has me feeling far more at ease. I have learned to quit freaking out when my child only eats meat and potatoes—she obviously needed it, because she shot up two inches the following few weeks and went back to normal eating after the growth spurt."
— Isobel, mother of Francine, age five years

Background
When I presented a staff workshop at an eating disorder treatment center, three *eight-year-olds* were in the inpatient unit with medical complications from severe eating disorders, and two of them were boys. The impression that eating disorders happen only to teen girls is false.

Experts feel that anorexia affects about one percent of Americans, with bulimia also at about one percent. The most common eating disorder affecting between two and five percent of the population is binge eating disorder (BED), which is expected to be included in the DSM V diagnostic manual as a distinct eating disorder as of May 2013. The diagnosis of "eating disorder not otherwise specified" (EDNOS) presents with a mix of symptoms that don't fall into the diagnostic criteria for anorexia, bulimia, or BED.

Most eating disorders are EDNOS or BED, and many also exist with "comorbid" (meaning also present), conditions like anxiety, depression, substance abuse, or obsessive-compulsive disorder. Although anorexia receives the most media attention, and has long been felt to be the most deadly of eating disorders, a 2009 study in the *Journal of Psychiatry* concluded, "Individuals with eating disorder not otherwise specified, which is sometimes viewed as a 'less severe' eating disorder, had elevated mortality risks, similar to those found in anorexia nervosa. This study also demonstrated an increased risk of suicide across eating disorder diagnoses."[19] Research is ongoing.

> Eating disorder diagnoses appear to be on the rise,[20,21] and in younger and younger children. A child or teen has a far higher risk of being diagnosed with an eating disorder than Type II diabetes[20]—even though diabetes is what we more commonly hear about, especially with the current interest in "childhood obesity."

Then, of course, there is the category of "disordered eating," which doesn't necessarily meet the criteria of an eating disorder but is not healthy or happy eating either. As a childhood feeding specialist, I am deeply concerned about the trends I am seeing with my young clients.

Children With Disordered Eating Behaviors

I believe that the focus on weight, the obsession with the thin ideal, the war on obesity, and ramped-up concerns around food in general—from additives, food coloring, and white flour and sugar—are contributing to children developing feeding problems and distorted eating behaviors. With an estimated one in five children struggling with eating to the point where it hampers physical, social, and emotional development (feeding disorders), we need to do a better job of supporting healthy feeding, starting at birth.

Instead of supporting healthy attitudes toward food, I hear from moms of six-year-olds who are encouraged in school to count calories and fat grams, schools giving extra credit for weight loss, and children judging one another's food choices in the name of healthy eating. Children are taught to fear sodium, fat, sugar, or anything nonorganic. I am concerned that as a country, we are raising kids who are not "eating competent," because the focus is on what they *can't* eat, the shame, and the extreme attention to body size, health, and nutrition.

> **Our current cultural climate around food raises kids who do not trust (note I did not say, *cannot* trust) their bodies around food.**

I don't treat eating disorders, and if I am concerned after my initial screening, I refer the family for an evaluation. However, I rarely refer, because what I see are families with small children who are struggling and not eating normally, but do not qualify for eating disorders. Sadly, however, I have received calls from parents of eight- and nine-year-olds who seem to be exhibiting signs of an eating disorder and have been struggling with feeding, sometimes in feeding therapy for years. Would earlier appropriate intervention have prevented the continuation and progression of their eating disturbances?

The most common worrisome behavior I see is children who are "bingeing." These children come in all shapes and sizes, which is not surprising, given that studies show that men and women with binge eating disorder (the most common of the eating disorders) also come in all body sizes.[22] Some examples include:

- A lean six-year-old girl who snuck into her neighbor's house and drank three juice boxes and ate most of a box of Ritz crackers before she was discovered. Her parents don't keep that "crap" in the home.
- A seven-year-old whose weight is "normal" but increasing. She's been on "portion control" and no treats since she was four years old because she "has no stopping place." She's not invited on play dates anymore because all she wants to do is raid the pantry.
- An "overweight" nine-year-old girl whose mother found a frosting container and candy wrappers under the bed. The girl had pulled the half-used frosting container out of the trash.

- An "obese" 12-year-old-boy whose mom, a nurse, has tried desperately to keep him on "green-light" foods and has followed doctor's orders to "not keep any junk food in the house. You're the parent, act like it!" So on his way home from school, this boy stops at the grocery store and eats a dozen donuts.

Here is a little of what we know about kids who binge, or as the studies say, "eat in the absence of hunger" (EAH):

- When "forbidden" foods are overly restricted, girls as young as age four report feeling guilt and shame and increased EAH.[23]
- Youth who have a history of dieting or restriction tend to binge or EAH with stress.[24]
- Parents who restrict and binge raise kids who tend to do the same.[25]
- Studies in young girls show that the more parents restrict, the more it correlates with increased weight gain, and EAH.[26]

Whether or not the children above are bingeing because they are seeking a "forbidden" food, they feel guilty, they are on an outright diet and are hungry, or a combination of factors—these kids are not "sugar addicts" nor particularly concerned with body image. While they may not qualify for "eating disorder" diagnoses, these children already have serious problems with food, and the feeding relationship needs to be addressed. Parents in these scenarios and others often ask if their child has an "eating disorder." In overly simple terms, I think of it like this:

It's probably a feeding disorder if:

- After the parents change the feeding atmosphere, the child's eating improves.
  - · The selective eater who branches out slowly in variety when the pressure is off
  - · The four-year-old who stops sneaking forbidden foods, like the half-used frosting container from the trash
  - · The child who stops vomiting when the pressure and force feeding stops
- The child is not overly concerned about body image, or worried about getting "fat."

It may be an eating disorder if:

- The child continues with worrisome behavior after parents have stopped counter-productive feeding behaviors, and support healthy feeding.
- A significant anxiety, obsessive-compulsive disorder (OCD), or depression component exists for the child.
- There is unexplained weight loss.
- The child who once enjoyed a variety of foods self-restricts her eating, calories, or types of foods.
- The child is preoccupied with body image or weight.
- The child is preoccupied with food (talking about it, looking through cookbooks, and cooking but not eating are examples).

- The child has required medical intervention for not eating or drinking. So the nine-year-old who has been to the emergency room for dehydration more than once may have started with a feeding disorder, but now is possibly experiencing an eating disorder.
- See page 185 for other warning signs.

I am deeply concerned for the children who are often small, selective, or "problem" eaters who have been pressured to eat, often with extreme behavioral modification or other therapies, and gag and vomit regularly. When a mother called about her six-year-old ballet-dancer who has gagged and vomited daily during recommended therapy meals since age two, I fear the repercussions for this little girl: the neural pathways (brain patterns) that are being laid down and her risk for continued struggles with food and possibly bulimia. Similarly, the call from the mother of a four-year-old boy who has been gagging and vomiting with feeding interventions for two years has me worried.

In a way, the "diagnosis," or debating about the definitions of when it is a feeding or eating disorder may not be helpful. The key is assessing *the child and the family* and finding the best resources and information that will help in each situation, whether it is working with parents to rehabilitate the feeding relationship, improving general parenting skills, working with the child on eating and anxiety issues, or all of these. (Alas, insurers are not so open-minded, requiring a "diagnosis" before paying for treatment.)

Parents Set the Tone

Don't underestimate the positive role you play in shaping your child's attitudes and experiences around food.

For a long time, "the mother" was considered the cause of most eating disorders—the mother who was too controlling, or was always dieting. The thing is, many children diet, and have mothers who diet, and few will develop anorexia. It is far more complex than blaming mothers.

However, many adults *were* raised in neglectful and even abusive situations around food, and I do not wish to diminish their experiences either. If you or your child experienced trauma, abuse or neglect around food, of course that plays a role in current eating and feeding behaviors. Again, it is a mix of many factors.

Children learn their eating patterns primarily at home. Mothers who diet and binge tend to have children who do the same. They may not qualify for a full-blown eating disorder, but are they healthy and happy? The good news is that children who grow up with the habit of family meals go on to feed themselves more reliably as adults.[27]

I ache for the mothers who call me in tears, who say, *"I know this isn't right, but every-one told me she would get used to normal portions,"* or *"because everyone said, don't let her have treats."* These moms and dads are doing what they are told, and they are not lazy, or cruel, or heartless; they are scared and are doing what they think is in the best interest of the child. Those of us who work with families, from physicians to speech therapists and early childhood teachers, must do better to partner with parents and support them with feeding and parenting.

The Trust Model and Raising Competent Eaters

Eating disorders are complex, with genetic and environmental factors at play. Based on the dramatic improvements I see in children with food preoccupation, bingeing, and se-lective eating, I have hope that with supportive feeding, we can raise competent eaters, and perhaps prevent some of the suffering associated with disordered eating and eating disorders. You have a better chance to raise a competent eater if you try for the healthiest possible feeding relationship with your child.

Guiding principles:
- Trust your child with eating.
- Teach him to trust his body.
- Teach her to feed herself good-tasting foods at regular intervals.
- Support her in relying on her internal cues of hunger and fullness.

Be a good role model:
- Eat meals together.[27]
- Make your home a no-dieting zone. "In this family, we don't diet."
- Don't label food as "good" or "bad." A balanced and healthy diet has room for all foods.
- Through the Division of Responsibility (DOR), and your words, teach your child that he can trust his body to know how much to eat. "Grandpa, that's silly! She doesn't have to finish her plate, Suzy knows how much she needs to eat."
- Avoid spending time with adults who make frequent comments about weight, calories, etc. If your family makes comments in front of your child, ask them privately to stop.

Support healthy body image. (Body dissatisfaction is a prime motivator for disordered eating behaviors):
- Don't talk badly about your own body. (If necessary, fake it at first.)
- You don't have to always love your body, but you do have to learn to *not hate* it. (Courtesy of Michelle Allison at The Fat Nutritionist.)
- No teasing or weight talk. "In this family we don't tease about how people look."[28]

- Normalize body-diversity, such as, "Daddy is bigger than Uncle Jim. People have different hair color, and maybe it's curly, their eyes and skin are different colors, and their bodies are different, too. I am taller than my sister, and I am rounder, too!"
- Look into Health At Every Size resources that support healthy behaviors and wellness for all bodies.
- Talk with your children, as is age appropriate, about "media literacy." That is, about how TV and retouched photos don't show how real bodies look. "You know, no one really looks like that." Think about the media (TV, movies, magazines, newspapers, Internet) you have in your home, and the messages your child sees and hears.

How to advocate:
- There will be plenty of opportunities. Stand up for what you believe in conversations, or write a comment on a body-shaming blog or Facebook post.
- At your child's school.
  · Ask to see the "health and nutrition" curriculum. Be on alert for messages that promote weight loss or health behaviors with the goal of losing weight or "not getting fat." Calorie or "energy balance" programs also focus on calories and are not consistent with the Trust Model.
  · Don't allow your child to be weighed at school.
  · Be vocal about supporting eating competence in the schools, and challenge the teachers who would have your six-year-old counting calories or lecturing about "good" and "bad" foods.

Mothers With a History of Eating Disorders

At least half the moms in the families I work with tell me they have a history of an eating disorder or disordered eating. This is of little surprise, as most American women struggle with eating and body image to some degree.[29,30] These moms describe an almost-paralyzing fear of passing on their eating problems to their children. *"I was scared to death I would make her crazy about food, but I also didn't want her to be fat. I didn't know what to do."* At one of my first workshops, the mother of a healthy nine-month-old girl cried, *"Every time I feed my daughter I feel like I am on the knife-edge between anorexia and obesity."* I give these mothers tremendous credit for reaching out for support with feeding.

> I write about *mothers* with eating disorders because mothers are primarily the ones who share their eating histories with me and who seem most concerned with the child's eating. Men also suffer from eating disorders, and I do not mean to diminish their experiences.

Even mothers who have recovered can feel triggered (the return of thoughts or behaviors related to the eating disorder) or anxious if a child's weight is "too high," or "too low," or if a child eats a particularly large or small meal. Mothers with an active eating disorder have perhaps the hardest journey, and their children will have an added obstacle to learning how to be competent eaters. If a mother can't have flour, refined sugar, or any other number of foods in the house, or can't sit to eat with the family, she will struggle to raise a healthy eater.

The good news is that children can be a powerful motivator for getting help yourself. Children eat several times a day, if you are doing your job. If your own eating is causing significant anxiety and struggles, and is affecting your feeding relationship with your child, please find help.

A Mother Shares Her Journey With Feeding and Her Own Eating Disorder

"Before I had children I was terrified that I would pass on my disordered eating. It was soul-destroying. Before I got pregnant I did therapy (again!) to get a grip on my EDs. When my kids were toddlers, I thought I was doing everything 'right.' I made everything from scratch, offered healthy snacks, only milk or water to drink, etc., and used to get very frustrated at the biscuits and squash they ate loads of when we were out (…no warning bells at this point for me though!). Before long I was hearing, 'How many spoonfuls of this do I have to eat so I can have pudding?' and, 'I've eaten everything on my plate. Is that good?' Suddenly all the warning lights came on in my head. My children were losing the ability to listen to their bodies and were eating to please me/to get pudding. All the things I had sworn I didn't want my children to grow up with.

I had to find a better way for my children, though I was still struggling with my ED. For example, I was deep down happy to have to restrict my own eating even further when my newborn had food allergies and I had to cut out dairy and wheat.

I tried Baby Led Weaning with my third, which led me to the Division of Responsibility. I give the term control freak a whole new meaning, so this was my worst nightmare. Three meals and two snacks a day, and no commenting on what they eat, or whether they eat at all. It was all so difficult for me! My daughter didn't go near vegetables for a few weeks. I had to sit on my hands at times and clamp my mouth shut so I didn't comment or ask them to try something. I had some great email support at this time, reassuring me that it was all normal (that was you, lovely Katja!).

Now, all three children love trying new foods. Again, often new things are served up a few times before everyone has tried them, but it's about familiarity and not feeling pressured to try anything they're not comfortable with. I leave it up to them.

I have finally, started to deal with my own eating and am currently almost three months into recovering from the eating disorder that has been with me for nearly 30 years. I am starting to apply these principles to myself. Starting with three meals and three snacks a day. Trying to listen to my body and relearn hunger and satiety. I will have to keep working at it, but for the first time ever, I am convinced that I will get there. Thank you so much again for all your support." —Mira, mother to Thomas and Emma

If you are doing pretty well with eating, watch and learn from your children. Be a curious and calm observer. I am told over and over again by clients that it was an "ah-ha moment" for them to see their child not finish a bowl of ice cream. After applying the DOR, watching their child eat in a natural and tuned-in way has helped give many parents the courage to take that final leap themselves and become truly tuned-in eaters. It can be magic.

As a parent, the more disordered you are with your eating, the more difficult feeding will feel. If you are pretty close to eating competence or on the journey, your kids can be powerful inspiration. If, on the other hand, you are mired in obsessive thoughts about your body or food, you are going to get stuck. Your kids can be your greatest motivation for change.

While you are working on your own eating, the following are a few thoughts to help guide you:

- Be open with your partner if you can; s/he needs to know what is going on.
- Find support and learn about healthy eating from books like *Secrets of Feeding a Healthy Family*.
- If family meals or certain foods are too triggering, or right now you can't participate for some reason, ask your partner or another trusted family member or adult to be there for family meals. One client who was getting help found that her husband was able and willing to support the kids with family meals when he realized how important it was for his children, and that for now, it was simply too much for Mom. He was able to sit at breakfast with Mom's trigger foods and allow his daughter to eat as much as she needed when Mom found it too difficult.
- Find help from trained ED professionals.

Your Child, Exercise, and High-Risk Sports

In addition to optimizing the feeding relationship and avoiding dieting, another issue that has come up with clients is exercise. Along with troubles with food, people with eating disorders frequently engage in excessive exercise, and many have a poor body image. If your child has a rocky time with eating or growth or is at risk for feeding problems for any reason, consider very carefully what extracurricular activities you will support. It may be wise to steer clear of weight or appearance-centered sports like gymnastics, wrestling, or ballet.[31]

If your child does have a passion for a particular sport, it is wise to be vigilant. Consider having a frank, confidential discussion with coaches to ask what they are talking about in terms of weight and nutrition. For example, one mom was shocked to learn that her daughter's high school track coach was recommending a weight-loss tea. You will need to be alert and proactive. There certainly are studios for dance or gymnastics that promote joy and health and don't shame bigger bodies; I'm simply advising parents to be aware of the issue, advocate for your child, and enjoy.

If You Suspect Your Child Has an Eating Disorder

Eating disorders do not discriminate between adopted or biological children, and they do not discriminate based on race, size, gender, or social status. Continuing family meals throughout early and late adolescence is important. With busy lives, it seems impossible to make family meals happen as kids get older. I have heard time and again how parents noticed early warning signs at the family table when a child suddenly started cutting out cheese and red meat, then all meat, then carbs, and so on.

If you are concerned, do not wait, talk yourself out of worrying signs, or let others dismiss your concerns without investigating further and seeking out an evaluation for your child and family. Eating disorder activist and "unwilling expert" Becky Henry, author of *Just Tell Her to Stop*, tells the heartbreaking story of trying for *two years* to get a diagnosis and appropriate treatment for her teen daughter. Her daughter's eating disorder (ED) was able to fool their pediatrician and two therapists (who were not ED specialists) into thinking she had no problems with eating.

**Early diagnosis and treatment greatly improves the chances
for a more rapid and full recovery.**

If you are concerned, the following may reveal red flags of an eating disorder:
1. Does it seem to you that your child has lost control over how she or he eats?
2. Does your child ever make her/himself sick because s/he feels uncomfortably full?
3. Does your child believe he is fat, even when others say he is too thin?
4. Do food and/or thoughts about food dominate your child's life?
5. Do thoughts about changing her body or weight dominate her life?
6. Are shared meals difficult because of your child's eating behavior or comments about food, eating, or body image?
7. Are you or others worried about your child's weight?

In this informal survey, two or more "yes" answers strongly indicate the presence of disordered eating. Adapted from the Scoff Questionnaire by Morgan, Reid & Lacy-BMJ (1999) excerpted from the Emily Program Website, www.emilyprogram.com.

If you are concerned, please listen to your intuition, trust yourself, and get it checked out. Have a list of your concerns ready and talk to your child's health care provider in advance, letting them know you want a referral for an evaluation by a specialist in eating disorders. Stay involved. Research is showing that family-based therapy is very promising in the treatment of eating disorders.

Summary

Heavy stuff, I know. The fact that you are reading this book means you are being thoughtful about how you want to raise your family around food. This discussion about attitudes, food, and emotions was meant to help you feel confident when you face your son or daughter across the family table. Hopefully, it will motivate you to do your best to provide a pleasant table, where food and family are enjoyed.

Chapter 7
Day-to-Day Feeding Challenges

What You Will Learn

This chapter will look at specific concerns based on feeding stages, such as transitioning to solid foods or unique situations like respite care or bringing home a new sibling. The adopted child may be developmentally behind, so when I use the terms "toddler" and "infant," I am speaking in terms of what the child can *do*, not his age.

The First Few Days

You may have months to prepare for the arrival of your child, or hours in the case of foster care.

Being curious, supportive, and mindful of all your training and preparation will help, but always be responsive to your child.

If you are able to know which foods your child is familiar with, having these on hand may help with the transition. However, you may not know your child's history with food. Assume it has been less than supportive, and be absolutely reliable about providing food. Your child won't know she can trust you yet, so *showing* her, with feeding and everything else, will help make her feel safe and begin the process of attachment.

"When Kiki first moved in at age two, I was very clear about making food available, and we had meals pretty much every two hours. Her first full day with us was Halloween, and I gave her pretty open access to her candy for the first few weeks. I think both of those things helped her trust at least tentatively that her food needs would be met."
— Carmella, foster/adoptive mother to Kiki

Even for the older child, you may want to initially offer a meal or snack every few hours. With a younger child, where you might not know her skills with eating, offer food in different ways. Be sure you have a bottle with a few nipple options, a sippy and a straw cup, some soft foods, and some finger-food options. Your child's reactions will help you know what foods she is ready for and what is comfortable for her to eat. Sit with your child and reassure her she can eat as much, or as little, as she wants.

If It's Only First Days: Feeding in Respite or Short-Term Situations
If a child is coming to you for only a few days, perhaps in crisis or for respite care, the immediate need is to help the child feel as safe and nurtured as possible. Inviting the child to participate in family meals is a wonderful opportunity for him to experience a loving and calm family meal, and maintaining routines is important if you have other children. Trying to offer foods that feel safe to him is a nurturing thing to do. Consider feeding the entire family his favorite foods. Maybe you order pizza and serve it with raw veggies and dip, or you make mac-n-cheese and serve it with canned peaches. Your job is not to make the child thinner or bigger or get her to eat her veggies, but to *nurture* during this difficult time. Overlook manners, such as eating with fingers or utensils. If she comes from a food-insecure home, reassure her before meals. This can be supported with comments such as:

- "You don't have to eat anything you don't want."
- "You can eat as much or as little as you want."

Infancy

The key in every stage is following your child's lead and learning her cues. Sometimes you will get what she is trying to tell you right away and sometimes you won't, but you will get better with time as you get to know one another. Some children who have experienced malnutrition, in-utero drug or alcohol exposures, or poor early care will probably not know what they are feeling or how to communicate their needs. She will learn to express her needs, and you will learn to read her cues over time by trial and error: trying the bottle, diapering, or rocking; feeding in a quiet room; or perhaps offering a pacifier.

If you are adopting or fostering an infant with feeding problems and you are anxious about figuring it out or struggling to read his cues, a lactation consultant can be a great resource. (Lactation consultants can help with both bottle and breast-feeding.) These professionals are experts at reading the infant's cues around feeding and can help you understand your baby. In addition, family and friends might want to help feed and care for your baby. However, you may need to be assertive while protecting your early bonding time with your child as you figure out feeding and sleeping and everything else, so ask others to support you as a *family*. For example, they can walk the dog, buy groceries, or bring meals. Once you are established with feeding and bonding, you can let others participate in feeding and nurturing—as your child allows.

If possible, whether you are adopting internationally or caring for a child in foster care, learn as much as you can about how the child is currently being fed. Observing feedings or mealtimes will often give you the most useful information.

- Is she being held? How?
- Is it pleasant?
- Is she fed on a schedule?
- What foods are being fed?
- What formula are they using?
- What temperature?
- What utensils is he using? (If possible, take some of the nipples, bottles, and formula your little one is used to, even the spoon if he is spoon-fed).

Again, every child will be different. Some older infants who are in less supportive settings become incredibly independent and advanced with self-feeding. One parent noted that, *"Suzie was able to feed herself completely independently from the moment she came home with us at six months."* Others lag behind with self-feeding skills if they were never given the opportunity or if there are other developmental concerns. You can't predict, so be prepared to meet your child where he is.

That said, it is not critical to know details about how and what your child was fed if you are prepared to tune in to the clues and information coming from your child. By following your child's cues, regardless of her history, you can feed in a supportive way.

Lucy shares that they had no information about Stella's feeding, and they did just fine. *"When she came home from China, we had no idea if she was still taking formula or had started eating table food. Since we had her escorted home, we were not able to talk to her nannies and find out her routine. So basically we gave her formula only for a few days, but it became clear she was hungry, so we just started getting her blended foods one at a time just like other babies."* Lucy didn't "get it right" in terms of guessing what Stella could do right away, but they figured it out together.

> Children who have special needs, are healing from infections or other illness, or have a history of challenging feeding may present with more subtle cues. She may get quiet or change demeanor, lose interest in toys or play, get flushed in the face, or become more easily distracted. It is okay to experiment and see if your child is hungry or needs a cuddle. Offer a bottle or solids as appropriate and take "no" for an answer. Even if you are eager for your infant to eat and gain weight, avoid getting pushy with a bottle. You can always offer again in a little while. And remember, it will get easier to read her cues.

The more you try to impose your ideas of timetables (remember that the infant is in charge of the *when*, unlike the older child, where parents lead with structure), specific amounts, and how much weight she needs to gain, and the more you fret, obsess about, and pressure and override her cues, the higher the chances are that you will struggle.

Cues an infant might be hungry:
- Crying or fussing.
- Screaming.
- "Rooting" in the young infant—turning the head toward a touch on the cheek or face.
- Sucking on hands or other objects.
- Continuing to suck or eat eagerly, or with attention and interest, even if she finishes a bottle.

Cues a child might be full or not interested in eating right now:
- Sucking has slowed down significantly or stopped; she seems distracted.
- She appears content when the feeding is over.
- Turns head away.
- Pushes nipple out of the mouth.
- Screams.
- Stops sucking, looks away.
- Arches body or tries to move away from the bottle.
- Apparent discomfort or pain with eating may indicate something else is going on and should be discussed with you child's doctor. See Appendix II: Medical Conditions That Can Affect Feeding.

Consider Fannah, who came home at age eight months from Ethiopia. At the 80th percentile weight for length, her doctor was worried that she was "almost overweight" and recommended specific ounces at specific intervals—and no more. Mom did as she was told and cut off feedings when the bottle was empty, even though Fannah screamed at the end of every bottle and still seemed hungry. Unfortunately, ignoring her cues that she needed more and needed to be the one to decide how much set this family up for major struggles with food (see Chapter 5).

> Avoid the temptation to interrupt feedings to check how much she is eating. Allow her to drink from a bottle until she pauses or appears uncomfortable. You can try burping her then, and after that you can check to see if she is still hungry by offering the bottle. You don't need to burp every ounce or two. Follow her cues. Stopping and checking how much she has had to see if she needs burping, or because you are curious, interrupts feeding and may be so upsetting to your baby that she eats less. A resource for infant feeding and sleep specifics is Ellyn Satter's DVD, *Feeding With Love and Good Sense II.*

Or consider Connie and her children, Alicia and Ric, adopted as infants two years apart. Both were significantly malnourished when Connie first met them. Connie was given all kinds of advice for specific amounts to feed the children, how often, and what foods. Connie instead decided to "trust" them (her word in recounting the story, not mine), and when she followed their cues, they thrived. One child at first ate mostly the yogurt and cheeses he was used to, while the other was more interested in vegetables and meats. They did not eat as much as they were "supposed" to at most settings, but sometimes they ate more, and as they settled in with Connie they both gained at a healthy rate.

Formula

All infants 0–12 months of age should be on formula (or breast milk, but I am not addressing breast-feeding in adoption here as there are other resources available if that is what you choose).

Ideally, if the formula your child is drinking is appropriate (not watered down or nutritionally inadequate), keep her on that formula.

If you are adopting internationally, buy some of the formula your child is on or have some brought over with your child. If you cannot get the same brand (or it is inadequate), over a period of several days, start by mixing small amounts of the new formula into the former, gradually increasing as tolerated until you have switched to the new formula. Some children will change easily to a new formula, while others may be more wary of new tastes. Follow your child's cues. (See www.adoptionnutrition.org for more information.)

All children adopted internationally should have a thorough evaluation, if possible, with an international adoption (IA) doctor or your local practitioner using the Academy of Pediatrics guidelines for IA (see online Resource appendix). If your child is not tolerating formula or appears to have problems, discuss options with your doctor. Initially, switching to a hydrolyzed cow-based formula might be a good step. Try not to swap formulas frequently to "see if it helps," as this confuses the picture. If your little one was started on soy-based formula, you can discuss continuing that with your doctor or switching to a hydrolyzed dairy-based formula.

If your infant appears ill or seems uncomfortable or in pain, have her evaluated. Signs of poorly tolerated formula are incredibly hard to interpret, since so many other things may be going on, from infection, to difficulty adjusting, to grief. Some signs may be:

- Fussiness
- Crying or colicky behaviors
- Constipation
- Distension and gas

After 12 months of age, if your child has made a successful transition to solid foods, you can switch to whole cow's milk. *Do not use whole cow's milk before twelve months of age.* If your child is doing catch-up growth or is developmentally delayed, or has not figured out solids quite yet, you may want to continue supporting her nutritional needs with formula for a few more months. Talk with your doctor or a pediatric registered dietitian (RD).

Cana was at the 10th percentile and growing steadily, but was only beginning to really explore solid foods. She had some developmental delay and poor overall muscle strength (tone), but she was improving every day. Cana's mom was offering her appropriate finger foods and helping her, but she took her time and didn't seem to eat as much as her older brother did at this age, or as skillfully. Cana's mom was a bit surprised when at Cana's 12-month visit, Cana's doctor advised switching from formula to two percent milk. Since we were already talking about Cana's feeding, and she was in that transition phase to solids and was still getting most of her nutrition from liquids, I advised her to continue with the formula for a few more months and see how things progressed. Cana was behind in her transition phase and needed the extra nutrition from the formula while she learned to eat and enjoy solids. By 16 months of age or so, Cana was enjoying a variety of solid foods and was switched slowly to whole cow's milk without a problem. I encouraged Cana's mom to discuss her plan with her pediatrician, who supported the plan.

Starting Solids

Starting solids can be an enjoyable introduction to family foods, or it can set the stage for problems down the road. Typically, this six- to 12-month period is called the "transition," when a child goes from getting most of her nutrition from formula or breast milk to most of her nutrition needs met by a variety of solid foods.

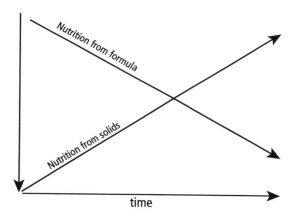

6-12 months in general for the transition

7.1 Schematic for transitioning to solids. In reality it is not such a neat, linear process, but the idea is that as intake from solids increases, nutrition from bottle or breast decreases.

It can take children *many* neutral exposures to learn to like new foods. They learn by watching you eat, by smelling, by squishing, licking, and spitting out. Don't give up. Here are some hints for starting on the right foot. Don't start much before six months of age. If your little one is already adept at feeding herself, is younger than six months, and shows interest in solid foods, follow her lead. Ask your child's doctor about any allergy concerns or supplements.

Guiding Principles:

- Feed based on what your child can DO, not on how old she is (see page 319).
- Follow the **Division of Responsibility in feeding:**
  - · You decide what, when, and where (which formula or breast milk, baby foods, or table foods to prepare).
  - · He decides how much and if to eat from what you provide.
- Approach feeding with a calm and pleasant demeanor.
- Have your child join in at family meal times. Eat with your child.
- Trying to get a child to eat more or less will not make them grow faster or slower. Pressure with feeding almost always backfires.

Be Responsive:

- Be prepared to observe and take cues from your child.
- Some babies intensely want to "do it myself!" and will reject the spoon. Help him with appropriate foods, load the spoon, and let him put it in his mouth.
- Don't trick, force, or play games. Allow your child to feed herself.
- Let him eat as fast or as slow as he wants.
- You can follow the *Baby-Led Weaning*[1] approach (see page 194) and skip spoon-feeding, or a combination of spoon-feeding and allowing your child to feed himself.

Some Specifics:

- Learn as much as you can about your child's feeding and eating before your child comes home.
- Be sure she is sitting upright, can open her mouth in anticipation of the spoon, and can close her mouth around the spoon.
- Aim to be feeding about every 2–3 hours by the time she is around 12–16 months of age, or by the time she is self-feeding with some skill.
- Be aware of choking risks; have her eat upright and stay close.
- Let him explore his food and make a mess.
- Let him play with and explore appropriate utensils.
- Serve different tastes and textures often, and don't assume she "doesn't like it" if she doesn't try it or she spits it out.
- When possible, avoid feeding your infant on a schedule.

The earliest feeding is about the experience. It is not about getting in food. She may stop after one or two bites, and that is okay. It is more about exploration and attitude than nutrition.

All parents should be trained in CPR. Tips to lower the risk of choking:
- Prepare foods that are appropriate for her skill level.
- Avoid foods that are a choking hazard, including popcorn, grapes, peanuts, candy, and hotdogs.
- Have the child sit down to eat, where you can see her.
- Don't eat in the car or on the go.

Baby-Led Weaning (BLW): A Brief Review

The Baby-Led Weaning (BLW) approach describes a way of starting solids and transitioning off breast or bottle. Basically, the British authors of the book, *Baby-Led Weaning*, say that healthy babies do not need to be spoon-fed—ever—and make the case that BLW is the right way and makes for less stressful feeding, with kids who are less picky and happier at the table.

The gist is that babies will show they are ready for food by grabbing it and putting it into their mouths. The authors write, "All you are doing (and asking them to do) is to miss out on the puree stage."[1] They advocate having the baby eat what the family is eating and join in with family meals while continuing to breast or bottle-feed.

I like a lot about this model, mostly because it is very familiar to the Trust Model. In my opinion, many of the benefits attributed to BLW are due to following the child's lead with feeding and maintaining the Division of Responsibility (DOR), which BLW does.

"Parents should do what they feel most comfortable with and do what is going to work best for their child. Some babies want to do it themselves. Others want to be, or need to be, spoon-fed. Either/or or both is just great as long as the Division of Responsibility is observed."
—Hydee Becker, Pediatric RD

However, here are some concerns I have with the BLW approach:
- They seem to endorse grazing for the older child as long as it's "healthy," i.e., letting the toddler help herself to "healthy" foods at any time as long as she sits down at the table. I believe grazing doesn't help most children do best with eating.
- Seems to recommend a one-size-fits-all approach in terms of foods to offer.
- May be falsely reassuring in terms of choking risks. I worry that if the child is on the mother's lap (as they seem to endorse) during meals, Mom might not notice right away if the infant is getting into trouble with choking.
- A study from *Maternal Child and Health Journal* indicates that children who develop more slowly may have nutritional deficiencies, particularly iron. The

researchers recommended, "combining self-feeding with solid finger food with traditional spoon feeding."[2]

Adopted and foster children are more likely to have developmental delays and nutrition deficits, particularly iron. Children develop at different rates with their oral-motor skills, and parents should tailor foods to each child. (See page 319 on feeding based on what your little one can do.) I know my daughter would chomp off huge bites of teething biscuits and have trouble with the pieces, while other infants her age happily would suck and gum the biscuits. Hydee Becker, a pediatric RD who has consulted with my clients, also had concerns about offering large chunks of meat as the authors recommend, in terms of choking. Again, BLW concepts may work wonderfully for some children, but not necessarily all.

Gagging

Occasional gagging in infants and young toddlers is the reflex that protects the airway and is part of normal oral-motor development. As children gag, they quite efficiently move food away from the airway to the front of the mouth. Infants have a gag reflex that is triggered in the front of the mouth, so they gag fairly often as they mouth toys, hands, spoons, and solids. Mouthing and teething is important to oral-motor learning and development, and even if a child gags herself with her hands or spoon, that is okay too. As children mouth objects and food, over time, the gag reflex weakens and moves farther back in the mouth.

Gagging is common for the older infant learning to eat foods with more texture. If your child gags frequently, offer fewer pieces at a time if he overstuffs regularly, or check that the flow of liquids isn't too fast from the bottle or cup. Gagging more than a few times a meal may also mean you are advancing textures too quickly: try pureeing or mashing foods a bit more and moving on with more texture again in a few days. Some infants like to take big bites (as my daughter did) and might not do well with teething biscuits or crackers, while other children may do just fine. Be responsive to your child.

If she gags or vomits repeatedly and is in distress or upset by the episodes, or not gaining weight or advancing with textures, mention it to your doctor (see Chapter 3).

Gagging can be disconcerting, but as much as possible, try not to overreact. If you hop up and hold a cloth under her or appear panicked every time she gags, she will feel scared, which may upset her and affect her eating. I have seen many parents misinterpret normal gagging as choking, and their fear leads to unsupportive feeding by not advancing textures appropriately.

Choking is different. The child will be in more distress, will not make any sounds or progress in clearing the food item, and may also change color. **Be sure you are trained in CPR so you can spot and know how to deal with choking.**

If your older child is gagging frequently with eating and/or you are engaged in feeding battles, you need help. This is a scary and very negative experience.

If It's Not BLW, is it Pressure?

The authors write, "Being spoon-fed by someone else means the baby is not in control of how much she eats." They infer that parents who spoon-feed all play games, pressure, force, don't expose the child to a variety of tastes, and have a miserable time with a child who will invariably end up picky. Not true. It *is* easier to push a spoon-fed baby, but a tuned-in parent lets the baby decide how much to eat, spoon-fed or not. Some children with delays or challenges may need to be spoon-fed to support good nutrition, and this *can* be done following the child's lead.

In a bit of a twist, in the one study cited in the book in support of the child choosing what to eat and how wonderfully the children did with it, many of those children were spoon-fed by adults, and all the children, even the spoon-fed ones, were willing to try new foods.[3]

BLW is not a comprehensive feeding resource. For example, the book does not offer advice on the following:
- Once children develop their own opinions and start saying "no"
- Dealing with different temperaments
- Other ways parents pressure beyond the spoon. Parents can still be pushy with enforcing rules about eating "this before that," pushing foods, etc.
- Normal eating and growth, which is so critical for many parents to trust a very large or very small child with eating

Trust Your Decision

I've spent some time on this concept because I get asked about it on occasion. There is more than one right way to feed a child, if you are following the child's lead. If you want to do BLW, go for it. Get the book, but also read *Child of Mine* for a more complete picture and more concrete help for transitioning into the next phases of feeding. I also recommend getting the BLW cookbook if you are following BLW.

Toddlers: The "Perfect Storm"

When children become toddlers, their growth rate slows and their appetites might too. Many toddlers seem to eat less than they did as older infants. Toddlers also go through a naturally finicky phase, where even if they ate a great variety of foods, they now approach new foods with caution, or "neophobia," which is literally the fear of the new.

This natural finicky phase may mean:
- Your child won't want different foods to touch each other.
- Her first, second, and often third response to a new food will be "no."
- She will show a preference for simple carbs and sweet foods.
- She will try to get you to serve her favorite foods. She may tantrum and throw foods she doesn't like. This is normal.
- Foods she used to love are suddenly rejected.

Review Chapter 1 about how kids eat in terms of erratic eating and learning to like new foods. This will help you stay strong during this wacky phase and not push your child to eat more, or less.

Tips for navigating through the "perfect storm:"
- Keep serving the foods you want her to like to eat. What they reject one day, or one minute, they may enthusiastically eat the next.
- Expect tantrums. It's what they do. Trying to feed her with the goal of avoiding tantrums will lead to trouble.
- Stick with structure and pleasant family meals.
- Stay calm and pleasant company.
- Have realistic expectations. A toddler may not be hungry and may be done with a meal after five minutes. She may get down, but once she does, mealtime is over. She should be able to play on her own or watch a DVD while you finish your own dinner. "Daddy and I are still enjoying dinner. Why don't you play with your Legos nearby? We'll be done soon."

The Early Years: Helpful Feeding Gear
Kids seem to need a whole lot of stuff these days, from baby swings to Skut bikes, helmets, and fancy toothbrush timers. Feeding is no exception. The following is a rundown of a few of the more common gadgets and tools that can make feeding easier, and also a few words of caution about unnecessary gear that can get in the way.

Highchair: If you use a highchair, look for one that is easy to clean and fits your space. IKEA has a cheap, bare-bones model. If your child is developmentally delayed or has weak core muscle strength so that she needs support while eating, ask your therapist for suggestions on how to adapt and alter your home seating. Rolled-up towels tucked in on both sides can give her stability so she doesn't tire quickly from simply holding her body in place. A free hand-me-down highchair is often the best choice.
- **Proper placement in the highchair:** The child should be at a 90.90.90 sitting—that is, 90 degrees at the hip, knees, and feet.

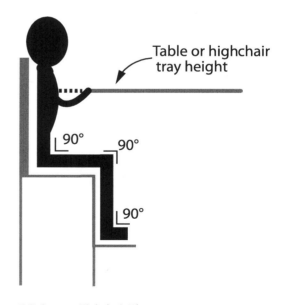

Table or highchair tray height

7.2 Correct Highchair Placement

- **Level of highchair tray:** The tray or tabletop should be at a level about halfway between the nipple line and the belly button. Many trays are often too high, which makes it harder for kids to feed themselves.
- **Foot support:** This can be critical, as dangling feet can be distracting for children, especially those with sensory issues. If you have to build your own footrest, do so.
- **Quality:** Consider the Tripp Trapp brand or other fancy adjustable chair, such as the OXO Tot Sprout. If you can spend the money or get one used, it may be worth it. I spent almost as much on various attempts at booster solutions over the years. These chairs have built-in and adjustable footrests. In the end, some children prefer kneeling, which is not ideal in terms of chair tipping, but can be okay against a wall, with one parent's foot on the chair for stability, or on a secure bench seat.

Plates with compartments: These can be useful for a time. You can go straight from no plates to these. When children go through that naturally selective stage (typically from about 15 to 36 months), it can help to separate the food in little compartments. Making a stew? Put some chicken, carrots, and potatoes into their own little sections if your kids are fussy about foods touching.

Silverware: Again, follow your child's lead. I have seen capable older kids struggle with forks that are meant for beginning eaters. Not having the right tools can be frustrating. Find a spoon with a deeper bowl than many "baby" spoons. Use a dessert or small fork to help kids eat.

- **Knives:** A great variety of knives are available to allow kids to help with food prep. One safe tool for little hands is a plastic lettuce knife or a dull butter knife. Kids can cut things like mushrooms, bananas, peeled fruit, and lettuce quite easily, and they often love to help. Small dip spreaders (we got ours at Target) are a great help with spreading butter, peanut butter, or hummus, and even cutting soft foods. IKEA also has great kids' utensils.

A mesh bag feeder: For example, the Baby Safe Feeder. These mesh bags can be a helpful tool if used properly. For example, this was nice for us when we would eat out with our daughter when she was between age six and 10 months. We would take her along and pop a piece of apple or avocado or other food into the bag, as well as mashed table foods as appropriate, and she loved to work on it. It can be a way to introduce new textures and flavors and can help with teething pain if you use ice cubes or frozen fruit, just be sure the bag is closed properly. Be prepared for the bags to discolor, and clean according to instructions.

Step stools: Get a few of these at different heights. We rotated three stools over the years from the small stool/kneeling pad that came with our daughter's baby tub, to a sturdy mid-sized model, to the tall one from the hardware store. As children grow, they will need different heights for different tasks. I would think we were done with one only to pull it out for tooth brushing or reaching the kitchen counter. Rubber bottom features will help them stay put.

Sippy cups: After your child has mastered bottle-feeding, and during the transition to solids (around six to 12 months of age for the typically developing child) introducing sippy cups or straw cups with handles is important. Ideally, sippy cups with a valve are used for a relatively short length of time, since the sucking pattern on the classic sippy cup is like bottle-feeding and can lead to oral-motor and speech problems if continued for too long. Offer and transition to a straw cup early on, when your child can hold the cup by herself. Ideally at 12 to 15 months of age, you can transition your child to drinking from an open cup at meals and sit-down snacks, and save the straw cups for snacks away from home. It's messier, but better for development. If your child has oral-motor delays, ask your therapist for ideas on appropriate cups.

Water bubbler or playful spout: With only water between meals, it can help to have a way for your child to serve herself. Have a collection of child-sized plastic cups where she can reach them and a way for her to get water that might be a little fun. We rented a "water bubbler" because I didn't like the taste of our home's tap water, but a great benefit was that our daughter could serve herself, and it was fun for her. You can often rent a unit for $10 a month, with water delivered to your door. It was also nice as a new mom to have the hot water spout so I could quickly make myself a cup of tea. You can also buy and install cute spouts on a faucet and set a step stool up so your child can reach and get her own water.

Sprinkle shaker: Use an empty saltshaker. You can make your own mix of cinnamon and sugar (ratio 1:2). Kids often really like sprinkling. Try it on applesauce, yogurt, buttered toast, and apples. You can even use regular sprinkles to help introduce new foods. Varieties of "natural" sprinkles are available without artificial food additives and colors if that is part of your routine.

Tea strainer: Again, kids like to sprinkle. You can add powdered sugar or cinnamon, or a mix, and make "snow" on pancakes, waffles, or fruit.

Teething rings: Offer a variety of teething rings and mouthing toys that have various textures, perhaps with nubs on them to help with mouthing skills (like Tri-Chew or similar).

Duo spoon or other dipper: This can also help with desensitizing and can give children a sense of control. Allow children to dip the spoon or teething ring into purees, yogurt, or mashed foods and suck or lick the food off the spoons.

Cooking or Food Prep Gear

Chest freezer: This can be really helpful for getting family meals on the table and saving money. Buy and freeze meats on sale, other pricey items like specialty (soy or other) milks for allergies, or a variety of convenience foods. You can also freeze batch-cooked meals or meals from friends. Every family I know with a chest freezer loves it.

Slow cooker: This gadget can also help to get meals going. Cook up a pork shoulder for pulled-pork BBQ sandwiches one day and pork tacos the next. Freeze servings for easy, quick meals. Young children often do well with the softer, slow-cooked meats.

Food grinder: These can be great to help introduce your little one, or your child with developmental delays, to your family's foods. You can use a hand-turned unit or a food processor. You can grind the meat at the table that you are eating for dinner. Be sure to add water, broth or sauce as needed to make it moist enough for your child to handle. Spread ground-up meat on toast or crackers or put a blob on the table or tray for your little one to feed herself.

Frozen pops: You can make your own frozen pops to support nutrition while feeding well, such as the BellyFULL make-at-home brand, which comes with recipe cards for nutrient-dense pops.

Gear and Products: A Word of Caution

Sometimes using no gear is best. Babies learning to eat solids don't need utensils or plates. You can use spoons if you are spoon-feeding, always following your child's lead. He may want to play with the spoon, or not. Sometimes using two spoons, so he can hang on to one while you load the other, helps. Put the finger foods on the tray or table directly. Plates are often a distraction.

 • **Pouches or "squeezies:"** These are relatively new and convenient, and even come in organic and a variety of flavors, but already I am seeing families getting stuck with these handy pouches with the nozzle and cap. The problem is, when a child is sucking down a squeezie of pureed pears, she is still sucking. Yes, it's "solid" food, but delivered in a way that is often developmentally not appropriate. When some parents worry about intake and their child readily eats a squeezie, I've seen them only offer squeezies at meals and snacks. They are appealing to children because the child can control the experience. They can often hold and take the food in on their own, which to the child may be preferable to being fed by the parent, who might be anxious or pushy with a spoon. I've also seen older infants who only eat squeezies, which also does not help advance the child in terms of texture. There is nothing inherently wrong with a squeezie, and it's a great choice to round out that snack at the park, or with one meal or snack a day, but be careful if you are reaching for the squeezie at every meal or snack "just to get something in her." The same advice goes for any food item, whether it's a smoothie, frozen pop, or supplement. If it's the only thing you are offering, beware.

- **Child-sized tables:** While these may be great for crafts and the occasional snack, the temptation may be too great to allow children to have all their meals and snacks at a child-sized table. Many modern dining tables are almost counter-height, requiring extra-tall chairs. These tables are not conducive to having family meals. Rather than have children eat separately, consider getting a standard table or shortening the legs of a taller table.

- **Sippy cups:** Sippy cups lend themselves to drinking on the go and between meals. Just be aware that your little one isn't wandering around with a sippy cup full of milk or juice between meals, which can lessen appetite and lead to decreased intake and increase cavity risk.

- **Snack traps:** The risk here is primarily to structure and appetite. It is far too easy to allow a child to carry around a snack trap of cereal or puffs, which undermines appetite and increases cavity risk. Use these for planned snacks on the go.

- **Mesh bag feeder:** I have also seen this gadget misused. That is, when a child is capable, but a parent has a misunderstanding of choking risk and relies only on the mesh feeder because of a fear of choking. It is not a substitute for learning to deal with increasingly complex textures. Relying too heavily on mesh feeders or squeezies interferes with a child's learning and development with eating.

> When I have worked with families where children eat at a separate table, because the child can get up easier or it's more convenient, the child misses out on the most critical "gear" at the table: *you,* the parent. Children should eat at a table with parents whenever possible.

The Older Child

Families with older children have told me that various adoption and feeding resources aren't helpful for them. One mom who adopted preschoolers says, *"Beyond bottle-feeding and starting solids, there just didn't seem like there was any information for our family out there."* My go-to resource book, *Child of Mine*, stops at kindergarten age (though I still think it's a must-read). The thing is, the Division of Responsibility holds true for older kids, but it does look different.

Just like with an infant, familiar food can be incredibly comforting during a time of transition. If your new-to-you child loves mac-n-cheese, find out what his favorite brand is and plan on incorporating that, at least initially. Making an effort to prepare familiar foods shows that you are honoring the older child and are paying attention, and can be a way to show affection that is physical without embracing or touching. The child who has experienced trauma and may need work accepting physical affection can get some nurturing needs met through feeding.

Every meal doesn't have to be mac-n-cheese or another favorite, but simply meeting his most basic physical need—hunger—and doing so reliably, without pressure or guilt, is a powerful way of saying, "You can trust me. I care for you. I love you."

You may remember Amy's story from Chapter 2, which demonstrates how critical food can be for establishing trust—no bottles needed. *"We had a 15-year-old boy in foster care with a history of runaway episodes,"* she recalls. *"He was gone for about 30 hours. When he came back, I decided there was no point being upset, so just told him we'd been scared, made sure he was safe and healthy, and quickly threw a box of mac-n-cheese on the stove to get him some comfort food. That floored him, because it turns out that he'd been denied food in his home after his running. I think it ended up bonding him to us much more than anything else could have. He's still a part of our lives and our 'family' even though he doesn't live with us."*

Family Meals and the Older Child

Family meals also present a reliable time for the older child to connect with parents and siblings. Being firm about eating together is important. They may not want to partake at first and may bristle at the no-texting or headphones rules, but they will often grow to enjoy and depend on this time.

Jennifer started with family meals and the Division of Responsibility when her girls were 13 and 16. She had struggled with selective eating with her oldest daughter, Yiseth, for a dozen years, and had basically given up. A former avid cook and "foodie," she had resigned herself to cooking the handful of dishes that Yiseth would accept. *"Not much changed until I did your Webinar. From age 3½ to 16, the number of foods she would eat stayed at about 25, and she added only new flavors of ice cream to the list of foods she would eat."*

Jennifer went back to work when her girls were in grade school. On Fridays, she would call them before she left work and ask what they wanted for dinner. *"Chinese? Subway? Rotisserie chicken?"* Everything was met with complaints and whining, and Jennifer admitted she thought, *"How ungrateful! I would have loved restaurant food when I was a kid."* Everyone was already in a foul mood before dinner was even served, and at least one of the kids found reason to complain.

After thinking about the DOR, she realized it was *her* job to decide what was for dinner. *"I stopped asking them and just brought home dinner. They almost never complained, and I even got the occasional 'thank you, Mom.' I think I was asking them to do something that was not their job. Just that change made such a difference."*

Jennifer now loves family meals, and within weeks of instituting the DOR, her notoriously picky teen was trying a few new foods. *"Dinner has become pleasant and relaxed, and it is not stressful. Yiseth feels respected at mealtime rather than hassled. She eats more at dinner than she used to before, which has cut down on the late-evening snacking. I am enjoying cooking again. I really don't pay attention to what she puts on her plate and also try to keep my husband from commenting. I wouldn't say that she has dramatically increased the variety of foods she eats, but it is in the range of normal now, and that is great. I think she will be able to go to college in 18 months and nourish herself independently with a dorm meal plan."*

Even teens enjoy being at the table. Jennifer admits that her friends think it's strange that her teenagers want to eat dinner with the family. *"We went through years of hell, and this is such a treat. I love that my children want to be there with me. It's really the sanctity of the family."*

Jack shared this story about a reluctant teen. *"My son is a senior in high school. He started dating a new girl who kept wanting to make plans over our dinner time. Family dinner has always been a priority, so we told him he could go out after, or she could join us. At first, she thought is was 'weird,' but pretty soon she was a regular and delightful guest at our table."*

My own brother, even in his somewhat moody and quiet teen years, would still come to the dinner table. Often, after the meal, he would recline on the upholstered bench and linger before he retreated behind his closed bedroom door again. Granted, we had always had family dinner, so it was easier to continue—but it's never too late to start having family meals.

Jennifer's tips for older kids:
- Serve foods family style. Pre-plating foods Jennifer wanted Yiseth to eat caused battles and never worked.
- Enjoy each other and try not to worry about who is eating what or how much.
- Stick with it. *"At first the girls complained, but now we all like to eat together."*
- You decide what is for dinner and cook what *you* want to eat. (See the section "Menu Planning: Consider Versus Cater" in Chapter 4, Page 106).

When the fighting is over, and the attention and negotiating about who is eating what and how much is no longer an issue, the family table actually becomes a pleasant place where kids really want to be.

DOR Over The Years: Helping Your Child Take Over the What, When, and Where

Ideally, the feeding relationship changes to acknowledge your child's growing maturity and independence. In the following, I use "infant" and "toddler," but in terms of development, not age. It is important to parent at the stage where your child is functioning. An eight-year-old who tantrums frequently and is unable to regulate or even recognize his emotions might be functioning emotionally as a toddler. He might need to be fed that way until he catches up. That eight-year-old might not be ready to be in charge of his snack, but another same-age child, who has mastered the previous stages, may be.

Feed based on your child's emotional age and on what he can do.

Infancy Through Preschool

Infancy: the goal is to keep the infant happy, feed on demand, and meet her needs.
>   Parent: decide *what* and *where* to feed
>   Infant: decide *how much*, *if,* and *when*

Older infant/young toddler transitioning to solids: over the time of this transition, you will include your child at mealtimes, and hopefully by the time she is good at feeding herself finger foods, she will be eating (and drinking formula or breast milk) roughly every 2–3 hours, with water in between.
>   Parent: decide *what, where,* and becomes in charge of *when*
>   Child: decide *how much* and *if* from what is provided

Toddler and preschooler: if your goal is to make your toddler happy every second, you might struggle. If you feed only his favorites so he doesn't get upset, you may be encouraging selective eating down the road.
>   Parent: decide *what, when,* and *where*
>   Toddler: decide *how much* and *if* from what is provided

Discipline

Many parents have a hard time with behavior around meals and eating, often beginning in the toddler phase. Discipline may be a big part of your feeding challenges. If you are terrified of your child having a tantrum to the point of wanting to always give him what he wants, feeding well with the Division of Responsibility (DOR) will be hard. For example, one mother of an only child said that when she got home from work, she wanted her son to always be happy. She felt guilty for working and only ever served what her selective six-year-old requested. "I just don't want to fight, I want us to connect," she agonized. This mom was confusing connecting and parenting, with letting her son do her jobs of deciding the *what, when,* and *where,* and he was really stuck with his eating. Another mother, fed up with her daughter's "overeating," admitted that when her child begged for treats while they were doing errands, she always gave in rather than deal with the fallout. The following are few tips for managing discipline:

- Discipline, redirect, manage, and teach around a child's behaviors as you normally would, but *not* because of *what* or *how much* he is eating.
- Get help. If you realize what your child is doing is a power play, like getting up to get chips in the middle of the meal or walking over to help herself to a granola bar after you told her the kitchen was closed, you need to get back in control of

the situation. (This is assuming you are otherwise following the DOR and feeding reliably with structure, and allowing the child to decide how much.) There are many resources to help with discipline (see "Resources" at www.thefeedingdoctor.com). If you are not confident or consistent, or frankly lost about how to discipline or understand and help your child with her behaviors, then you will need to take measures such as learning more, talking to your social worker, or getting further outside help.

- Remember, it is a child's job to test limits and push your buttons. If they always get what they want and are allowed to break the rules (as in, "This is what's for dinner and you may not get up and get other food," but he gets up anyway), you may struggle with turning feeding challenges around. This problem also sets a pattern for other limit setting.
- You also have the choice of giving in. If your child rages with FASD-related impulse-control issues and the rest of your family is okay with him having peanut butter and jelly at dinner, that may be the best approach for your family at this time.
- If you are dealing with a child who has experienced trauma, FASD, or other behavioral concerns, ask the professional working with you for suggestions.

Grade School/Middle School Years

When she is ready, your child can begin to take on more responsibility. If you have been at this for a while, she may already have wonderful skills with self-regulation and enjoy a variety of foods. For the most part, though, your jobs are still:

Parent: decide *what, when,* and *where*

Child: decide how *much* from what is provided

Continue to eat primarily at the table. Though he may seem like he doesn't need you, provide company at meals and snacks if you can. As he's ready, your child can take on more tasks, such as:

- Choosing more often what he will have for snack. He should still be done in time so he has an appetite for dinner.
- Becoming more involved with menu planning, if he is interested. Keep it simple and think about covering food groups.
- Helping more with cooking and food prep. Remember, though, just because he can fix his breakfast and scramble his own eggs for dinner doesn't mean he should do it alone and eat alone.
- Beginning to decide more of the *what* when eating out. You might suggest food groups, etc.

What About Family Meals and Eating Out?

Family meals aren't always at home; many families eat out on a regular basis. Know that if you do it together, it's a family meal. Go into the restaurant and enjoy the food and each other. With small children, waiting for food can be hard. Choose your restaurants wisely, especially when you are new to the Trust Model.

When my daughter was small, my two ideal criteria for restaurants were if they had booths and a buffet. Our favorites were Ruby Tuesdays and local Chinese and Indian buffets, which always had mild options and a variety of fruits, veggies, proteins, sauces, and starches. Salad bar buffets are a great way to introduce veggies, fruits, sauces, and more with little risk. Grab a plate or two, load up lots of options like cherry tomatoes, green beans, sunflower seeds, and pasta salad, add a few containers of different dressings for dipping, and put it in the middle of the table as "appetizers." Kids might be bored or hungry and be willing to try something new—without pressure. You may need to get him his own plate, but the child who is healing from restriction and food preoccupation will see that there is plenty of food.

Division of Responsibility and Ordering Food When Eating Out

How you will guide your child with ordering depends on how frequently you eat out. If you eat out often, you may need to be more involved in helping your child achieve balance. If eating out is a rare treat, you can feel better about letting him order what he wants.

With young children, you are still in charge of what is on offer. I find that in restaurants, it works well if you give choices from the menu with a goal of balance: "So, you want fries, would you like the chicken or the shrimp with that?" The following are some guidelines:

- Allow one fried choice; for example, fries with lean meat, or chicken tenders with rice.
- If you allow soda, consider letting them choose soda or dessert, or lemonade or dessert.
- Share a dessert or ask for an appropriate-size dessert, showing the wait-staff the size of ice-cream scoop you would like, for example. About half the time, you might get what you ask for.
- If there aren't many balanced options—and frankly, many veggies at restaurants are not very appealing (although Ruby Tuesday's regular broccoli side is one of the better restaurant veggies I've had)—aim to make up for balance the rest of the day or week, offering more fruits or veggies with the afternoon snack for example.
- Teens who are eating competent may be given more leeway choosing what to eat. See the section below on high schoolers for ideas.

Check out my YouTube channel for a three-minute video on eating out and the Trust Model, in addition to other short and helpful videos: http://www.youtube.com/feedingdoctor

---

High School

As your older, adolescent child is able, you are now preparing her to live independently. Your child does not have to be cooking entire meals at this point. Having family meals and allowing her to see you plan and cook is important. Try not to force an uninterested child into cooking. Stick with family meals as much as possible. We tend to think of teens as "too old" for family dinner, or they think it's "lame" or don't need their parents as much, but they do. Meals are a neutral, dependable time to touch base with your child.

- Allow the teen to get her own snack after school.
  - · Have a variety of options available. It seems that with teens, convenience is the most important factor when choosing food. You may want to have chilled water in the fridge or cut-up fruit and veggies, or yogurt if it seems that your teen is only choosing quick, prepackaged snacks. It may be too much effort to peel an orange, but grabbing cut-up melon with those crackers and cheese might do the trick.
- If he's mastered self-regulation and enjoys a variety of foods, you can allow the older teen more freedoms—for example, ordering on his own at restaurants or having seconds on dessert.
- If interested, the teen can perhaps take on some grocery shopping with a list that you have reviewed beforehand. Find fun ways to include her if you can.
- If interested, he can take on planning and cooking one meal a week. Boiled pasta with a jar of marina sauce, a veggie, and bread is a great start.

For information about feeding through adolescence,[4] you can find excellent resources online at the Ellyn Satter Institute.

Forcing or Pressuring a Child to Cook With You (Hello Power Struggle) May Backfire

When my brother left for college, he was a decent cook. He had the patience and interest to help my mother in the kitchen. I, on the other hand, had a short attention span and "better" things to do, like climb trees or watch *Happy Days*. My father expressed his worry to my mother, as I was heading off to college, that I did not know how to cook. My mother's reply: "I'm not worried. She likes to eat. She'll learn." As I moved into my first apartment, I called home for tips for making teriyaki chicken or mashed potatoes, and began cooking with her at home during visits. When my own daughter was two and three, I would ask if she wanted to help, and she mostly declined. At age six, however, she suddenly seemed to enjoy pitching in. Offer opportunities, take "no" for an answer, and try again. You never know when a child might come around.

Remember as you move through the stages with your child that some children will master skills before others. Follow her lead and be responsive and respectful. At any stage, there will be challenges, big and small, and they will affect how you parent and feed. Let's look at some common challenges.

Bringing Home New Siblings, and Other Big Changes

If things have been going relatively well and now have fallen apart, it is helpful to remember that factors outside of the feeding relationship can affect eating. Is a new sibling coming into the home? Is there anxiety over a move, a new school, or a big leap in development like learning to walk or run, read, or make that cognitive leap to logical thinking? Any of these may be exhausting her emotional and energy reserves.

Many factors can precipitate or intensify food battles. On your part, perhaps an article about eating more fish has you feeling guilty, you are grappling with a decision to return to work or stay home, or there is a new worry about weight, either high or low. Things can also change from your child's perspective, like worry about school, conflict with a peer group, or adjusting to a new sibling.

Seven-year-old Gavin's story illustrates how factors not related to eating can worsen feeding struggles. Around kindergarten, Gavin seemed to want to eat more bread and pasta. Carol, Gavin's mother, became concerned about his weight, which had been stable for years at the 75th percentile, but because he asked for bigger portions, Carol got nervous and changed how she was feeding. She began strictly limiting portions, asking Gavin to eat more fruits and veggies ("green-light foods") and wait 20 minutes before having seconds. During this time, Gavin was having more behavioral problems at school and was grappling with his feelings about learning more about his adoption history. Gavin was also getting used to full days in school, dealing with peers, and more focused work time at school.

Gavin's behavior at school and at home worsened dramatically, and meals became tearful and regular battles. Gavin was constantly whining for more food, and before long, he was food preoccupied and sneaking food in his room, and consequently his weight was accelerating. Interestingly, when I reviewed Gavin's growth in more detail, within a few months of his initial interest in bigger portions, he grew about 2½ inches.

With the behavioral and feeding challenges coinciding, it was miserable overall. Meals seemed to be the place where their difficulties played out most dramatically. There was a lot going on with this family, who really felt stuck: Mom had Dad on a diet; she was also very slim, often forgetting to eat, and seemed annoyed that Gavin needed to eat regularly.

As it happens occasionally, this mother did not follow up after the initial evaluation. Some parents just don't feel comfortable with the Trust Model, and I suspect that Carol couldn't trust that Gavin could self-regulate and was too worried about his weight to let go of control. Still, there is a great deal to be learned from their story, as it powerfully demonstrates the spiral of control and resistance, as well as how Gavin's other challenges may have intersected with the feeding battles.

Perhaps if had Gavin had been supported and trusted with his eating, his increased energy needs may have been understood as preparation for a growth spurt. Reducing the stress at meals and instituting the DOR would have helped address Gavin's food preoccupation and weight acceleration. Helping this family get their feeding relationship back on track might not have addressed the behavioral concerns at school, but it would have been a significant start as family meals could have been a safe haven to connect, rather than a flash point for more conflict.

I have had some families reach out for help and then not follow up initially, only to get back in touch several months or even a few years later. My hope for Gavin and his family is that by learning about the options for feeding, this mother may be better able to observe what is and isn't helping Gavin and make positive changes in the future. And, as I tell my families, this is a process with ups and downs, and my door is always open.

Change and Regressing

In the introduction, Jennifer shared that bringing home her youngest daughter seemed to be a particularly difficult transition. Yiseth, her oldest, who struggled with selective eating for years, was adopted at two months of age and came through early feeding joyfully, eating a decent variety of foods without a struggle. It's common for some children to sail through early feeding stages but get stuck during a developmental transition, such as the toddler years or during a major transition in the home.

> Major changes like travel or the addition of a new member to the family are common triggers for worsening feeding challenges for *all* families. The toddler, or a child who is developmentally at that stage, will often have a difficult time with travel, new foods, change in routine, and new time zones. Problems with behavior, feeding, sleeping, and constipation are not uncommon.

For Jennifer's family, the tricky toddler phase was compounded by a traumatic six-week trip overseas to bring home her little sister. There were issues with constipation, stressors of unfamiliar foods, smells, people, etc. Understandably, Jennifer obtained the foods that Yiseth needed to be well while in Guatemala, racing around town to find fruits or the few foods she *would* eat. Several simultaneous changes contributed to their getting stuck in some counterproductive feeding patterns even after their return home:

- Jennifer began to cater to Yiseth's food requests out of worry, and gradually offered fewer and fewer options.
- She cooked separate foods for Yiseth that she knew she would eat and got into the habit of feeding herself and her husband after the girls were in bed.
- The routine fell apart (understandably) with a new infant in the home.
- They continued to struggle with constipation.
- Mom quit her job to stay home.
- Mom realized that cooking from scratch was not working.
- Mom lost her joy of cooking.

I told Jennifer that although her story was her own, I have heard variations on the theme from mothers everywhere: biological, adopting, working, and stay-at-home. Something happens—a sibling, an illness, job stress, whatever it is—and families understandably go into survival mode. Combine those life stressors with a lack of feeding understanding and support, and they lovingly turn to feeding strategies that seem to help in the short term, but get stuck.

When I shared the universality of her experience, Jennifer's smile broadened. *"That makes me feel so much better. I always thought it was because we took her with us. I look back and wish we had done it all differently. I blame myself for so much of this. Knowing that other moms are going through the same thing really helps."*

Even without a trip overseas, knowing that things often get worse with major transitions can help you hold steady, or get back on track, when it happens. Sue experienced similar challenges when she brought home daughter Mary's half-brother. *"Mary backtracked slightly around the time her brother came home (age 2½ for her), but we had been prepared for regression as a possibility in a variety of areas when a sibling was added to the home. She got back on track in due time."*

Being kind with yourselves as parents, knowing there may be a time where you rely on takeout or letting some things slide because you are dealing with bigger fish, is okay. Forgiving yourself and getting "back on track" with how and what you want to feed will be easier with the DOR, and without the guilt. Having a healthy feeding relationship can provide that cornerstone, that comforting center, with reliable time to connect and come together when other areas in your lives are more chaotic.

"I have been amazed when we go around the table and share our favorite part of the day, how often they say, 'Dinner is the best part of my day,' or how often they reference our meals and eating in their writing at school. It is clearly such an important part of their lives. Now that I'm not so worried about nutrition and my son's weight, and I know about family-style meals and the DOR, I can honestly say dinner is often the best part of my day as well. What a nice surprise!" — Jacqueline, mother of Matthew, age seven

Summary

Throughout all the stages and challenges described in this chapter, having a strategy and philosophy to help guide your responses to your child and help her mature and develop with her eating will prove invaluable. Remember to:
- Follow your child's lead.
- Be responsive.
- Do your jobs, and let your child do hers.

Chapter 8
What About the What

"I wish someone had told me not to worry about trying so hard to only offer the 'healthiest' foods. It made it all so much more stressful with our picky eater. Perfection is the enemy of the good, you know?" — Lori, mother of Stan, age four, adopted from Russia

"We changed to gluten free and casein free (GFCF) as a family. I don't know how you could do it otherwise. It is incredibly hard to have one set of rules for one child and another for the adopted child. These kids are often already so different, with meds, IEPs at school, and therapy. I just said, 'This has to be all of us.'"
   — Lara, mother of Brian adopted at age two years

Choosing *what* your child eats is your job (although through adolescence it slowly transitions to the child). Under the best of circumstances, planning for, shopping, storing, preparing, and serving three meals and two to three snacks a day is hard work.

What You Will Learn
What happens when there are special circumstances? When your child can't eat what others eat due to allergies, your child decides he wants to be a vegetarian, or you decide to trial a GFCF diet? This chapter will begin to address some of those situations.

In this chapter on the *what* we serve children, I will also briefly touch on a few nutrition "worries" that come up over and over, including protein needs, sodium, sugar, and a discussion about iron and dairy.

What About Vegetarianism?

When You, the Parents, Are Vegetarians
You can raise healthy, happy kids on a variety of diets, including a vegetarian diet. It may take a little more planning, but it can be done. If you choose not to eat meat or fish, offering dairy, egg products, and legumes, like beans and lentils, will help round out harder-to-get nutrients. Become educated about nutrition, take a bit of extra care, and enjoy those family meals.

The good news is there are abundant resources, from Websites to cookbooks, for planning nutritious meals and snacks. Most vegetarians I know are very thoughtful about nutrition, and do just fine. Some I know however, particularly tweens and teens, become "carbovores," eating only carbs, with little fruits or vegetables, in addition to avoiding meat and fish.

Some vegetarian parents I have worked with think a lot about nutrition, and find themselves struggling with food battles and children who sneak "forbidden foods," and tend to eat them in larger quantities when they have access. My friend tells a story about being in the basement playing with her son and hearing a noise upstairs. When she went to investigate, the uninvited six-year-old neighbor girl was sitting in their pantry eating crackers and drinking juice boxes, and lots of them.

"I Don't Eat Meat. Should I Give It to My Kid?"

Many vegetarian families handle the issue differently. Some vegetarian parents allow their children to choose meat when eating away from home; others do not. Some vegetarian parents will also prepare meat for their children if asked. Some families consume a lot of "meat analogs" like Tofurkey, while others do not. Find what works for your family.

For families where animal welfare, or concern for the environment, is the reason behind the choice, the increasing options of free-range, organic, and grass-fed meats and eggs allow more choices than a decade or so ago. These may be more expensive than conventionally raised meats, so families may choose to prioritize the food budget or eat smaller portions. Less premier cuts of these meats may be more affordable, like chicken thighs or ground beef. Bringing your own cartons to co-ops and packing your own eggs can also save a bit of money. Again, this is a personal decision.

I do not recommend a vegan diet (no dairy, meat, fish, or eggs) for children, but if you choose it, I highly recommend researching the topic and doing a full intake analysis for your child with a dietitian who is familiar with vegan nutrition to look for possible lacking nutrients, particularly if your child has experienced malnutrition with growth delay or catch-up growth.

What if We Eat Meat, But My Child Wants to Be a Vegetarian?

I've talked with several moms who fretted about telling their kids about meat. A typical scenario is the four- or five-year-old who has just put together where meat comes from and refuses to eat meat.

My thoughts on this come from personal experience and from helping clients. My daughter enjoyed eating meat—though this was not always the case, as she was almost three years old before she really started eating the typical dinner-type meats like chicken or beef. At around age four, she asked, "Mom, where does chicken come from?" I answered, "This is chicken that lived on a farm, and now we are lucky to enjoy it for dinner. Isn't it yummy?"

I said this in a pleasant way, no apologizing, very matter of fact, and I changed the subject while enjoying the delicious dinner. She seemed to accept this, asking a few questions about the chicken dying—"it was quick." She asked, "Is that blood?" My reply, "Yes it is. Some people like to eat that part." (We were eating a roasted chicken with a red spot near the bone.)

The topic was revisited on occasion to establish that pork was from pigs—"we are thankful to the farmer and the pigs for this delicious meal"—and that there were no eyes in our chicken or on the shrimp because most people we know don't eat that part.

In addition, when a small child looks up to someone who talks about being a "vegetarian," they may also be intrigued and want to explore the topic with you. My daughter's interest came up again when the oldest girl in her class, as well as one of her teachers, made comments about being vegetarians. When she casually said she wanted to be a vegetarian like her teacher, I replied, "In this family, we eat meat." She sat at the table and helped herself to a variety of foods, including the meat.

Shortly after, we ate artichokes (twice in one week; she didn't eat any the first time, but did the second), and she asked, "Are artichokes *real*?" Upon further questioning, she asked, "Well, they have *hearts*, are they alive like animals?" It was a reminder that children this young are not as rational or cognitively developed as we sometimes think. Generally, this type of interest in vegetarianism will blow over.

What's This I'm Eating, Momma?

The *"What's this I'm eating, Momma?"* talk went smoothly for us. The following are some ideas for addressing the meat question:

- Being prepared in advance with how to deal with this topic will help you feel confident, rather than doubtful.
- Watch nature TV (such as the Discovery Channel's *Life* series or ABC's *Walking With Dinosaurs*) that shows the sometimes cruel side of nature. After a few tears shed over the baby Diplodocus getting eaten, you can explain that it's why the mommy dinosaur lays so many extra eggs, and how some animals get eaten by other animals.
- If you can, visit farms and orchards where there are turkeys or chickens running around. "Yes, that's what we eat at Thanksgiving," you can say. Again, be brief and make unemotional, matter-of-fact statements.
- Avoid fretting or apologizing, and don't launch into lengthy discussions about how sad it is.
- Friends tell me that their older kids love to watch *Bizarre Foods* with chef Andrew Zimmern. He is always so respectful of other cultures and their culinary traditions, and the kids get a kick out of the "yuck factor" of eating bugs.
- Small kids don't need nutrition information. Keep it simple and don't lecture about health, nutrition, or protein. After almost a year of my daughter's preschool teacher asking the kids what "protein" was in their lunch each day, she asked, "Is melon protein?"
- Ask yourself questions to clarify your own position; for example, if you had to, would you kill a chicken to eat it? Again, these are all personal decisions. We like eating meat as a family. I find when I eat meat-free, I feel less satisfied. I have made peace with it myself.

You don't need to lie, but you can spare the details. "Is there meat?" he asks, as you hand him his lunch box. "You have noodles and steak and mushrooms," or, "Just shrimp stir-fry today," or, "rolled-up turkey with Miracle Whip, plus cherry tomatoes, crackers, and cheese." That may satisfy him. Always start with less information. Your child will let you know if she is asking or ready for more.

If your response of, "In this family, we eat meat," takes care of it, great. If not, continue to cook the foods you want to eat; learn a little more about vegetarianism so you can plan choices with higher protein and iron, like beans or nut butters; and leave the door open for your child to return to meat. Don't push her to eat it or fight over it, which will make it harder for her to find her way back to meat if she wants to. (See below, "Cooking When Only Your Child Is a Vegetarian.")

What About the Older Child?

When your 13-year-old asks to be a vegetarian, it is different than the four-year-old, and the discussion needs to be age appropriate. Telling a teen, "In this family, we eat meat," will sound like you don't value her decision-making skills and acknowledge her growing independence. Ask her to explain her interest, and listen. If she talks about weight loss or calories, or you notice other warning signs associated with disordered eating or an eating disorder, act on your suspicions and pursue an evaluation (see page 185). Vegetarianism, veganism, or any change in eating (boys too) that excludes foods or food groups may be a warning sign for unhealthy eating attitudes.

Assuming you sense no cause for concern, and your son has explained his reasons, look at this as an opportunity. If "ethical" reasons are his concern, explore eating less meat or meat raised with more animal-friendly practices. Some stores like Whole Foods have a rating system for how the animals are treated, and specialty butchers and co-ops are increasingly available. To my surprise, I have found that our local co-op has regionally sourced meats that are cheaper than the "organic" or "grass-fed" meats at the grocery chains. Choosing a cheaper cut of premium-raised meat, like chicken thighs or ground beef a few times a week, could allow him to feel comfortable eating meat as long as you are okay with that arrangement.

If your teen chooses to eat a vegetarian diet, he can begin to take responsibility for his choices. You can help by purchasing a book on nutrition or having him see a dietitian, particularly if he is also an athlete or you have any concerns. Be sure to talk to the dietitian first, then accompany your child to the initial meeting to be sure that your child will be supported and that no food choices, including meat, are demonized. Again, your level of involvement will vary depending on your child: his age, abilities, and maturity. Follow his lead. Many young people experiment with vegetarianism for a time but return to enjoying meat.

Cooking When Only Your Child Is a Vegetarian

How do you plan family meals when one child is a vegetarian? Remember the concept from Chapter 4 of "consider versus cater"—that is, to think of your child's likes and nutritional needs when menu planning, but not letting them dictate the menu. If your vegetarian child is allowed to eat peanut butter and jelly every meal or is treated differently than your other children, you can imagine where that is headed. "Why does Sam get to eat peanut butter, and I have to eat casserole? It's not *fair*! I'm not eating this, it's gross!" Consider nutrition, learn a few vegetarian dishes to serve, or be mindful about including vegetarian choices such as beans for lunch or peanut butter toast at breakfast.

A Word About Dietitians

Like any professional you work with, you may need to do a little digging to find someone who fits your needs. Registered dietitians get a standardized curriculum in their training, with specialization earned through practicums and work experience, such as work with a feeding clinic or a diabetes practice. I believe it is important to work with someone who is a *pediatric* RD. Some general RDs are not aware of the Division of Responsibility and the Trust Model in feeding, or have little experience with it. For example, if your RD recommends calorie restriction or specific portion limits, or encourages you to push your child to eat more, this shows a lack of experience with the model. As with any professional working with your family, trust your gut, ask questions, and get recommendations from other parents or a trusted member of your health care team.

Questions to ask your RD:
- Are you aware of the Division of Responsibility and Ellyn Satter's work?
- Do you believe that children can self-regulate, that is, he can know how much to eat if I do my jobs with feeding?
- Do you think my child needs to be taught portion control?
- Do you believe that pushing my child to eat more will make him grow better?
- Will you talk about meat or fat being "bad," or about "red-light foods?"
- Will you talk to my child about his weight? What do you plan to say?
- Can you help our family support my child's nutrition following a vegetarian diet while not being negative about meat?
- Do you belong to a pediatric practice group or a vegetarian nutrition practice group?

Try www.eatright.org to find a dietitian that is right for your family.

Milk, other dairy products, and eggs will help to round out nutrition. If your child chooses to only have milk, fruit, and pasta for several dinners each week, but eats protein and iron sources at other times, he'll cover his nutritional bases. If you are concerned, you can find a dietitian to do an intake analysis to see if there are any substantial holes that you may be able to help support with a few additional offerings. See protein and iron in the section "While We're at It, Let's Deal With Some Common Nutrition Worries" on page 224 for more information.

Be sure that everyone in the family is respectful. That means no one gets to tease the vegetarian, and the vegetarian also doesn't get to make mooing noises or go on about poorly treated animals if others are enjoying meat.

"Healthy" Eating: Pleasures and Pitfalls

In addition to choosing to avoid meat, some parents also choose to avoid other types of foods, such as anything with artificial coloring, "processed" foods, or "white" foods, including sugar, flour, and rice. (See the section on "What About Food Allergies?" on the next page for more suggestions if you are avoiding entire food categories.)

The families who do this successfully preserve the positive relationship with food. The parents are calm, and they focus on the pleasure and joy with the foods they eat. The way they talk about and engage with food is critical. For example, while shopping recently at the co-op, I watched children help their mother pick out fruit. The children were sniffing the fruit and they were all marveling at the pretty colors. If you chose to feed this way, and your child is thriving, then enjoy and feel free to skip to the end of this section.

When parents are highly invested in their children eating "healthy" (this means different things to different families) it can set up conflict around food. As mom Lori said, *"For us, the 'perfect' became the enemy of the good."* I see this challenge more commonly in my vegetarian families.

> For some children, avoiding many commonly available foods can lead to intense interest in "forbidden foods." If you have one child who does well with your food choices, and another who is preoccupied with what she *can't* have, realize that temperament plays a role, too.

When the feeding relationship is negatively impacted with this kind of eating, I most often observe a lot of talking about nutrition with a focus on the foods (and their perceived health risks) they must avoid. Occasionally, when these families find me because of a child's selective eating or sweets "obsession," there is a history of disordered eating for the mother.

One mother was so restricted that her daughter had never had breakfast cereal or bread. The little girl was extremely selective and anxious to the point of panic attacks when faced with eating out or situations where she might not find a food she liked. She was anything but happy, and she had major deficiencies in her intake. This mother, on further reflection, had carried many of her disordered behaviors and thinking from her anorexia into a more acceptable way of avoiding foods—sometimes known as "orthorexia." Mom was unable to have any breads, pastas, or cereals in the house because these would trigger binges for her. This is not common, but it happens.

Orthorexia is not an officially recognized eating disorder, but is characterized by an unhealthy obsession with "healthy" eating. It results in intake that cuts out whole groups and types of foods, often leading to inadequate energy and nutrient intake.[1]

Some children with anxiety or a genetic susceptibility to eating disorders find this kind of eating, with the negative food talk, particularly difficult and stressful. One client's four-year-old son only ate fruits and vegetables labeled organic because all others were "poison." In general, he avoided fruits and vegetables, so perhaps he, too, was using his mother's concerns about pesticides and organic foods as a power chip in his battle for control, as he was pushed to eat the dreaded fruits and veggies.

It comes down to Ellyn Satter's statement, "When the joy goes out of eating, nutrition suffers." Whatever foods you provide for your children, keeping the feeding relationship and the joy in mind is key. If you sense that your child is really struggling with forbidden foods for whatever reason, you may benefit from ideas in Chapter 4, in Chapter 6, and in the "Sweets and Treats" section later in this chapter.

What About Food Allergies?

A food allergy occurs when the body's immune system reacts to a certain food. The body's immune system actors (antibodies), most commonly IgE, react with the food and trigger the release a host of chemical mediators, including histamine, that lead to the symptoms of food allergies: hives, tingling and swelling in the mouth and throat, difficulty breathing, vomiting, diarrhea, a drop in blood pressure (kids look pale and clammy), and very rarely, death. Food allergies seem to be on the rise, but parents also often overestimate how common food allergies are. In one study, parents overestimated by twofold the actual incidence of food allergies in their children.[2]

And it is confusing. Part of the issue is that many reactions that may actually be skin sensitivities or intolerances are interpreted as an allergy, when they are not. For example:

- Citrus and other acidic foods can irritate the skin, causing redness around the mouth and bottom, particularly if the child is still in diapers.
- Some kids have looser stools in response to fiber. Parents tell me they limit the child's fruit intake due to loose stools, and that the child is "allergic." This is not an allergy, and other than the mess, is not necessarily problematic.
- Lactose intolerance can have unpleasant symptoms, but is not an allergy.

Recommendations are changing all the time in terms of food allergies and when to introduce foods, and what foods to avoid. Some studies seem to show that early introduction of foods means less allergies, while others seem to show that waiting until after six months of age decreases incidence of allergies. As an adoptive or fostering parent, you can't control the past. If you adopted an older child, you had no control when solids were introduced and what kind, and you had no say in whether your child had breast milk or formula and what kind. You *can* control how you feed your little one now.

> The 2011 guidelines from the National Institute of Allergy and Infectious Diseases (NIAID) state, "There is no evidence that supports delaying the introduction of solid foods to an infant beyond 4 to 6 months of age to prevent allergic diseases from developing. This includes giving an infant a food containing milk, eggs, peanut, tree nuts, soy, or wheat."[3]

If Your Child Has Food Allergies

Decide if your child has the temperament to not eat the same foods as the rest of the family, or if you will *all* follow the limited diet. Perry, who has one child with severe tree nut and peanut allergies as well as dairy and gluten allergies, feeds the whole family the same way. Avoiding nuts is a safety issue, but it was important to cook one meal for the whole family and not have her daughter feel different or left out. Though Perry really doesn't like cooking, she has researched Websites and found cookbooks for dairy-free cooking and baking, finding that easier than the alternative. Perry has worked hard and succeeded with preserving the joy around food for her family in spite of serious challenges. Here is what has helped Perry:

- Focus on what your child *can* eat, rather than on what she can't.
- When your child goes to parties, bring a treat for him. Perry has learned to send along her gluten-free, casein-free (GFCF) cupcakes for her child. She bakes and freezes them for special occasions.
- Find support groups and online forums for more information and help.
- Learn about reading labels. For example, "milk" may appear on labels under "whey, rennet, quark, nougat, lactic yeast, nicin, ghee…" There are printable cards and multiple resources and support groups if you are dealing with food allergies. Starting with the National Institute of Allergy and Infectious Diseases (www.NIAID.nih.gov) might help.

Other Tips About Feeding and Allergies

Official advice changes frequently, so check with your child's doctor. Before you cut out any food groups due to allergy concerns, be sure that you have seen a reputable allergist (pediatric if possible) and a pediatric RD.

- Introduce solids when your child is ready; for typically developing children, this is usually around 5–7 months of age. For children who are delayed, which is more common for children who have lived in an institutional setting, follow their cues and talk to your doctor or dietitian about supporting appropriate intake.
- You often won't know any family history around allergies, so try to stick with introducing one new food at a time. Wait three days or so before you introduce a new food to watch for any reaction. (This does not mean that you have to only

serve the new food or have to serve the new food every day for three days. If kiwis are new, offer kiwis and watch her for a few days for any signs of reaction while not introducing other new foods.)

- If there is evidence of allergies, asthma, or eczema ("atopic" signs), talk to your doctor about when to introduce what foods.
- Even for peanuts, the 2011 NIAID guidelines quoted above (at the time of this writing) say you can introduce them after six months of age if there is no known family history of peanut allergy. If there is a family allergy history, check with your doctor, and consider waiting until age three. Without knowing the history, it is best to check with your child's doctor. Most guidelines say wait until one year.
- Rule out parasites and other infections if your child is adopted internationally or has unexplained gastrointestinal symptoms. Infections make it harder to look for reactions or signs of discomfort.
- Let your child be your guide. Do not pressure her to eat foods. Sometimes even young children know when a food has made them feel poorly, and they will choose not to eat it.
- Eosinophilic Esophagitis (EoE), a rare inflammation of the esophagus, or swallowing tube, is associated with food allergies. Symptoms can mimic reflux. (See Appendix II, Medical Issues That Can Affect Feeding, for more information.)

Eczema might not be enough of an indication to cut out entire foods groups, particularly if you can manage the skin condition—and if you are already dealing with selective eating or nutrition concerns. (See "eczema" in Appendix II, Medical Issues That Can Affect Feeding.) Colleagues who work in allergy and GI clinics explain a typical scenario: a fussy child, or a child with mild eczema, gets the blood test (RAST) for allergies from the primary doctor. The test shows possible allergies to one or even several foods. The parents are told to eliminate the foods, but with no further instructions. They panic, scramble to find foods the child can eat, cater, feel guilty, and then see the allergist a year later for follow-up. The fussiness and eczema may or may not be better. A year later, the child has had no exposure to the foods, and now when even small amounts are reintroduced, the child has a *severe* reaction. In addition, the worry and lack of support has introduced a counterproductive dynamic into the feeding relationship. Many children do outgrow mild food allergies, and perhaps these children were robbed of that natural process. It is important to pursue a thorough evaluation, and have expert support before eliminating foods. Note, blood tests vary in accuracy with the child's age and other factors. This is part of why seeing a specialist is so helpful.

What About "Therapeutic" Diets Like Gluten and Casein Free (GFCF)?

When a child is struggling, whether it is with stomach upset, constipation, behavioral rages, or learning problems, parents want to do everything possible so the child can be healthy and happy. Increasingly, more attention is being paid to how nutrition affects children, including not just physical needs, but also their cognitive and other neural processes such as impulse control. In addition to traditional therapies and medications, many parents are also considering dietary interventions as part of a treatment plan for children with drug and alcohol exposures, cognitive delays due to prolonged malnutrition, or other behavioral problems associated with ADHD and autism spectrum.

The general research I have seen on dietary interventions seems unclear either way.[4] However, I do know that many families feel that following certain nutritional regimens have helped their children. I also know parents for whom the trials did *not* help. I will use GFCF as an example, as it is the most common therapeutic diet that parents undertake. If you research and chose to pursue any elimination diet, having a healthy feeding relationship will be key to the success of the trial.

How can what a child eats affect how they behave and think? Beyond the obvious blood sugar connection and the effects that macro (protein, fat, carbohydrates) and micro (vitamins, minerals) nutrient deficiencies can have on behavior, there is another possible way that diet can effect behavior: the "leaky gut." A lot is written about the "leaky gut" theory, where for some individuals, the digestive system is not functioning properly, perhaps damaged from in-utero alcohol exposure, frequent antibiotics, or a genetic susceptibility to gluten. The theory is that the undigested gluten or casein (milk protein) molecules cross into the blood through the "leaky" gut, and from there into the brain, where they "affect the brain like an opiate drug."[5] (Opiates, or "opioids," are drugs like morphine.)

As always, you know your child best, so if a therapeutic diet helps, great. If you are curious to try it, it's reasonable. However, these restrictions do limit what you can offer your child, and many children come to their foster or adoptive homes with limited intake already. Often a child's favorite foods are high in gluten and casein: macaroni and cheese, pastas, breads, and milk. If you contemplate an elimination diet, don't do it lightly.

Lara's Journey with GFCF

Lara's two children with FASD had extreme impulse control problems. Her adopted son, Brian, had rages to the point of police intervention. Lara explains, *"Brian acted out, and our daughter, Grace, acted in."* Grace, meanwhile, had a known family history of celiac disease (intolerance to gluten) and was on two GI medications, including a stool softener and an acid blocker. Lara recalls seeing information about GFCF years ago. *"I had been seeing posts in parent support forums for years, and I would delete it. I wasn't ready. I will try not to beat myself up over that. I think our son was ready sooner, but our daughter has more severe trust and attachment issue, so I don't think she would have been ready earlier."*

What Lara explains is that pursuing elimination diets while the child is still struggling and working on attaching can provoke intense feelings of anxiety and worsen power struggles.

Lara warns, "*I think it is absolutely critical that there is a secure relationship and attachment and that there aren't food struggles before you begin any elimination diet.*"

Lara and I share a reluctance to talk about dietary interventions because we know that so many families are already feeling absolutely overwhelmed and simply can't take on another "should." Sit with the decision for a time, focus on building your relationship, learn what you can and, when and if you feel ready, consider giving it a try.

Therapeutic Diets and the Trust Model

Therapeutic or elimination diets are hard work at first; they require learning new ways of cooking, meal planning, and other tasks. Recognize that. Be kind with yourself through the process, and ask for help and support when you can. Remember to focus on what your child *can* eat, not on what she can't. Lara described loading the countertops with clear containers of all the things they could eat, like cashews, dried fruit, and rice, and made homemade potato chips on the first day. Some families have observed that going "dye-free" helps with attention and behavior. Regardless of the type of therapeutic approach, any dietary intervention trial should be followed for a minimum of three to six months. Any time you are removing food groups or options from a child's intake, check in with an RD or your doctor before you begin.

If you decide to pursue complementary therapies, including dietary interventions, look for a physician or provider with some familiarity or at least an open mind about complementary treatment options. Increasingly, medical centers have Integrative Medicine departments, and more doctors are trained in or have a special interest in integrative or complementary modalities, including dietary interventions. I think it is still important to have a physician or dietitian involved in your child's care, and be wary of unscrupulous companies and practitioners who prey on the fears of desperate parents to sell pricey and often questionable supplements.

If you want to pursue a specialized diet, how do you do that within the Trust Model?
- Try not to feel sorry for your child. Approach it with a positive attitude. When we feel sorry for our children, we tend to give in, cater too much, and allow guilt to govern our food choices. For example, we think, "He can't have so many things, I'll let him have treats whenever he asks to make up for it."
- If at all possible, the whole family should follow the diet, but find what works for your family. Is the whole family going with it? Are others feeling deprived? Can you find ways to consider the child with dietary restrictions without being too obvious, but still meeting the needs of others? (For example, Lara's biological son enjoys cheese and pizza when he's out with friends.)

- Be matter-of-fact about what she can or can't eat. Lara called it a "plan." She laid out the new eating "plan" for the whole family and never presented it as a "diet."
- Try to link it back to how the child feels, not just labeling foods. "Regular milk from cows makes your tummy feel bad, and we want you to feel good. Let's try this milk today." (May be lactose-free or other alternative.)
- Stick with the Division of Responsibility. That means keep the structure, say no to requests for food between planned meals and snacks, and allow just water in between.
- Have family meals. Serving your child his GFCF special foods at the kitchen island while you graze on other foods isn't very supportive.

Dr. Linda Black has written on this topic as a mother of three children adopted from Russia who benefited from the GFCF diet. "Do not try to change your whole diet at once; adapt your normal recipes to GFCF so that you continue eating familiar comforting foods," she advises. "Begin gradually in order to minimize the withdrawal from opioids, but try to be completely GFCF within a month."[6]

The good news is that there has been an explosion of resources online, as well as products in grocery stores, for families who feel better on GFCF diets. Take some time to peruse those resources (some are in the Resources section at www.thefeedingdoctor.com.com), and experiment with recipes. Consider a potluck, find a local group of parents who have the same concerns and restrictions and have a potluck/recipe-sharing party, or host a taste-test party where everyone can buy one or two items but you can try 10–20 new things and not break the bank. If your kids are old enough and are excited by the process, invite them along. Make it a party.

If you are laughing at this section because your son only eats mac-n-cheese and French toast fingers, treat him first like any other selective eater. Begin with family meals and structure. Serve his mac-n-cheese and French toast fingers from a bowl in the middle of the table along with bowls of what you are eating (see Chapter 4). He needs to see what he will learn to eat and be comfortable around it. Introduce GFCF versions of his favorites.

"I am hesitant to talk about the success we have had, because I know that there are families that will try this and not see significant improvement. I don't want to give anyone false hope, that this is a magic bullet, but I think many children could benefit from a trial of GFCF. Our son's sensory experiences have improved greatly in the last year since we have been doing GFCF. Ironically, we initially did it more for our daughter, but Brian has seen the most dramatic improvement."

— Lara, mother of biological and adopted children. (Of note, Lara's daughter Grace was able to stop her GI medications, but Lara hasn't seen as dramatic an improvement in Grace's behavior as in Brian's.)

With these elimination diets, I wonder if the success is due to the actual removal of certain foods or sometimes just the fact that these ways of eating tend to mean families pay more attention to overall balance, preparing meals, and eating together. If it helps your family, I suppose the "why" is unimportant. My medical school professors would be upset to hear it, but really, you'll know it's helping if your child is happier and healthier— so trust your instincts.

Tips to promote gut health that won't hurt:
- Consider a probiotic supplement (good bacteria that support a healthy gut system).
- Use a probiotic supplement during and after antibiotics or with diarrheal illness.
- Offer yogurt or kefir drinks with live active cultures as choices in the meal and snack rotation.
- Consider a fish oil or flax oil supplement. Some fish oil brands are chewy and don't taste too bad. Some of my patients and clients didn't like that they could taste fish oil hours after taking the supplement. In this case try giving it right before bed, or switch to flax oil, which has almost no flavor and can be mixed into smoothies or oatmeal. You can also look for foods fortified with DHA and omega fatty acids. You can even buy milk with added DHA.

What About Religious Requirements or Restrictions?

If you decide to follow a religious code of eating, ideally the whole family would eat that way. Hopefully, you will also have family and community who share your eating style. However, some clients have difficulty with religious eating requirements, such as menu-planning or meeting nutritional needs while keeping kosher, or the teen with disordered eating who feels best when she eats regularly and does not easily tolerate fasting.

You may find some resources within your religious community for guidance. For example, the issue of eating disorders in the Orthodox Jewish community is getting increasing attention, with some treatment centers offering kosher foods. The topic is no longer simply swept under the rug, but is being dealt with more openly.

In regard to fasting, if your child is small, or doesn't deal well with low blood sugar levels, or going without food is scary due to a history of food insecurity, expecting him to fast may be too much. Fasting can be particularly terrifying and trigger binges for those who have experienced restriction or are repeat dieters. Explore your concerns with your religious leaders and with your conscience. Seek out support and understanding from others in your religious tradition who may be willing to listen and consider your situation.

The following guidelines can assist you in incorporating religious guidelines into your feeding routine:
- Focus on what you *can* eat. Your child can eat pizza, maybe only with cheese or only meat.

- Celebrate the cultural and family connections.
- Celebrate the reasons behind the food rules. For example, talk about how it makes you feel closer to God and that it is important for your family.
- If you are struggling, find a therapist to help with behavior and transitions.
- When your child first comes to live with you, you may want to accommodate him and the diet he is used to, first working on attachment and healing and then gradually shifting to your way of eating.

While We're at It, Let's Deal With Some Common Nutrition Worries

Nutrition worries, often unfounded, are the second most common reason, after weight worries, why parents pressure and get stuck with feeding. Here are some of the most common nutrition concerns I help families resolve so they can focus on feeding.

Protein

Protein seems to be the number one nutrition worry for the parents I work with, most of whom greatly overestimate how much protein a child needs. Almost universally, when I see an intake analysis for even a selective or "underweight" child, the protein the child consumes exceeds the minimum recommended amount. For example, a toddler drinking a cup or two of milk throughout the day, part of an egg, and a slice or two of deli meat gets *more* than adequate protein. When parents understand how relatively easy it is to get enough protein, they can relax and not pressure, and also not cater.

> During a workshop, a mother of a 12-month-old shared, *"I give my son chicken nuggets every night because I know he'll eat them and he needs protein."* She was overestimating how much he needed and limiting his chances to learn to like a variety of protein sources. He was not an unusually selective child, nor did he have any delays or special needs. Limiting the foods he is offered to his favorites, out of her unfounded protein worry, makes it more likely that he will refuse other protein sources and demand chicken nuggets. This mom needs to keep offering many different sources of protein.

The following are some general protein needs:
- One- to three-year-olds need about .55 grams of protein per pound of body weight. A 29-lb. boy would need roughly 16 grams of protein, or about the amount in two cups of milk. Clearly, a small one-year-old will need less than a larger three-year-old.
- Four- to six-year-olds need about .5 grams per pound of body weight.
- Seven- to 14-year-olds need about .45 grams/pound of body weight.
- 15- to 18-year-olds need about .4 grams/pound of body weight.
- Girls older than 15 and boys older than 18 years of age need about .36 grams per pound of body weight.

Non-meat protein sources (amounts given to show how it adds up):
- Milk: 1 cup = 8 grams
- Cheese: 1 ounce = 6–8 grams
- Yogurt: 1 cup = 8 grams
- "Greek-style" yogurt: 1 cup = up to 18 grams (check labels; protein varies)
- Nuts or nut butters: 2 tablespoons = 7 grams
- Eggs: 1 egg = 7 grams
- Fish and shellfish, like shrimp: 1 ounce = 7 grams
- Beans and lentils: ½ cup cooked = 7–10 grams
- Edamame soybeans: ½ cup = 14 grams (edamame, which the child can shell, is a fun snack)
- Tofu: ½ cup = 20 grams
- Veggies: ½ cup cooked = 1–3 grams
- Grains: ½ cup cooked pasta, 1 slice of bread, ½ cup oats = 2–4 grams

"I want to feed my son meat lasagna tonight, but I heard that too much protein is bad for his kidneys." If your son is otherwise healthy, it would take massive amounts of meat lasagna to affect his kidneys, amounts he simply could not consume. The only time in my medical practice I saw a healthy young person get into trouble with protein and kidneys was when a teen took too much protein powder supplements (to "bulk up") and dehydrated himself on purpose for a weekend wrestling tournament. He chewed gum and spat, rode exercise bikes in plastic bags, and used other drastic tactics to make his weight category. The combination of excessive protein load, dehydration, and extreme exertion with muscle breakdown of several wrestling matches led to temporary and reversible kidney problems—all totally avoidable with common sense (something notoriously lacking in the average teen). This mom's question is another case where an unfounded worry was interfering with a joyful feeding experience.

Iron

While many parents fret over protein, they forget about iron. Don't forget about iron! With a vegetarian diet, iron is often harder to get in adequate amounts, versus protein. If your child is not eating meat, it will be important to offer iron-rich foods. this may be a question for your RD or doctor in terms of supplement needs.

Children who experience catch-up growth have a higher risk of iron deficiency; therefore, they probably need supplements. A significant portion of internationally adopted (IA) children with a history of poor nutrition and growth also have iron-deficiency anemia and will need supplements for some time. Again, iron is often more difficult to get than protein, and iron deficiency has serious consequences, from affecting IQ to energy. It is important to recheck iron levels after beginning any supplements to be sure your child is getting enough. This is not something to be taken lightly.

Here are some common iron sources:

- Red meat.
- Poultry, like chicken and turkey.
- Other meats.
- Egg yolks.
- Dark leafy greens (spinach, collards).
- Dried fruit (prunes, raisins).
- Iron-enriched cereals and grains (check the labels).
- Beans, lentils, chick peas, and soybeans.
- Artichokes. Surprisingly, many children like to eat artichokes, peeling the leaves and dipping them in sauces like balsamic and olive oil. Again, don't underestimate what children will like. I had my first artichoke at a neighbor's when I was 10 years old, and I loved it. My daughter has enjoyed them as an occasional treat since she was about two and a half years old.

> Hydee Becker, RD, suggests giving iron supplements during bath time, since iron can stain clothing. The fun of the bath also helps distract from the taste. You may notice a temporary staining of teeth.

Salt

One mother of a girl being evaluated for growth hormone replacement therapy fought with her daughter about salt. Mom would go to the trouble of cooking a balanced, from-scratch meal most nights, but argued with her 10-year-old about adding salt. The girl preferred salty foods, but mom worried about sodium—one *more* thing to worry about. Or maybe not?[7]

Salt is the latest bogeyman. I can quite calmly say, don't worry about it. If it helps a child enjoy foods, by all means pass the salt. The health claims about following a low-sodium diet are not conclusive, and they are certainly not a compelling-enough reason for engaging in battles with your child over food. A recent independent Cochrane Review of the research[8] found no difference in health outcomes with low-salt diets (largely in white males since they were most commonly studied), and a large Danish study showed that the folks who had the highest urine sodium (correlating with intake) had the *lowest mortality and health problems.*[9]

So unless your child has a known kidney problem where he can't process salt, it is difficult to overdo it, particularly in a family where most of the food is cooked from scratch. Processed foods are a large source of salt, and even that doesn't worry me too much. Again, focus on supporting joy and flavor, and enjoy the relief that this is one battle you don't have to fight. In addition, when you stop trying to limit or control salt, your child may become less interested in it.

Nitrites

Nitrites are often added to meats in the curing process or for preservation, as it was found to be the active ingredient that stopped bacteria from growing in salts that were traditionally added. The research on nitrites/nitrates is mixed, with some suggesting increased cancer risk when consumed in large amounts. Since there are now plenty of nitrate/nitrite-free options, if you are serving hot dogs or lunchmeats more than a few times a week, choosing "nitrite/nitrate-free" may lower the risk.

Sugar

Small children like sugar. Duh. Sweet-sensitive taste buds are at the tip of the tongue. One of my favorite studies looks at children's versus adult's preference for sweet taste, and when the shift to adult tastes happens. Through various ages, study participants were asked to add sugar to a drink until it got too sweet.

For children, there was pretty much *no such thing* as "too sweet." They continued adding sugar until it wouldn't dissolve any more. Adults stopped at about the sweetness of soda, finding anything sweeter to be "too sweet." Interestingly, the point the shift occurred was not by age or from something the children learned in school. The shift to adult taste for sweet tended to happen just after the growth plates in the long bones fused,[10] meaning the children had reached close to adult height, or stopped growing. What that suggests is that there is a biological drive behind that preference for sweet taste. Children are growing, and it makes sense biologically that they would be attracted to sweeter, and therefore higher energy, foods to fuel growth.

Think back to your own childhood. I loved sugar-sweetened cereals at hotels or sleepovers, but I was not allowed them at home, and tended to enjoy large amounts when I had access. However, now as an adult, the thought of that pink, oversweet milk, "marshmallows," and cereal is off-putting. Children's tastes mature, and they will do so more readily if we don't interfere.

> Sugar blowouts usually occur when many kids are around and on a special day. Talking about how sugar makes kids hyper can be a self-fulfilling prophecy or carte blanche for crazy antics. The child can claim, "The sugar made me do it!" as I saw on "treat" day at out daughter's "sugar-free" preschool. The teacher repeatedly and loudly lamented, "See, I knew it. You are all totally crazy on sugar day!"

But Sugar Makes My Kid Crazy

I hear this a lot, and it is commonly accepted "truth." Though many studies have tried, none have shown that consuming refined sugar affects behavior. You know your child best, but consider this: Often, when your child has "sugar" blowouts, he has little balance, with no protein or fat. Remember the graph about energy, blood sugar level, and time on page 39? If your child only gets sugar or simple carbs, as in the party with candy and juice, there is a rapid blood sugar peak, followed by a rapid fall. Often, the *drop* in blood sugar, rather than the peak, explains the behavior.

> ***We were told diet soda and Crystal Lite were "preferred beverages" by the pediatric RD at a university children's weight loss clinic, for our two-and-a-half-year-old food-obsessed daughter! I don't want her drinking diet drinks, what about juice?"*** asks Cami. The current quick "fix" for "obesity" is to blame and ban sugar-sweetened beverages, including fruit juice, with many experts recommending diet drinks with artificial sweeteners. An article on artificial sweeteners from the Mayo Clinic Website had this to say, "…numerous research studies confirm that artificial sweeteners are generally safe in limited quantities, even for pregnant women."[11] While that statement is meant to be reassuring, there are a few too many qualifiers for my taste. As there is conflicting evidence on studies involving artificial sweeteners, I personally prefer that children go the natural route and avoid artificial sweeteners. As part of structured and balanced offerings, they can enjoy beet or cane sugar, honey (after one year of age), maple syrup, or foods sweetened with fruit juices, and even high-fructose corn syrup. I encourage parents to become educated consumers and make decisions for their own families.
>
> Just the sweet taste in diet drinks releases insulin, which makes blood sugar drop and can lead to hunger. If you do choose to serve diet drinks, try to do so with meals and snacks.
>
> If you want to avoid artificial sweeteners, as Cami did, a reasonable approach is to shoot for around four ounces of juice or sweetened drinks a day. I recommend that parents serve about half water and half juice. There are even juice boxes with diluted juice that you might consider if you serve them often. Recognize that on some days there will be more juice, and other days there will be less. I like fruit nectars or cloudy apple juice too. Served within a healthy feeding relationship with meals and snacks, I don't believe that fruit juice contributes to problematic weight gain. I do think that children should not regularly drink soda, and that between meals, water is the beverage of choice.

The following suggestions will help avoid blood sugar crashes, and hopefully the "crazy" too:

- If you are offering high-sugar foods, also offer protein, fat, and some foods with fiber. Pour a glass of milk or add some crackers, cheese, and fruit to the spread. (At a WIC food supplement tasting event I attended, the kids all made a beeline for the colorful fruit kebabs, over the muffins and other choices.)
- Consider candy that has fat and protein. I love Snickers bars for that reason, with nuts and chocolate, or Peanut M&Ms.
- Kids will learn that if they only eat candy, they won't feel so good afterward.

Those "mistakes" are how they learn to listen to their bodies. It is far more useful for them to learn how it feels than to just hear lectures about it.

- Some parents who avoid food dyes have observed that the behavior issues improve. This begs the question: Perhaps the child is reacting to the food dye in candy and sweet foods, rather than the sugar? (I also don't think this is a common finding, but something to consider, especially with increasing options for natural food dyes.)

Is Sugar Addictive?

I don't think so. There are scientific papers and theories that argue "yes" and "no." Of course, the pleasure centers that are involved with addiction do light up with certain foods more than others, particularly foods with high sugar, fat, and salt, but those pleasure centers light up with sex, too. Anything that promotes survival will be tied in to those reward pathways, and food certainly is critical to survival. But a recent review published in the *American Journal of Clinical Nutrition* concluded, "There is no support from the human literature for the hypothesis that sucrose may be physically addictive or that addiction to sugar plays a role in eating disorders."[12]

With that said, the thing that has convinced me most that sugar is not addictive is that *permission* to eat sugar often cures the "addictive" behaviors like craving and overconsumption. When the food-obsessed child is allowed matter-of-fact access to sugar within a framework of supportive feeding, she learns to handle sweets. She enjoys them, but forgets about them in between opportunities. She might pester you for them like any other child, but she is no longer "obsessed" and, on her own, might even leave her Halloween candy after three or four pieces.

That is not the same experience as with cocaine or heroine, where permission and purposeful inclusion of the drug does not lead to learning to handle it, being healthy, or moving forward. Moving forward in a healthy way, and helping kids learn to manage sugary foods and other "treats," is a topic most parents wrestle with, and one that we'll tackle next.

I recently saw a phone app for "obese" teens using the addiction model. How sad. These young people are told they have a disease they will have to manage, like alcoholism, for the rest of their lives. It uses abstinence, support groups, and the language of the 12-step program. The "addiction" or "addict" label has the potential to do great harm. This tells the child he is incapable, he is damaged and sick, and can never learn to have a healthy relationship with food. Words matter. If thinking of sugar as an addiction has helped you with your eating, that is fine, but I would caution against using addiction language with children and teens around sugar, or food in general. These common examples model addiction language and may not help with your goal of raising a competent eater: "I can't control myself around bread!" or "I can't stop until I eat the whole bag; I have no self-control," or, "I am having a major *snack attack,* a craving *I can't handle.*"

Sweets and Treats

You may have picked up by now that sweets, candy, and desserts are limited and treated differently than other foods. This is the one area where *the adult decides* how much. Why? Because sweets are so appealing that they are difficult to learn to manage without a little more direction. If a child is allowed unlimited sweets with every meal and snack, the sweets tend to displace more nutritious foods, making variety and balanced nutrition harder.

However, in order to deal with the potential "forbidden-food" phenomena, where the child becomes unduly interested in sweets, the child needs fairly frequent opportunities to learn to handle "forbidden foods." With the strategies of 1) serving a child-size portion of dessert with the meal and 2) allowing regular "treat snacks," dessert will lose its power and be dethroned from its place of glory, becoming just another food to be enjoyed among many others.

Step One of Your Treat Strategy: Serve Dessert *With* the Meal

Serving a small portion of dessert with the meal creates an even playing field. You put the roasted cauliflower out at the same time as the Popsicle or pudding, eliminating the hierarchy. Food is just food. It's all wonderful. At first, he will stare, dumbfounded. With older children, you may want to prepare them. "Max, we haven't been enjoying meals very much because we are always talking about dessert and not much else. We are going to start serving dessert with the meal. You can eat it whenever you want, but that is your share."

If you have wielded dessert as a tool for getting veggies in, it will take him a while to understand. He will eat dessert first, for a few days or even weeks, but eventually you will see him lick a Popsicle, maybe eat a bite of chicken, then lick the Popsicle and poke at a carrot. During the transition, he will eat dessert first and probably won't eat those two bites of veggies, so remind yourself that bribing with dessert wasn't teaching him to learn to like veggies. This is a process that may take some time, and things will seem worse before they get better.

Dessert With the Meal Helps Selective Eating and Self-Regulation

Serving dessert with the meal makes it just another food and frees up all the energy and focus from dessert to the other wonderful options at the table. It helps with selective eating. The other piece is that it helps kids eat the right amount for them. Dessert is so yummy that if you serve it at the end of the meal, even if the child is stuffed, he will shove it in, essentially learning to overeat.

Hydee Becker, RD, tells the sad story of a little boy she observed at his daycare. He was being seen for accelerating weight gain, but the rule at daycare was that he had to eat every bite of his lunch before he could have his M&Ms, which they called his "clean plate treat." Becker recalls him saying, "but I'm full," only to be reminded of the rules.

The Problem With Bribing With Dessert

Allowing dessert with the meal is usually the thing parents struggle with most. *"But I won't be doing my job if I don't make him eat some of his real food before dessert."* And, *"How will I ever get him to eat veggies if I can't use dessert as a bribe?"* I ask parents to reflect:

- How is it working for you to bribe with dessert?
- Is it pleasant?
- Has it taught your child to learn to like a variety of foods?

Because bribing with dessert generally has several unintended consequences, it:

- Teaches kids that dessert is the only good food.
- Teaches that all other foods are a distasteful hurdle they have to get through to get to the good stuff.[13]
- Sets up nightly negotiation sessions.
- Might train the child to overeat (see below).
- Studies show that when kids are bribed or rewarded to eat a new food, they may eat it on that occasion, but they *like* the food less.[14]

> **When we bribe kids, they are suspicious. They learn, "Huh, this stuff must be really bad if Mom and Dad have to bribe me to eat it."**

Similarly, consider the emotional piece (See Chapter 6). A scene I witnessed at a Chinese buffet illustrated how setting up the two worlds of "must eat" versus "treat" was not helpful. At a table near ours, a family of three adults and a preschool-aged child were sitting with frowning faces, all the adults were staring at the child, chiming in one after the other, "Colton, you have to eat those two bites of chicken before you can have the donuts. You know the rules, two bites…" This grim scene, with Colton's grimacing, whining, and negotiating, and all the grown-ups pretty much doing the same, finally came to an end when Colton choked down the two pieces of chicken. Then, it was like a cloud lifted. All the grown-ups transformed into delightful, supportive companions, while one went to bring back a plate of donuts. The boy was praised, and everyone cheered when the donuts showed up. They had a grand time eating those delicious donuts.

We know that the combination of sugar and fat is particularly yummy and lights up those pleasure centers in the brain nicely, but equally as reinforcing was the attitude of every single adult at the table. When the "real food" was out, it was torture, but when the donuts showed up, it was rainbows and puppies. This child is learning a powerful association with the different kinds of foods, and it is not helping him learn to eat and enjoy *all* foods.

She watched him for 40 minutes, slowly eating his entire lunch *and* all his M&Ms. He was taught to ignore his body's signals, and he overate—twice. This is another reason why I am against school rules where the child has to eat a certain amount or certain foods before dessert.

For the first several months (to years) of the transition, I recommend serving dessert with the meal. As your child gets older and more skillful with eating a variety and knowing how much to eat, you can gradually move the dessert to the end of the meal.

An important point is to let your child know when there will be dessert. I made this mistake only to have a child who was too full and then disappointed she didn't have room for dessert. That was powerful to see. My daughter, who was four at the time, had eaten a lovely meal with friends. When the unplanned dessert came out, she was full, and cried while others enjoyed it—but she had listened to her body. I reassured her that she could have the dessert with lunch the next day.

No Seconds on Dessert

"But I want more ice cream. Why can't I have more ice cream?" Dessert is one portion, and you can be very matter of fact. Avoid bargaining or over-explaining. "We all get one share of dessert, and if you are still hungry, you have other choices." Some days, dessert might be fruit salad or a bowl of grapes. Avoid anger or apologizing for your limits, but you *can* acknowledge emotions. "I'm sorry you're upset, but we had ice cream yesterday. Dessert is grapes today, and we'll have ice cream again soon."

What if My Partner and I Don't Eat Dessert?

I didn't grow up eating desserts with family meals, but my husband did. After reading *Child of Mine*, I started serving desserts three to five times a week after our daughter was about age two. Before that, she didn't really know what she was missing, and none of us missed dessert either. Once she went out in the "real world" more often and was exposed to treats like ice cream and cookies, I felt I needed to be purposeful about helping her learn to manage those foods.

At most dinners, my daughter is the only one eating dessert. When she first noticed and asked why, I simply explained that I would prefer to eat more steak, potatoes, or soup than dessert. This is something that families need to work out for themselves, but if your child is really struggling handling sweets, you may want to start having dessert for a while.

What About Desserts That Melt?

Seems minor, but I get this question a lot. With an older child, you can put the Popsicle or ice cream in a little bowl and let her choose when she wants it. Sometimes it comes out at the beginning of the meal. If they are distracted and it is melting, offer to put it in the freezer. For older children, pre-scoop the ice cream in a bowl and put the bowl in the freezer. Let your child know it's there, and she can help herself when she is ready. The older child who has pretty good skills with eating can wait until the end of the meal.

Step Two of Your Sweets Strategy: The "Treat" Snack

About one to two times a week, serve a snack where a treat or formerly forbidden food (FFF) is included, and he can eat as much as he wants. When I get a call from a parent whose child is sneaking certain foods like candy or cookies, we have to find ways of bringing those high-interest foods into the meal and snack rotation.

Serving one or two as dessert, or a plate full of cookies for snack, is how. It is scary, because if your child has been limited and is craving and sneaking the FFF, he will eat lots of it initially. He may eat so much he even makes himself sick. That is part of learning how to manage the foods. Hovering and warning him not to eat too many is not the point.

It might look like this: after school, make together and serve a pan of Rice Krispies treats. Sit down and enjoy it with milk. Allow him to lick the spoon. You can serve it with a favorite fruit so he has the option of getting a little more balance. I recommend trying to offer some fat and protein as well, which is why one or two percent milk is so nice. Another option is to make the treat a trip to the local candy store to buy a bag of candy. Pour out the candy, serve with milk, and enjoy. When he only eats the candy and is hungry sooner, don't lecture or punish. (Put leftovers in your candy jar in the cupboard to enjoy here and there with meals and snacks.) Consider allowing an appetizer before dinner, commenting once with, "Yeah, when I only eat candy, I get hungry really fast, too." Let him know he can choose a few pieces of candy for his lunch the next day.

The "treat" snack can be hard for many parents. If it is for you, start with something that feels safer, like homemade oatmeal-raisin cookies with milk, and go from there. With time, you should see your child eat a little less, perhaps slower, and possibly choosing a banana or other options. I remember being amazed after we did this for a while that my daughter, after one or two Rice Krispies treats, milk, and half a kiwi, would stop. Just like that.

Halloween, Valentine's Day, Easter, St. Patrick's Day...

Every year before Halloween, I would re-read the Halloween section *in Child of Mine*. Handling the candy stash is particularly anxiety provoking for many parents, and it's not just Halloween anymore. It seems that at every holiday gathering, my daughter came home with a bag of candy. We have had many opportunities to deal with the candy stash with a strategy we have successfully implemented for years, always with a little surprise on my part.

On Halloween, my daughter gets to bring her stash home, dump it out, and take out the stuff she doesn't like (luckily for me, she doesn't like peanut butter, so I look forward to my Reese's). She can eat as much as she wants. We usually sit at the kitchen table with a glass of milk. She samples a few, spits out many she doesn't like, and usually ends up eating from three to six pieces of candy and is done.

We put it away, and the next day, she again gets to eat as much as she wants, at snack time with a glass of milk—a treat snack. After that she gets to choose one or two pieces to go in her lunch box or as dessert with dinner. Usually within a handful of days she forgets it is there, and we add it to our candy container in the cupboard. It has been remarkably painless. If you are new to the process, your child might eat a lot more, but he might also surprise you.

> *"I was tired of negotiating. The whole 'How many spoonfuls of this do I have to eat to get my pudding?' thing is so tiresome. (Pudding is dessert in Australia). The first time I let Thomas eat his Easter stash, he ate and ate until I was sure he would be sick. And then he stopped two pieces before he'd eaten it all. Just like that. It was almost as if he had to test if I really meant that he could have as much as he wanted. My daughter didn't even want that much. And now, a couple of years on, their Easter chocolate lasts until the summer. Not because I'm restricting it. It's there and available, but they don't often feel like eating it."*
> — Mira, mother to Thomas and Emma

Hydee Becker, RD, does this with her son, and in past years he followed a similar pattern. The year he was age five, he ate the entire haul before bed, with nothing left even for treat snack the next day. I loved how Becker approached it with curiosity. "I wonder what he'll do next year?" If they do eat a whole lot, avoid the temptation to intervene. Let the process play out; if overconsumption is routinely a problem, reassess if you are allowing enough "treat snacks" or are interfering in some way, such as lots of commenting.

Putting "Formerly Forbidden Foods" (FFF) Away

Think of sweets as a learning opportunity for you and your child, and be curious. I learned a lot the year we ended up with two gingerbread houses, one we made at home and one made at school. Sitting in the middle of the dining room, they were always in sight and on my daughter's mind. My competent eater was pestering me about it several times a day, occasionally taking a nibble or two when she thought I wasn't looking. (NOTE: The occasional sneaking of food is normal at this stage, but habitual, secretive bingeing is not.)

On December 26, we had a "treat" snack where she had some milk and got to eat as much of the candy from the gingerbread house as she wanted. She had about the equivalent of one to two teaspoons of scraped frosting and four or five pieces of candy with some milk. She had wanted some gummy bears, but said she was full. I didn't want her only choice to be to eat them now or throw them away (which would trigger the "scarcity effect" and make her more likely to overeat), so I told her she could have the handful of gummies with her snack that afternoon. We tossed the rest without incident.

This story illustrates treat handling, but also the concept of keeping foods put away and out of sight. With my clients who have kids transitioning to the Trust Model, I recommend putting food away. Most kids who see candy or cookies will ask for it, regardless of hunger, especially those who have been restricted. Keeping these treats in a cupboard and purposefully serving them at fairly regular intervals at meals and snack times will help children learn to incorporate these foods into a normal, balanced diet.

Michelle Allison, a nutritionist who writes at www.TheFatNutritionist.com, says this about putting food away, or "in its place:" *"Now, it's one thing to think: 'Yeah, some cookies would be awesome right now,' and you go and get some cookies, and indeed they are awesome. It's another thing entirely if you pick cookies by default because they were there and you didn't have any better ideas."*

What About Dairy?

I get asked a lot about milk. Low fat? Organic? Soy? Here is a quick rundown of my thoughts on dairy.

Milk, yogurt, and cheese can be a really easy, delicious choice to help you offer your child balanced nutrition. Dairy makes providing snacks and meals easier. Regular, reduced- and low-fat milk and yogurt provide carbohydrates, protein, and fat. Cheeses provide protein and fat, and all provide calcium.

Milk and other dairy foods provide nine essential nutrients, including vitamin D and A and calcium and riboflavin. The USDA defines an "essential nutrient" as a dietary substance required for healthy body functioning.

> Ultra-pasteurized milk boxes are now in stores in both chocolate and white milk at one and two percent fat, and are a great way to balance out a snack on the go and cover protein and fat needs.

About Lactose Intolerance

Lactose intolerance is higher in children of African, Asian, and Central American descent versus those of northern European descent. Many parents assume their child will be lactose intolerant, and ask about going straight from formula to soymilk, "just to be safe." Universally, infants are born with the ability to digest lactose, the sugar found in human or cow's milk, so infants should be able to digest lactose even if they lose that ability as toddlers or young children.

Lactose intolerance is usually characterized by a set of symptoms:
- Abdominal discomfort
- Bloating
- Gas
- Abdominal pain
- Decreased appetite
- Loose stools

Lactose intolerance does not necessarily mean that your child can't tolerate any dairy, and it is not the same thing as a dairy *allergy*, where you would want to carefully read labels and avoid milk or milk products entirely. (Remember, a true allergy is an immune response, often to small amounts of the trigger food, with common symptoms related to histamine release, including hives, mouth and throat tingling, and swelling.)

Humans living in cultures that evolved along with domesticated cattle over the last several thousand years had a survival advantage if they could use dairy as a nutrition source beyond early childhood. A genetic mutation allowed some individuals to produce the lactase enzyme and benefit from dairy, a great source of calories, fat, and protein that may have otherwise been scarce. These individuals survived at a higher rate and passed that genetic mutation on until more than 90 percent of Northern Europeans now have that gene. China, for example, didn't domesticate cows until relatively recently, so there was no advantage to pass on any genetic mutation that allowed for lactose digestion; therefore, we see higher rates of lactose intolerance in those of Chinese descent.

Studies have demonstrated that many adults diagnosed with lactose intolerance can comfortably consume the amount of lactose in one cup (eight ounces) of milk with a meal, or two cups divided over the day with food.[15]

If your child has stomach problems or upset, it is reasonable to attempt a dairy-free trial. (See special "therapeutic" diets on page 219 for more information.) Stomach upset or loose stools are a tricky thing to figure out, particularly if 1) there is a language barrier, 2) your child is pre-verbal, 3) there have been infections or parasites, or 4) he's had multiple rounds of antibiotics, in which case you may also want to supplement with probiotics and a fish or flax oil supplement.

Reintroducing Dairy

Natalie had been off all gluten and dairy for almost a year to see if it would improve her low energy and loose stools. Mom had been careful to be sure she had not taken in any dairy or gluten. Unfortunately, her symptoms did not improve, and Mom felt that reintroducing dairy slowly would help her to meet Natalie's nutritional needs and make snacks and meals easier. She started with small amounts of hard cheeses a few times a week and watched for any changes. With no change in her daughter's behavior, stools, or activity, Mom gradually increased the amount of cheese offered and also introduced yogurt. Natalie had not yet chosen to drink milk, which may mean she just doesn't like it right now, or that she is lactose intolerant and it would make her uncomfortable. While we worked to rehabilitate the feeding relationship after years of food battles, Natalie's energy and activity began to improve.

Consider these options as well:
- Studies have shown that chocolate milk is better tolerated in some people with lactose intolerance.[16]
- More aged cheeses like Cheddar, Swiss, Parmesan, and Colby tend to be better tolerated since they are lower in lactose.[15]
- Yogurts with live, active cultures can be comfortably consumed by some.
- Lactose-free milk.
- Lactaid helps digest the lactose and reduce symptoms.

What If My Child Can't Drink Cow's Milk—or We Choose Not To?

Goat's milk, cow's milk, and soymilk have roughly similar protein and calories, though soy has lower fat content. Rice milk, on the other hand, is not nearly as nutritious, and I do not recommend it as a standard dairy alternative. Almond milk has one gram of protein, versus eight grams in cow's milk. Almond milk does have added calcium, vitamins and minerals, but is also lower in fat and calories. Almond milk is made from crushed almonds and water, so it is clearly not appropriate for persons with tree nut allergies.

If a child has allergies or intolerances and needs to have any food groups removed, whether they include dairy or gluten, a consultation with a pediatric RD is in order. This is particularly true if your child has experienced malnutrition or catch-up growth with increased nutritional demands.

The Official Recommendation on Dairy

The Dietary Guidelines for Americans (DGA)[17] encourage all Americans to increase intake of low-fat or fat-free milk and milk products to the recommended daily amounts: 2 cups for children two to three years of age, 2½ cups for children four to eight years of age, and 3 cups for those nine years of age and older. Milk is the number one food source of three of the four nutrients the DGA identified as lacking in the American diet: calcium, vitamin D, and potassium.

The following are some thoughts on serving dairy:
- Try not to focus on serving recommendations. Aim for an average over several days. If you try to push a certain number of servings every day, that invites pressure, and you know what that does.
- No studies show that fat-free dairy for small children lowers body mass index (BMI), and there is concern that fat-free dairy tactics cause some young children to not get enough fat.[18] Infants and toddlers less than two years of age need 30 to 40 percent of their calories from fat, and dairy can help provide that. Another study showed that the kids who drank whole milk actually had the lowest BMI scores of the children studied.[19]
- After age two, children need about 25 to 30 percent of their calories from fat. The recommendation is to switch to 2 percent or 1 percent milk at that time.

- Diets too low in fat can result in vitamin deficiencies, as vitamin A, D, E, and K are fat soluble, meaning they need to be ingested with some fat so they can be absorbed by the body.

The bottom line is to enjoy what tastes good. If your teen will only drink 2 percent milk or even whole milk, but it is within the framework of a healthy feeding relationship, I believe you can feel good serving those choices.

An aside about fat: For years, "low fat" was the recommendation, and we weren't supposed to eat eggs, red meat, or cheese—and as a country, we got bigger. In place of the fat, many food manufacturers simply increased the amount of sugar and simple carbohydrates. I am comfortable saying that one should avoid trans fats (hydrogenated fats), but there is controversy about how much saturated fat (from animal sources like meat or dairy) is "ideal." Many of the health concerns around saturated fat are now understood to be largely attributed to highly processed trans fats.[20,21] With that said, there is a lot we don't know. In general, with my "nutrition recommendations," if you follow the goal of variety, you will be fine. Some fat sources come from meat, fish, dairy, and eggs, and plan to offer some plant sources like avocadoes, olive oil, nuts, and nut butters.

He Won't Drink His Milk

One of my most popular blog post series was about my daughter not drinking milk for almost a year. Avoid pressure, even over milk. You can meet nutritional needs without milk, though it may take a little more planning.

When my daughter declined milk, I continued to offer milk with meals and snacks, and looked for ways to support her calcium intake from other food sources, such as yogurt. This was when I bought Go-Gurt for snacks (sometimes she would eat three at a time) and cooked with evaporated milk and additional broccoli, which has a good amount of calcium. There are great online resources about boosting calcium, and a whole appendix in *Child of Mine* devoted to the topic.

This was also a time when I got to experiment and observe my child. I reached out to colleagues with my concern, and one suggested I just serve milk to everyone at the table, and calmly say, "We are all having milk." My stubborn child was having none of it, and it resulted in a battle and lots of complaining. Lesson learned. I knew she felt that approach as pressuring because of how she reacted, so I backed off and let her come back to milk, on her own time, which she did.

It was a good reminder for me that this is a process that parents and kids figure out together.

"He Hardly Drinks Anything!"

The child who will refuse to drink to the point of dehydration is extremely rare, but it happens. If you are battling over drinking liquids, it can interfere with his tuning in to thirst cues. (Urinary tract infections or dark urine need to be evaluated by your child's doctor.) Also keep in mind that some children do fine on less liquids than others.

One client used to bribe with a favored food to try to get her son to drink liquids, with the predictable results of him engaging in battles and drinking *less.* The point is to identify a need and find ways to offer choices that meet that need.

The following are some ideas to boost fluid intake without getting into battles:

- Stop pressuring.
- Change the delivery: use a fancy cup or straw or a water bottle with her favorite cartoon character. As one mom recently said, *"It's amazing what she'll drink if I just put a straw in it."*
- Add ice if she likes it cold, or try it at room temperature.
- Have a tea party at snack time, with teacups and caffeine-free fruit tea. And go ahead: let her add some sugar or honey (if she's more than a year old). At a tea party, my then four-year-old daughter loved pouring the tea into her tiny teacup so much that she drank two pots. This can also work with diluted lemonade, water, or milk. Expect spills.
- Let them pour when possible. Use a small pitcher or creamer and give them some control.
- Enjoy hot chocolate together. Pretend not to notice if he doesn't drink much. Float a few marshmallows on top if he likes them.
- Find a way for your child to be able to help himself to water (see drink gear on page 199).
- Serve fruits, veggies, or other foods with high water content. There is a surprising amount of fluid in many foods, and sweet fruits like watermelon, other melons, or strawberries are often accepted. Try cherry tomatoes (cut in half if you have a young child) or cucumbers with or without dip. Serve fruit frozen occasionally or pack fruit with snacks, like those little cups of sliced peaches or mandarin oranges.
- Serve soups, Jell-O, pudding, or smoothies. Consider frozen fruit treats; you can make your own, too.
- Offer juice. Juice is not the enemy it is made out to be. If you haven't tried it, juice is an option with meals and snacks (see page 228).

He Drinks Too Much Milk

Some toddlers take in a lot of milk (more than 16 to 24 ounces a day), and it interferes with appetite and nutrition. When I see this, other things are usually going on. These kids most often are allowed to drink milk throughout the day and carry it around in a sippy cup. Or, the child is "picky" and pressured to eat or is struggling with variety. For the child, sometimes it is easier to get calories from milk than to fight with Mom and Dad.

The following are some options to manage milk intake:
- Offer milk or water with meals and snacks.
- Only water in between.
- Stop pressuring with foods, if you have been.
- Change to serving milk in a cup if she is able to drink from it (usually between 12 and 18 months of age.)
- If your older child still has a sippy cup of milk before breakfast, replace that morning ritual with something else and move the milk to breakfast time.
- Consider getting a water bubbler so she can serve herself water.
- Consider occasionally offering watered-down fruit nectar or juice with meals and snacks.

Flavored Milk

While my daughter shunned milk, I offered her chocolate and strawberry milk, even syrups she could mix herself, none of which appealed to her. When I get asked about flavored milk, it's usually over a concern about calories, sugar, or corn syrup. I would rather a child drink and enjoy chocolate milk versus no milk, and we have no conclusive evidence that flavored milk contributes to weight acceleration in children.

Many brands have been reformulated to have less sugar, and no high-fructose corn syrup, if that worries you. Many of my RD colleagues are very happy to see their children enjoying chocolate milk. As always, you choose what to offer, but this is another area where I feel the hype is exaggerated. If flavored milk is offered in the context of a healthy feeding relationship, with variety and structure, I think it's a good option.

What About Hormones and Organic?

The decision of what milk to buy is a personal one. Many moms I talk to want to buy organic but can't afford it, as it is usually several dollars more per gallon. One mommy blogger, who is also an RD, has admitted that she feels fine buying conventional milk, but is self-conscious about this controversial topic. Many moms feel guilty if they don't buy organic milk.

Let go of that guilt. Standard milk in the United States is highly controlled and safe to drink. On a tour of a family-run Minnesota dairy farm, I saw cows that seemed unstressed, walked themselves calmly (single-file) into the milking stalls, and chewed their cuds on clean hay.

Dairy cows are not routinely treated with antibiotics, like some chickens, hogs, and farmed fish are, though this practice is changing, too. If a cow is sick, perhaps with mastitis (an infection of the milk-producing glands), she is treated with antibiotics, and her milk is not put into the milk supply. Milk is tested both on the farm and again at processing centers for any traces of antibiotics. If antibiotics are found, the farmer pays a large penalty, so they have a vested interest in keeping the milk free from antibiotics.

Do you need to buy milk from cows not treated with rBST (artificial Bovine Somatotropin) to be safe? The milk from cows treated with rBST (which increases production) and untreated cows is identical on testing. In other words, you cannot detect any different levels of the hormone in the milk.[22] Milk does contain hormones that are made naturally from the cow, but rBST and dairy in general has not been proven to affect hormones in children or early puberty, if that's your concern. Bottom line: If your choice is no milk versus rBST or organic, I believe you can feel safe about the standard milk.

But, again, *what* you serve is up to you, the parent, and is a personal choice. I purposely steer clear of recommending certain foods or commenting on food politics because every family I interact with is doing the best they can to feed their families. For many families, organic, or even fresh quality produce, is not an affordable or practical option (try lugging your groceries home on the bus with children, no sidewalk, and limited kitchen space).

If it is important to you, learn more about your food choices and do what you feel is best. The above information was intended to help decrease some of the worry and anxiety around these food choices.

Chapter 9
Taking the Lead:
The Feeding Relationship Dance

You can either feed to support and nurture your child's inborn cues of hunger and fullness, or feed in a way that sabotages and buries those skills. The choice is yours.

Having worked with clients in their homes and by phone, the thing parents struggle with most is making the transition from their current counterproductive feeding practices to the Trust Model. On one blog forum on picky eating, a mom asked about the Division of Responsibility (DOR), "How is this stuff supposed to work?" This chapter is intended to help with the transition. Because for many struggling families personal support is not possible, I've given additional ideas and support as you work through those common stumbling blocks to show you how this "stuff" does indeed work.

As Ellyn Satter says, the feeding relationship is a dance between the parent and child.

To feed in the Trust Model, the parent and child have distinct roles. The parent observes and responds to the child—the parent *leads* in this dance, but is tuned in and responsive to cues from the child. You lead, but you are in tune with your partner, your child. Is he pushing back? Is he going with the flow? Are you enjoying yourselves? You might have to fake the confidence at first, as you will stumble a few times as you learn; but with time, you will get more comfortable as you build your skills, and it will be more fun.

Are you ready to lead or do you feel driven by your fears, your child's demands, and/or advice from doctors, family, and friends? If you've been using feeding practices that are simply not helping, and are interested in transitioning to the Trust Model, get ready. This is a leap of faith.

What You Will Learn

This chapter is informative, but hopefully also a little fun. Read it, go through the exercises, and do the role-playing with a partner, friend, or book club. This is the "homework" that can help you move forward.

I work with my individual clients through their blocks as well as reassure and support them with phone calls or emails during the transition (detailed in Chapters 3, 4, and 5). I can help them make it through the hardest parts—the buffets, the vacations, the pushy grandparents, the worries about size and nutrition—until they see their child's capabilities with eating begin to emerge. Those capabilities show up when a food-preoccupied child leaves food on his plate for the first time or goes to play with friends instead of eating for an entire party, or when a selective eater happily munches a few of the meal offerings rather than fussing for a favored food, or tries a new soup out of curiosity.

Make no mistake: If you have been pressuring, and you take that pressure away, *your child's eating will seem to get worse before it gets better*. This is normal and expected. He is testing the new rules and learning to tune in to those perhaps long-buried cues of hunger and fullness.

As we reviewed in the topic chapters:
- If you have been restricting, it's almost certain that she will eat far more than you feel comfortable allowing her to eat.
- If you have been pressuring him to eat more, he will eat less for a time, or he may even eat nothing on occasion.
- If you have been threatening or bribing to get certain foods in—like protein or veggies—he won't eat them, perhaps even for a long time.
- Your selective eater may even eat *fewer* foods for a while.

Scary stuff.

Early successes reinforce and strengthen a parent's resolve to feed in the Trust Model—when you begin to see that your child *can* be trusted. But waiting for those early signs is the hardest part. I help parents hang in there until it happens. I am that coach, cheering and pointing out successes along the way, but I also *challenge* parents to observe and look critically at their feeding. I hope that this book, and the advice and successes that families have shared, will help you hang in there while you wait for signs of progress. In the meantime, challenge yourself:
- Do you really trust your children?
- Are you really being reliable with structure and offering balance?
- Where are you getting stuck?

How Long Will This Take?

This is the number one question I get asked. We all want results, right now! Some feeding clinics and therapists promise results on a timetable; in fact, they are often required to produce results for insurance purposes. Be aware that progress in the clinic setting may not translate into progress in the real world (as many of my clients have experienced), and the pressure to see results can lead therapists and parents to pressure the child, which slows the process.

Sue says it took about seven months for her toddler with oral-motor delay and sensitivity, and her son, who was older when he joined their family, took almost a year to begin to increase his food choices. Nora, whose daughter was age five and ate less than 10 foods when she came home, had slow progress—with fits and starts—until about four years in. Nora says today, *"I actually think she is a better eater now than most of her peers."*

Some selective eaters don't really branch out until they are teens or leave for college. One mom told me her that 15-year-old son starting trying new foods because he was interested in dating, and didn't want to be "ordering off the kiddie menu." Another dad told about his selective daughter who learned to try all kinds of new foods in her first year of college.

Getting the Division of Responsibility (DOR) down can take time. Some folks already have the structure, variety, and family meal habit and only need to work on serving family style or backing off on pressure. Other families are starting in a more difficult place, with challenges such as grazing, intense conflict, and no family meals. If there are growth concerns or nutritional deficits, trusting this process is *even harder* and tends to take longer, and you may benefit from additional support.

Once the DOR is in place, which may take days or weeks or months, the time it takes for a child to begin to tune in to hunger and fullness cues, or branch out in terms of variety, depends on age and other factors such as the severity of restriction or pressure or the intensity of the child's history around food.

> Pam Estes, RD, and Patty Morse, RD, CDE, are registered dietitians with more than 30 years of combined experience with the Trust Model working with families with feeding tubes, complicated medical and developmental issues, weight worries, and selective eating. They describe how they, too, initially had to make that leap of faith. At first, as they helped families transition to the DOR, they admitted their own doubts, wondering, "Will this work?" It wasn't long before both transitioned from, "Will this work?" to "How long will it take?"

For neurotypical children with problems such as "overeating" or "picky" eating, a toddler might take four to six weeks; a grade-schooler, six to eight weeks; and a high schooler, three to six months. Adults tend to need much longer—from months to years—depending on the severity of the original problem. The process can take longer if one has developmental or oral-motor delay and if there is a prolonged or traumatic history with feeding. I have seen a 10-year-old feeding clinic "failure" with selective eating branch out and rehabilitate his attitude toward food in a few weeks, and "food-obsessed" toddlers learning what "full" feels like in less than a month. Other clients have taken six months or more than a year to really see an improvement in variety or volume.

According to my clients, another valuable resource is Satter's DVD, *Feeding With Love and Good Sense II.* When you are in the thick of it, it can be hard to be objective about what is going on in your own home. Watching dozens of other families struggle and figure out feeding, all with insightful narrative, is an incredible gift. Let's face it; life is busy, so watching a DVD with your partner may be more practical than reading another book. Antonia shared, *"My husband and I watched the DVD together, and it was amazing to see in all these families how the kids reacted to the pressure. It made me look at what I was doing from my kid's point of view."*

Even if you have a teen or a seven-year-old, watch the DVD from the beginning or read *Child of Mine*, which covers infancy through kindergarten age. Even if you weren't with your child or don't know his history during that age, you are learning a new way of thinking about food and development, and it's all relevant. Also, even though your child may be two years old with her physical development, she may be more like an "almost toddler" when it comes to food or her emotional and psychosocial development, so learning about typical stages and development with feeding is helpful.

Compare your child only to herself, not to other children her own age.

Now I will veer into what may seem like sexist territory. In my professional experience, almost every time, the moms are the ones who read the parenting and feeding books and the dads pick up whatever information filters through by osmosis. This was the case in my own home where the parenting, sleep, and feeding books crowded my nightstand, while *Autoweek, Cycle World*, and *Smithsonian* magazines were on my husband's side. Luckily, he was more than willing to listen to my explanations and follow my lead. Ideally, anyone who is taking part in the feeding of the child will learn about the model. This leap of faith is tricky, and the more you can learn, challenge, understand the research, and read about other parents' stories for yourself, the easier this process will be.

Leap of Faith

You are either reading this in preparation for your child's arrival, already at your wits' end, or somewhere in between. Here is how this process usually unfolds with my clients.

You have known for a while that things aren't right with feeding. You feel conflicted, confused, and not competent. I've been there, too. Something has to change, but you don't know what or how, and everything you have tried hasn't helped. You've done an Internet search, a book arrives, and you (usually Mom) read a few sections or look in the index for a particular concern, and you try a few things. At this point, this is what I hear:

- *"I don't know how to make this work in our family."*
- *"I tried this for three days, but our three-year-old ate more than my husband, and I got scared!"*
- *"If I don't bribe with dessert, he'll only eat bread."*
- *"Well, we're trying a 'modified' version, but he still eats only five things."*
- *"This was supposed to take a few weeks; we've been at it for over a month and we're still fighting all the time."*

- *"We experimented with the dessert with the meal, but still insisted he had to eat his vegetables. It was still miserable."*
- *"My husband just can't let them eat dessert if they don't eat at least some of the meal."*

These families continue to struggle. Maybe things are *a little* better, maybe they are worse because now they feel they have failed again, or the skeptical partner (after three days) uses it as proof that the Trust Model *"just won't work for our child."*

Take the dad (please) who challenged me during a workshop. It was the second time I had talked to this dad's group, and in front of all the other dads (most of whom had not heard this message before), he said, *"This doesn't work. I'm doing everything you say to do, and my daughter is still really picky, and we are still fighting at meals. It's been a year!"*

I asked him a few more questions. It turns out he and his wife were so worried about calcium that they still forced their daughter to drink a glass of milk with every meal. So no, they hadn't quite made that leap of faith, nor trusted the process. They believed they were doing it all right, but were missing a big piece. And they were still engaging in a power struggle at every meal.

Or take Sue, who admitted she had serious doubts after she read Satter's *How to Get Your Kid to Eat: But Not Too Much*, recommended by the nurse practitioner at her international adoption (IA) clinic when her son's eating and tantrums were an issue. *"I read the book before seeing the speech therapist. Since I had already worked with her with our daughter, I trusted her. I read the book and went in feeling, frankly, it was a bunch of baloney, and not how things work in my home. Never mind the fact that I also knew at the time that 'the way things work' in my home was not working. I went to the appointment and discovered the high regard in which the nurse practitioner held this book. I got quiet and listened."*

If you can believe in and go *all the way* with the Trust Model, you and your child can truly reap the benefits of a healthy feeding relationship. When someone says to me after a workshop, "I'm going to try to serve dessert with dinner tonight," it doesn't bode well. When parents pick and choose one or two pieces of advice from a workshop and don't take the time to understand the model, they usually find that it doesn't "work" the way they hoped and they quickly give up. Learn as much as you need to, read the testimonials and blog posts, watch a video, get buy-in from your partner, and believe in your heart this is what you want to do *before* you jump in. Rome wasn't built in a day, and you won't rehabilitate a difficult feeding relationship over one meal of mac-n-cheese.

Why Bother?

What are the benefits of a healthy feeding relationship? You are more likely to:

- Look forward to eating with your child.
- Have confidence in your feeding choices.
- Enjoy more variety and rediscover your joy of cooking and eating.
- Feel free to love your kids with less worry about weight or size.

- Stop worrying about who is eating what or how much. As one mom put it, *"I get to be a mom again, not a food cop!"*

Your child is more likely to:
- Have stable and healthy weight
- Learn to eat based on internal (from her own body) cues of hunger and fullness
- Eat a variety of foods and enjoy better nutrition, and feel confident and competent in all aspects of his life
- Be "eating competent" and avoid dieting and other disordered eating behaviors

Letting Go of Control

**To make that leap of faith, you also have to let go of what you can't control.
Or rather, let go of the illusion of control.**

Many religious traditions sum it up in so many words: *We suffer when we fight against that which we cannot control.* If you are a spiritual or religious person, this can feel like a test of faith or a spiritual journey. For the spiritual person, thinking of it in these terms and leaning on your faith tradition can help. My serenity prayer for feeding is really about letting go of control.

Serenity Prayer for Feeding
Grant me the serenity to accept the things I cannot change:
- My child's genetic weight
  - · It might be bigger or smaller than average, but it can be healthy
- My child's temperament
  - · An easygoing, curious child will more easily accept new foods than a cautious or strong-willed child
- My child's history with feeding
- My child's allergies
- *My* temperament
- My own feeding history
- My dieting or eating disorder history
- Factors that are not changeable in the immediate future, such as finances or kitchen setup
- Other? _____

Grant me the courage to change the things I can:
- Feeding without pressure
- Being reliable about family meals and structure

- Providing a pleasant atmosphere at the table
- Working toward offering a variety of foods
- My attitude about my own and others' bodies
- Appropriately managing behavior at the table, but not what or how much my child eats from what is offered
- My general parenting skills
- My communication with my partner
- My cooking skills
- My own selective eating
- Focus on healthy behaviors, not numbers on the scale

And the wisdom to know the difference:
- I am learning by:
  - Trusting
  - Looking for those little signs of progress and building faith
  - Reading books, resources, and attending workshops
  - Getting help

What Are *You* Bringing to the Family Table?

To understand your role in the feeding relationship, as with all aspects of parenting, you may need to take some time exploring your own past, particularly as it relates to food. Many American adults have a difficult relationship with food, and this makes feeding more complicated.

One dad shared that he didn't want to do family meals because they were too "formal," and he wanted eating to be fun for his kids. He recalled as a child not being able to talk at the table, and lots of pressure to eat. Exploring his feelings about meals being formal helped him get past a block. He learned to accept that having the ketchup bottle on the table, serving from take-out containers, and having fun together during meals were all okay—in fact, they were great. He found that he really liked family meals once he freed himself up from his image of what they should be.

Another mom says she hated being forced to eat veggies growing up, and that's the main thing she remembers—always being the center of attention as the picky eater. She had a great wariness of pressure because she didn't want her kids to feel the same way, but her husband wanted to make them eat veggies. She just needed a little reassurance that no, she wasn't overreacting by not wanting Dad to pressure, and that as long as she had family meals and provided them with lots of pleasant opportunities to enjoy veggies, she was feeding well and giving her kids the best chance to learn to like veggies. She and her husband needed to have some long talks and get a little reassurance from me as they tried to reconcile their different approaches. They both agreed that what they were doing wasn't working and were willing to change.

Consider Your Expectations

"I never realized how important it was that I not raise a 'picky eater' until I was strug-gling so hard to get him to try new foods. I had to question what the worst outcome could be. Would my mothering be a failure if my son never liked vegetables? I had to learn to lighten up my ideal of how I wanted him to eat, and just take things one bite at a time." — Sue, mother to Marcus

"Almost all of our meals growing up were eaten together around our dining table and were cooked by my mom. This instilled in me a routine of serving nutritious meals. While this was a positive, it was also a stumbling block, as it fed my frustrations with a child who refused to eat in a well-rounded manner."
   —Brigid, mother of Mena, adopted from India

"I am not a picky eater at all, and quite frankly, adults who are picky eaters annoy me, so I have not wanted my daughter to grow up and be picky."
   —Jim, father of Ava, adopted from Russia

Once you are aware of your expectations, hold them up against what you learned in this book about this process and how long it takes. You can then reevaluate whether your expectations are realistic or not. Being aware of the range of experience with these problems may help you readjust your expectations and move forward with more appropriate and attainable goals. Often, expecting too much leads to less than supportive feeding.

Reflect on Your Own Feeding Past

Our past informs how we parent, and this is true for feeding as well. Do we simply do as was done to us, or seek out the complete opposite? Perhaps somewhere in between is the way to go?

- How were *you* fed as a child?
    - What does a "family meal" mean to you? _____

      _____

    - Did you have family meals as a child? _____
    - What do you remember fondly about family meals? _____

      _____

    - What did you dislike about how you were fed? _____

      _____

- How do you think your relationship with food is now? _____

  _____

- How has it been in the past? _____

  _____

- Have you struggled with an eating disorder? _____
- Have you struggled with your weight? _____
- Did you have times growing up when you didn't have enough food?

  _____

- Have you dieted? _____
- Other? _____
- Additional notes: _____

  _____

  _____

Are any of the following tactics familiar to you from when you were a child? In other words, were any of these done to you? (Check any that apply):

_____ Bargaining

_____ Bribing (a sticker, toy car, extra TV time if you ate a certain food)

_____ Rewarding good behavior with food

_____ Promising a special food, such as dessert, for eating something or trying a food

_____ Persuading you to eat ("Come on, you want to grow up to be healthy and strong, don't you?")

_____ Playing a game to get you to eat

_____ Forcing

_____ Withholding food as punishment

_____ Taking over and feeding if you refused to eat (spoon-feeding a capable five-year-old)

_____ Threatening punishment for not eating

_____ Making you clean your plate

If any of these tactics were attempted with you, do you think they hurt or helped *your* eating? How did it make you feel?

Now look at the list above, but this time think about how you are feeding *your child*.

- Do you use any of the tactics to get your child to eat? If so, which ones?

  _____

- How long have you been using the tactics? _____
- Do you find you have to constantly "up the ante," as in negotiate longer, give better bribes, etc.? _____

If you are using pressure tactics, are they "successful?" (Note that most feeding tactics work a little, for a while at least.) _____

How do you define "success" with feeding? (Check any that apply):

_____How much your child eats?

_____Your child's behavior?

_____What he eats?

_____How he is growing?

When you think about what you have learned about the transition process, can you think of other ways to define "success" moving forward? _____

_____

If your child is used to eating *what, when,* and/or *where* he wants, what could happen if you start with structure and family meals?_____

_____

Consider Personality—Yours and Your Child's

The following is a quick refresher and description of the basic categories of temperaments or personalities around learning to like new foods:

- **Outgoing (or easy-going) and curious:** Generally likes to try new foods; a "no-thank-you-bite" rule may be fine with this child. "Hey, I *do* like this!"
- **Cautious and sensitive:** The initial response is almost always rejection, and it may take years before this child learns to expand his tastes.
- **Somewhere in between:** May not try a food the first few times, or like it when they do, but over the years learns to like the family's foods.

Think back to your personality, childhood, and your family of origin.

- **Which type describes you as a child?** _____

  · Did it change? Were you "picky" as a child but branched out in high school, for example? _____

  · Which one do you think describes your child? _____

- Does understanding your child's food "personality" help you feel more calm and patient with the process? _____

It's Important to Take Care of *You*

Prolonged problems of any kind, particularly with a child, are incredibly stressful. Aside from the adjustment of adding another family member, as well as a number of other things you might face—dealing with a traumatized child, financial burdens, navigating the foster care system, and behavioral or school problems—the additional worries about health, growth, and nutrition all make it worse.

When feeding isn't going well or there are concerns about growth, parents say they feel like they are failing at parenting and nurturing on a most fundamental level. When friends, family, and doctors pile on and imply that you aren't doing enough or aren't doing the right therapy, you're doing it wrong, you "aren't compliant" with a diet, or your child is "obese" or "failing to thrive," it feels awful.

Clients I work with have often struggled for years with feeding and weight worries. Many mothers have cried during sessions, sharing feelings of hopelessness, anger, regret, and an overwhelming sense of failure and guilt. The December 2011 *Infant, Child, & Adolescent Nutrition Journal* devoted to pediatric feeding problems acknowledged, "Many families have developed a negative pattern of feeding that is so pervasive it can result in clinically significant mental health symptoms for parents. Anxiety and depression are very common and can leave parents feeling hopeless, afraid, and unable to make changes in the mealtime patterns."[1]

Indeed, on our third call together, Maxine, mother of Asiah, cried, *"I've just been dealing with this for so long, I feel like I am at the bottom of a dark pit."* I highly suspected that she was to the point of being clinically depressed, and urged her to seek counseling and an evaluation.

You can't take care of your kids if you are falling apart.

Maxine *had* made impressive changes, but was still struggling with instituting the DOR. Her assessment, from her dark pit, was that *"Nothing is better; she is still so obsessed with food, and I feel like there is no hope that she will ever get this."* I gently pointed out that in the same call, Maxine had shared at least five stories where they had made major progress, such as the successful transition of the morning bottle to breakfast time, and that her daughter had on a few occasions left food on her plate and left the table without fussing—things she had never done in the years since she had joined the family.

From her "dark pit," it was hard for Maxine to see the light. She had trouble seeing and acting on the positive changes, and was sliding back to old counterproductive practices (pulling a screaming Asiah out of her highchair to end a meal) because she thought, "nothing was working."

Nurture Your Bond With Your Partner

If you are married or in a committed relationship, these struggles can wear down your bond with your partner. It is well known that in general, marital satisfaction plummets when small children enter the picture. Consider the stress on your partnership from perhaps years of fertility treatments, the months and years of paperwork and hoop jumping to complete your adoption, or the precious little time you had to prepare for the siblings who came to you through the foster system in the middle of the night. Add on possible medical and growth concerns, uncertainty, and frustration at doing everything you are told, only to continue to suffer. One mother, stuck in an incredibly painful and dysfunctional feeding relationship for more than two years, says that the feeding and weight worries were *"ripping our family apart."*

It may be a generalization, but I have often observed that it's the mothers who are more consumed with this topic, while the dads in these families have the more traditional role of coming in for dinner and not seeing or being part of the day-long turmoil. Many do not understand "what the fuss is all about." Mothers have often shared that they feel incredibly isolated and their marriages suffer as a result.

I am not dumping on dads or the partners who seem less worried. Often, they simply don't see the extent of the struggle or judgment from others. In general, male partners seem to worry less, and let's face it, most men have had an easier history with food and body image than women. This can be an asset when the other parent is more anxious or stuck in that dark pit.

Different parenting styles and personalities can be a gift to a child.

Dads and partners, if your partner is staying home and dealing with "I'm hungry!" non-stop, or "I'm not eating!" for hours on end, he or she is the one who is bearing the brunt of the accusations of parental neglect or incompetence—from what feels like *everyone*. Try to be supportive, compassionate, and help your partners get their needs met. If you can't be that sounding board, find a way to get someone who can: parent support forums, therapists, and support groups.

Parents: How to Support One Another With Feeding

If your partner is primarily the one planning and serving meals, there are ways you can help. As early as possible, participate in feedings, sit close when your partner gives bottles, and give some too as your child permits. Join in with meals and snacks and be as active a participant as you can. Make family meals a priority. Help with menu planning or shopping, thank your partner for cooking and shopping, and clean up after meals. If he or she asks you to be involved in feeding therapies or appointments, make every attempt to go along, at least initially. Read the books together or at least be willing to discuss what your partner is reading, and support the efforts of the other person taking the lead. I encourage moms and primary caregivers to cut your partners some slack, too. Let the little things slide, and support all efforts to be involved. We are all doing the best we can.

Many mothers have shared that just having someone listen helps the most. This is often a role I play with parents. I can empathize with their pain and the tremendous worry and effort they put into feeding, often with little "reward." As Meredith says about the trusted listener in her life, *"Being able to cry and be honest with one person about what a failure I felt like as an adoptive mom for having such miserable meals (when people kept comment-ing on how happy we must be to finally all be home together) was so important. And for that trusted person to just listen and say, yes, this was absolutely difficult. No solutions, no judg-ments, no fairy-tale view making me think I was crazy. Just accepting how I was feeling."*

Find that person who will just listen. Get help. Get a therapist or a couple's coun-selor, and try to have date nights where you *don't* talk about your child or your feeding challenges.

To help your child, you have to help yourself.

Many of these lists abound, but the following are some ways you can take care of your-self. You might laugh at some of them if you are in those early months and/or have a child literally clinging to you 24/7.

- A spa or girls' night might not be an option, but consider something that will help you get through the day or hour. Lean on your faith (listen to sermons online if you can't leave the house), and reach out to friends and family to support you either with meals, lawn mowing, or a sympathetic ear.
- Sing or find some music you can play, or like to listen to, during the day.
- Look at favorite family photos of happy times.
- Find a "mantra," something that soothes, that you can say to yourself when things are hard. Sylvia Boorstein is a favorite writer and meditation expert of mine. I have found a mantra from her book, *It's Easier Than You Think*, particu-larly helpful. "Everything is as it should be," is a great reminder not to struggle against what we can't control.[2]
- Find an aromatherapy oil that soothes you, perhaps lavender or lemon.
- Look into respite for your child for a weekend if you really need it.
- Laugh—at anything you can find. A video on YouTube, a book of jokes, even the absurdity of life sometimes.
- At the end of day, write down anything good that happened. Aim for five things. "The sun was shining. Lisa smiled at me today. I enjoyed a hot shower without interruption. I didn't burn the pancakes. I held hands with my husband before the alarm went off..."
- Brew a cup of tea or enjoy a cup of coffee with some good chocolate. (Is there any other kind?)
- Add your ideas: _____

How to Deal With Meddlers: Family, Friends, and Others

Don't expect others to understand the Trust Model. Between 85 to 90 percent of Amer-icans don't feed this way. It's countercultural, so don't wait for understanding or sup-port from family or friends, the media, or even your doctor. It goes against our very cultural fabric to suggest that children can be trusted to eat a balance of good foods, get nutritional variety, and eat the right amounts of foods. But they can—IF we do our jobs with feeding.

> *"One of the most difficult parts of instituting the DOR with a special needs child is handling the pressure from health care professionals who neither understand the Trust Model of feeding nor know about the research that supports the DOR. After a few session of verbal dueling, I came up with my own 'coping' mechanisms to get through the appointments without reverting to the pressure model. A few days before appointments, I practiced my 'ignore and smile' motif. I thought through a bulky outfit so our son's weight would be on the higher end of the scale. And then I just suffered through the session, not getting real help and hoping it did not harm—because it is hard—very, very hard to withstand the pressure of doctors, psychologists, nutritionists—and my husband, who is often swayed during these appointments. In the end, what helps, though, is that I KNOW nothing else works. Any pressure at all backfires. The only time our son does well with eating and weight is when I trust him and leave him alone to do what he is supposed to do: decide what to eat and how much."*
> —Rachel, mother of Andrew, age two years with complex medical needs, including severe GI involvement

"I know that some friends and family quietly questioned my methods and wondered if it was necessary."
— Sophie, mother of Quinn, adopted domestically with sensory integration challenges

"Well-meaning friends with biological children were not generally helpful. They offered a lot of anecdotes and made lots of attempts to minimalize potential differences between feeding the adopted child and the biological child." — Sue, mother of Marcus and Mary

"I gave her teachers a letter saying that I don't want her ever to be bribed with food or refused food if she doesn't eat something else." —Rose, foster mother to Amari

The reality is that many grandparents and relatives won't understand what you are doing, won't make an effort to understand *why* you might be doing it, and may actively try to undermine your feeding strategies. For example, my friend's son had a dairy-contact allergy (meaning even touching dairy caused a reaction), but her in-laws didn't believe in it, and once snuck him ice cream—with predictable results.

I'm not suggesting that you panic if Grandma offers extra desserts or an extra snack or two. For the occasional visit, a more lax structure, and less balance or more sweets, is fine. It may be a way that family tries to bond with your child, and having that time at Grandma's where the rules don't always apply can be very special.

However, if extended family or others who care for your child are actively and routinely undermining your feeding and parenting philosophies, it is your duty to advocate for your child.

"I got the occasional, 'We're going to slip her an M&M when you aren't looking' comment. This felt hurtful because it undermined my parenting intentions to do what I knew was best for my child. And it proved my family just did not understand what we were working with. I didn't offer M&Ms at 18 months because it was a choking hazard with her compromised swallowing ability, not some nutritional concern."
— Leah, mother to Elise, adopted from Russia at 13 months

When you eat with your extended family, your feeding (and thus parenting) may feel in question. Patricia shared how hurtful family comments can feel. *"My parents made subtle remarks implying that I was overreacting. After an extended stay with them, everything changed. My dad made some comments that really bothered me—like I was causing the problem, and I should make her eat everything on her plate."*

Knowing When to Intervene
If your own memories of eating at home were traumatic—such as if you dieted or were taunted, forced to eat, or weighed daily—that's a pretty good clue that you should not leave the relatives to do whatever they want with feeding. It is tricky dealing with family, particularly if you rely on them for childcare, and you don't see eye to eye on feeding. Do the best you can and ask your social worker or a family therapist for help if you need it. It isn't always clear when you should speak up for your child and when you can let things slide, but the following are a few scenarios in which I feel strongly that the child needs to be protected:
* If your parents/relatives force your child to eat or try foods.
* If they make your child eat something to the point of tears or vomiting—and certainly if they make the child eat the "gagged-up" foods.
* If they are yelling or angry at meals about who is eating what or how much.
* If they are trying to get your child to lose weight, feeding and talking about food or the child's body in harmful ways.
* If they are trying to get your child to gain weight by pushing or forcing food.

If you are working hard to establish the DOR with feeding and have extended visits, it is reasonable to ask relatives to try their best with it. In our early years with the DOR, I often reminded my parents (as we had done some mild "portion control" in my daughter's early months) to be sure to let her decide when she was done eating. I would say, "Even if she seems to eat a ton—or nothing—I don't care what you feed her, just let her eat until *she* is done."

How to Advocate

Ideally, before you leave your kids with relatives, share a few meals together. Observe and listen. Let the small stuff slide, but protect your kids—not from cookies or calories, but from comments like, "Look at your tummy, you've obviously had enough," or "You have to eat all your food before you can watch TV," or "You're too skinny," and other pressure with feeding.

Some Other Doozies You May Hear:

"What are you feeding him?"

"Just make her eat it, she won't let herself starve."

"Don't you think she's had enough gravy?"

"Here Lori, have some more celery if you're still hungry!"

Let's anticipate your next family holiday table. Maybe Grandma Eve raised six kids, and they are all "fine," so she is, of course, a feeding expert. Uncle Sam just lost 30 pounds at his company's Biggest Loser contest, so he knows everything there is to know about weight loss and is eager to share. Betty actually force-fed your three-year-old mashed potatoes last year (he threw up) because she is convinced he'd "love potatoes if he just tried them."

Other than bow out of the family Thanksgiving this year, which *is* an option, the following section will give you ideas on how to handle well-meaning, but unhelpful and unsolicited, advice. Your family will intrude, saying or doing the opposite of what you are trying to accomplish with feeding, eating, or body image.

"Follow My Lead"

The phrase I have found particularly useful with my own family and for my clients is, *"Please follow my lead."*

Your family doesn't have to understand, agree with, or actively partake in your feeding philosophies, but you can ask them to "follow my lead." If you have a meddling family with a pattern of trying to get your child to eat more or less, try foods, pressure, shame, or bully, step in with a polite but firm, *"Mom, please follow my lead with this."* Try not to explain or draw more attention, or argue the issue during the meal.

Ideally, you will find a moment beforehand to talk with your family and prepare them for this. "Mom, we are trying something with Maya's eating. She is expected to be polite and participate, but we are allowing her to choose what foods, and how much she will eat, from what is on the table. Please don't ask her to eat more, and also, don't make a fuss or praise if she *does* eat something new. I know it's not how you would handle it, but I hope you can *follow our lead.*" Use those words in your preparatory explanation. A brief reminder when they slip up should be enough.

They *will* slip up, and that's not the end of the world. With repeated reminders, hopefully they will back off. This way of feeding is so different from anything your family members may know, and "follow my lead" also gives them the opportunity to observe what you are doing and hopefully pick up on how the DOR works. And remember, it's what happens all the other days of the year in your home that matters the most.

The following are a few more examples of what you might say. Practice these phrases in advance or find words that work for you:

Grandpa: "If you take that piece of toast, you have to finish it all."
You say: "Actually Dad, that's not how we do it. Please follow my lead. Billy, why don't you start with half a piece, and if you're still hungry, you can have more."

Waitress: "You can't have dessert Sweetie, until you finish your broccoli!" (This really happens.)
You say: "You are getting no tip." (Just kidding.)
Try: "We're doing just fine here. Please bring her dessert now, thanks."

Grandpa: "Let's hide his bottle. He's distracted. He eats too much. Haven't you heard that obese babies will be fat adults and die before you do, and get diabetes and, and, and…"
You say: "Grandpa, we like to let little Timmy decide when he's done eating. He'll let us know. May I have his bottle back, please?"

Uncle Bob: "You'll hurt Aunt Betty's feelings if you don't eat any of her sauce."
You say: "Oh, Bob, that's silly! We love Aunt Betty, and thank her for making dinner, but we don't eat anything we don't want to. *I'd* like some sauce, though, please."

What to do when the talk turns to calories, fat, dieting etc. when impressionable ears are listening? You can try to divert with, *"Hey, let's talk about your trip to family camp this summer. We're thinking about going next year!"* I liked this post from Margarita Tartakovsky on her "Weightless" blog at Psych Central, on having a fat-talk-free Thanksgiving, particularly this practical line:

"I'd rather not focus on weight and food, but I'd love to hear about _____" *(fill in the blank with whatever interests you). Your goal is to refocus the conversation in a way that will allow you to connect with those around you."*[3]

The adage of "do as you would have others do unto you," and your child, also holds true. I make it a point never to comment on someone's weight. In my pre-enlightened days, I would compliment someone who had lost weight. I have been clued-in when colleagues and friends shared difficult stories about the holidays and eating disorders. You never know if someone is losing weight by dieting, over-exercising, bingeing, purging, severe restriction, or as the result of a serious illness. Because commenting on someone's appearance is so automatic, it took me a while to come up with something else.

Skip the looks, the clothes, and the weight. How about a sincere, "I am so glad to see you!" or "I missed your smile!" and "Tell me about school, or New York City, or…"

"There were eight of us for dinner at my parents' house, including my son and his girl-friend—both seniors in high school. Mom sat next to poor girlfriend (probably normal weight, if not thinner), and announced that Girlfriend wasn't eating anything green, and told her she needed to add more nutrition to her diet. Triggering my past issues, of course, I responded, 'It's Thanksgiving, we all get to eat what we want.' Which seemed to resolve the issue." — Tammy, a blog reader

Daycare or Schools

This is a tough one. The people who care for our children should, and mostly do, love them and want what is best for them. Finding affordable, safe, convenient, nurturing childcare is hard. Many parents I work with feel conflicted, because while parents often love their nanny or daycare provider, they may not agree with feeding practices and policies.

- While you are researching childcare, ask about feeding. I toured one facility and saw a single pretzel stick with a Dixie cup of water for snack. When I asked what they would do if my child was still hungry, they assured me, "Don't worry, we won't let her have any more because we want to do our part against childhood obesity." That center, though well respected, got crossed off my list immediately.
- Often, childcare providers make the same mistakes as parents—they pressure, bribe, and enforce two-bite rules. They do not encourage eating based on internal cues.[4] To be fair, many parents ask childcare staff to work hard to get their children to eat more, or certain kinds of foods.
- Many childcare centers have a policy that children eat "real" or "growing" food before any desserts, even if you pack the meal. As I've explained, this is not consistent with the DOR.
- Some staff can cross the line, and this needs to be addressed. Several parents wrote to me about children's lunches being inspected in front of the class. One kindergartner's snack-size candy bar (in an otherwise balanced and "healthy" packed lunch) was held up in front of the class as an example of a "bad" food kids should not bring to school.

How to advocate for DOR-friendly feeding at your childcare or school:
- Copy, fill in, and laminate the "lunch box card" in the Appendix (also available online at www.thefeedingdoctor.com under "Resources"). Place it in your child's lunch box and tell him that if an adult asks him to eat certain foods, he should hand over the card. This is hard to ask a child to do, but it may work for some.

- Have a private meeting with the daycare director and teacher. Print out DOR-friendly feeding policies for schools, which you can find online at the Ellyn Satter Institute.
- Reassure staff that this means less work for them, not more. You are simply asking them to help your child open containers, as they would for any child, then allow him to eat from what you pack, in any order and amount.
- Thank the staff for their efforts if they have been trying to get your child to eat more, or different foods, or less, but inform them that you are working on the issue at home, and that the pressure will slow the process down.
- Ask them not to report, in front of your child, on what or how much your child ate. If you must know, ask for an email or text.

If the staff simply won't do as you ask, consider finding an alternative. One mother told of her son's teacher, who seemed to take on his eating as her personal mission. The teacher would sit next to him until he ate his entire "main dish," and he was not allowed to go out for recess until he did. This greatly increased her son's school anxiety, but he would gag the food down so he could go out to play.

The Media and "Research"

Most science and health reporting in mass media today is junk. The headlines are for ratings and shock factor and to instill fear. Most reports in the press are almost verbatim from press releases. The headlines shout alarms such as, "New Treatment for Eating Disorders in Children!" or "Weight-Loss Program in Inner Cities Works!" or "Why Your Fat Baby Will Grow Up to Be a Fat and Miserable Adult. News at Eleven!" Or this actual misleading headline from the "Top News" Website, "Doctors Warn: Generation of Children Could Die Before Their Parents Due to Unhealthy Lifestyle."[5] (See page 144 for the story on this one.)

When I look at a study, even my initial review of the study's design and conclusions often results in three pages with 20 bulleted points of reasons why I question the results. Good studies are hard to do—they take time and money, but much of the studies being conducted are poorly designed, and then authors make sweeping statements that are picked up by the media because of buzzwords. Many articles written about eating and weight on the Internet, and even reputable newspapers, are full of inaccuracies.

Why does this matter? Because I know when I was learning to trust this process, and as my clients go through this, they will hear the daily bombardment of "childhood obesity" articles and new studies about tricks to get picky eaters to eat. Friends will send links to Websites that warn of the horrors of canned foods and food coloring, or imploring you to eat more kale or walnuts. Reading those "studies" created more anxiety and chipped away at my trust in the process, and ultimately in my trust in my child. One mom shared that an article about eating more fish threw her off track. *"Fish? He won't even eat chicken. I tried pushing fish sticks. I knew it was wrong, and I knew how much progress we were already making, but it just brought up that old anxiety."*

Tune out. Turn it off. Don't click on the link. If you do get sucked in, talk yourself down. Re-read and say the "Serenity Prayer for Feeding" (page 248) out loud. Look back at your journals from before you started the process to now. Remind yourself of your successes. If you've written about how you enjoy meals, how serving family style means no more fighting and better attitudes at the table, it will help you stay firm when someone on TV promotes the "two-bite rule."

Family and friends who aren't following the same approach as you are will also whisper, or even shout in your ear, "You're making her obese!" While another mom might hear, "Why can't you get him to eat?" It is easier to deal with those comments when you feel confident with what you are doing. But when your mother's doubts play on your own and you hear her voice in your head—"she's obese" or "he's too skinny"—even then, it's about them, not you. If you do things differently than your mom and dad did, they may take it as a personal rejection of how they raised you. If your neighbor strictly limits all sweets, on some level he will feel threatened when you feed your child differently. It's about them, not you.

You are not in the mainstream if you feed this way. Be prepared to tune out the voices of doubt. Observe your child and your family, see the successes, document them, and let them give you strength.

Your Safety Net for Your Leap of Faith

Family Meals

"Daily life requires some structure and routine so that everyone in the family knows what to expect and can move through the day with some comfort and predictability."
— Fred Rogers, *The Mister Rogers' Parenting Book*[6]

Family meals really are *that* important. Without the structure and reliability of the family meal, this process is going to be very, very hard. Family meals will help your child learn to trust you and give him the opportunity to learn to trust his body. As authors Gregory Keck and Regina Kupecky explain in *Parenting the Hurt Child*, "Children in the foster care system or who have been institutionalized have likely missed out on many cycles of attachment." About completing the cycle, "This should be done over and over again—in ways that build trust, decrease anger, and meet the child's real needs."[7] Feeding is the most obvious and natural way to concretely complete cycles of attachment.

In modern times, making family meals happen is hard, but family meals are a better predictor of a child's overall healthy eating, happiness, and success than the socioeconomic status of the parents or extra-curricular activities.[8,9,10]

From the time your child is first with you, make that extra effort to sit down and eat together. Here are a few questions and ideas to help build toward family meals.

1. If you are not having family meals now, what is stopping you?
   _____ Time?
   _____ Lack of cooking skills?
   _____ Money?
   _____ The chore of menu planning?
2. Look at your list of obstacles for family meals. Are there any ways you can begin to work toward your goals? For example, if you don't know how to cook, can you take a cooking class, find some easy recipes online that make use of convenience foods, or search through cookbooks from the library for inspiration? Also remember that take-out and convenience foods also make a family meal—if you eat them together.
3. For a few days, write down what you and your kids are eating now.
4. Bring those foods to the table, or on a blanket on the floor if you don't have a table, and eat them together.

Menu Planning

It seems that every resource that talks about kids and getting food on the table has a menu plan, from a spreadsheet to tear-offs to subscription Websites. I have tried to plan menus in these organized ways, using the printouts and the books, but it simply doesn't work for me. I read a book that even had menu planning based on ethnic cuisine: Monday is Tex-Mex, Tuesday Italian... For me, menu planning is the part of the process I least enjoy. Thus I would skip it and find myself fairly often with no idea of what we were having for dinner, or throwing more food away than I liked.

The following are some primary obstacles for the traditional spreadsheet-style weekly-menu planning:
- It doesn't take into account what is fresh at the market.
- It doesn't take into account what is on sale. Searching for coupons takes time (and most of the from-scratch grocery items don't have a coupon). Being flexible means that if cabbage or pre-cut cabbage is on sale, you can make coleslaw one night.
- It doesn't take into account what kind of day you are having or what the weather was like. If you've had a crappy day or an unexpected call from school to deal with a behavior issue, you might not want to cut up all of the root veggies for that roasted side dish. Or, it's a sunny day, and you want to let your son play at the park, not rush home to brown the meat in the stew pot.
- Menu planning itself takes time. If it feels like an added burden, not a tool to save time and money, you may need to reconsider your approach.

While traditional "menu-planning" didn't work for me, it works well for many families. (Parents share what worked for them on page 265.) Here are some advantages to planning menus:

- If you stick to a menu plan, one person can shop and the other can cook. (With no plan, the person cooking usually has to be the person doing the shopping.)
- It helps families stick to a budget.
- Many parents enjoy the process and the predictability.
- It can lessen food waste.
- It can help you plan and provide a variety of foods.
- Online and smartphone apps now organize menus and even shopping lists.
- The number of shopping trips can be reduced, which is critical if transportation and time are challenges.
- Plans are particularly helpful if you use a grocery delivery service.
- It can help get food on the table after a long day.
- If you are new to cooking or family meals, it can be a useful tool to keep you on track and avoid last-minute grazing because you couldn't think of an alternative.

What has been working for me is "the list." I go to the market, usually with two or three meals in mind. I see what looks appealing or is on sale. I buy three or four veggies for sides, fresh fruit for snacks and dessert, and a couple of proteins. At home, I write what I have in the fridge. One column is for veggies, another is for fruits, and on top right of the list, I make tentative meal plans: Turkey curry with broccoli for Monday, pork chops with green beans on Tuesday, etc.

When we eat the cabbage or green beans, or the figs or grapes, I cross them off. I don't worry that I will forget about the corn in the crisper and be angry with myself when I throw it out a week later.

If you're new to planning meals, start with what you are eating now, serve it family style, and sit down and eat together. Next try to plan, maybe before you leave for work in the morning, what you will eat that night for dinner. Next try a few days in a row. Don't try to force a method to work, but do give it a chance.

The key is to go slowly and see what works for you. If weekly meal plans spoil the experience, and you feel guilty that you couldn't or didn't do it or stick to it, keep searching for a solution that works. Have some convenience foods in the freezer you can rely on and some quick recipes. It can take time to build a repertoire. When I was building mine, if I tried four new recipes and one was worthy of regular rotation, I was pretty happy.

I cook mostly without recipes, the way my mom did. I have five or six ways I can cook most proteins, a handful of starchy sides, and ways to prep veggies and fruits. (See my blog archives and search "recipes" for ideas at www.thefeedingdoctor/blog.)

While my system works for us right now, and you may be happy with what you've worked out, perhaps another approach will work better down the road. But just like with eating, don't let the "shoulds" spoil the planning and getting food on the table. As my blog readers share, families find many ways that are right for them.

How Do You Get Meals on the Table? Stories From My Blog Readers

- *"I make a weekly meal plan and really enjoy it. It gives me a sense of sanity in a crazy week. I do it on a white board so if I get a wild hair and want to switch Tuesday's green beans with Wednesday's broccoli; one swipe of the finger does it. The kids, I think, like being able to see our week laid out like that. Dinner is such an extraordinarily important part of their day. Meal planning also helps me clear out the fridge and the freezer. Most importantly, planning out a week helps me balance our meals. I can see that, okay, I've got one beef meal, one chicken meal, one bean meal, one starchy meal, etc. And, once again, if I want to, one swipe of the finger, and I can get spontaneous."*

- *"Right now we live a few blocks away from a co-op. I go once a week to Target to get non-perishables, and every few days I walk to the co-op with my son and we shop for the fresh items like fruits, veggies, and meats. We enjoy the outings, and I can cook what appeals to me that day. When I go back to work, I know this won't work for us, and I'll miss it."*

- *"I do make a menu and buy from the recipes, but I also have some staples always on my list that I can use to make last-minute things if something on my menu doesn't work. But I've found that being in school has really messed up my menu planning/grocery list because my schedule is so unpredictable and time-pressed. Now I'm buying more convenience foods, and we're grabbing take-out more often. I used to soak my own beans and make my own bread, but we're eating canned beans and buying bread these days. Sometimes it's homemade lentil soup and sometimes it's take-out pizza, but at least we're having good family time eating together, so that's all good. I'll go back to cooking from scratch again when my time allows."*

  Author's note: I love how kind this mom is to herself. Guilt never helps, and realizing that sometimes you will rely more on convenience foods, and that that is okay, will help you stick with family meals and get back to it when life allows.

- *"I have a round of about 12 entree recipes—some with meat and some without. My kids and husband don't care if we have quiche every week, so we often do. Other items in the rotation include sloppy joes, homemade pizza or calzones, black bean burritos or quesadillas, split pea soup (in winter), roasted chicken, scrambled eggs, and baked pasta. Things that don't include protein/vegetable/ starch are rounded out with bread, frozen or fresh vegetables, noodles, or rice. The freezer means I can buy meat and frozen vegetables, and I can 'shop' in the freezer in weeks when money is tight or I don't have any big ideas."*

- *"My husband and I do weekly meal planning together. It's part of our Sunday mornings: a nice leisurely breakfast followed by meal planning over coffee. It's more than meal planning; we both look at our schedules for the next week and know who's picking up our son. That tells us how many meals need to be super quick to prepare, and how many we can take more time preparing. We don't eat meat, so I like to look at our meals over the week to see that we have a variety of protein sources. I try to balance out meals that may be challenging for our son with meals that are a sure hit. And we try to get at least one meal, like a soup or a casserole, that will provide leftovers. All of us go to the grocery store together. We make a list of meals, but we don't plan it out that Monday is X, and Tuesday is Y, so there is some flexibility. We always have staples for some quick meals (scrambled eggs, spaghetti and jarred sauce, or bean burritos) for nights that we just don't feel like cooking. Now that my son can read and reach a lot of things at the store, shopping together is becoming fun."*

Another obstacle parents face is keeping kids busy while getting dinner on the table. Here are a few ideas:

Keeping Kids Busy While You Cook: Ideas From Moms
- *"A bag of pom-poms (the bigger 1½–2 inch diameter ones) from the craft store provides endless hours of fun for the young toddler. They can put them into boxes and bottles, take them out, sort them, shoot them through paper towel tubes, etc."*

- *"This is such a crazy time of day that I save our TV watching until before dinner so I can get dinner going. We've had a chance to connect after school, and the TV winds the kids down and gets us all ready for dinner."*

- *"We have a counter with barstools in the kitchen near an "art supplies" cabinet with paper, crayons, colored pencils, paint, Play-Doh, stickers, and activity books. Also, refrigerator magnets—we have letters, numbers, dinosaurs, and now poetry magnets."*

- *"I filled a lower cabinet with plastic bowls, containers, and other unbreakable items. They loved taking them all out, stacking, and sorting while sitting on the floor."*

- *"I let my kids roll their cars through my legs while I cook, let them play with Tupperware and, most of all, let them "help" me cook with their stools pulled up to the counter."*

- *"Sometimes my daughter (age 2½) is fine sitting on a chair out of the way. If she's content to do that, I talk about what I'm cooking and what's going into the pot/ pan (which she loves to recount when it comes time to eat it). I let her participate as much as possible (helping me count as I measure, dumping things into a mixing bowl, bringing eating dishes to the table, etc.). She loves this because she's in a really independent phase right now. Other times, she has playtime with Dad or sits at the table with crayons."*

Also see "Saying Grace" (page 99) and "Rehabilitating Feeding" (page 97) for more getting-to-the-table ideas.

When in Doubt, Don't Blurt It Out

I'm a talker, and lots of my clients are too. I often get asked, "Is it okay if I say X?" We are smart, we try hard, and our kids may be bright and highly verbal. On one recent call, a mom realized, *"I talk to him like he's 40, and he's only four! My family never talked about anything, so I think I went to the other extreme."*

We are encouraged to narrate our days for language development, many of us use positive attention and reward (such as the Nurtured Heart or Love-and-Logic approach), and we all seem to be talking, talking, talking. I was at a playground with my daughter when a little boy stepped over a stick and his mom said, "Good problem-solving!"

Clients do this around food with kids *all the time*. It is hard to turn off. Maybe you shouldn't turn it off if it is working for your family. However, most of the talking around food is *noise* that makes it harder for your child to tune in to messages coming from inside her body, and tends to increase anxiety and resistance.

- Don't talk nutrition with young kids. A three-year-old doesn't need to know the word "protein," and won't understand it anyway.
- Don't go on and on about how pretty a food is or how delicious. One comment about a red berry or a sweet taste is okay.
- Don't talk about portions or weight.
- Don't talk about "green-light" or "red-light" foods, or "growing foods" or "fun" foods. All of those other names really mean "good" and "bad" to a child. The child who eats "bad" foods thinks he is "bad" too, inviting guilt and shame into the relationship with food.
- Don't ask questions that invite negativity or refusal:
  - "Do you like it?"
  - "Is it too hot?"

I have found the word "soon" to be particularly helpful when talking to kids. Remember, young children don't have a notion of time, so saying, "40 minutes," or "the day after tomorrow," makes little sense to them.
- "Dinner will be soon."
- "We'll have mac-n-cheese again soon."
- "I'm sorry we're not having ice cream again for dessert. We'll have it again soon. Aren't we lucky we get to eat so many wonderful different foods, like ice cream and potatoes and red peppers?"

We don't need to explain constantly. The wisdom is *within*, and our children have a better chance of learning to *listen* to that wisdom if we support them well with eating and stop yapping all the time. One mom wrote on my blog that it was "irresponsible" not to teach nutrition to young children, for example, and that they will feel ill if they eat too much "junk food." I suggested that it is far more meaningful if the child learns that through experience, and they will, if we trust them. When a child on occasion chooses to eat only candy for a snack, she will learn that she is soon hungry. If she chooses only to eat the Cheetos for lunch, she may not feel so good. It amazed me on the day after Halloween one year when my then three-year-old turned down candy, saying, "I've had enough sweet today." And we saved the candy for another day. (Remember that this is in the context of regular and balanced meals and snacks.)

Things you *can* say, and may need to repeat in a calm and gentle manner, include:
- "You don't have to eat anything you don't want to."
- "Is your tummy full, or do you want more?"
- "There will always be enough."
- "You can have as much as you want" (when reassuring the child who has experienced food scarcity or restriction).
- "You don't have to eat it, but you do have to be polite. Instead of 'Gross,' please just say, 'No thank you.'" (One blog reader shared her delightful phrase, "Don't yuck my yum.")
- "I'm sorry we're not having mac-n-cheese (insert other favorite) tonight, but we'll have it again soon. Tonight we're having _____."

Making it Through the Transition to Trust

Reminders
- Consider putting a note on the fridge with the DOR:
  1. My jobs: what, when, where
  2. Susie's jobs: how much and if

- Writing a little note that says, "Trust _____" [your child's name] can be a simple and poignant reminder that our children are trustworthy, and parents need to follow their lead.
- Write a note that says: "Follow her lead," or whatever helps inspire you or give you confidence while the DOR feels new and scary.

Celebrate Success

Not in front of your child, but when you are alone, pat yourself on the back for getting dinner on the table, for not pestering him to eat his pasta, or for letting her eat until she is done. Celebrate changes in your child: perhaps he put broccoli on his plate, tolerated a dish sitting next to him, or asked for more chicken, or she asked for seconds and stopped after one or two more bites.

> Remember, the early successes will be yours: getting the kitchen table cleared off for family meals, getting dinner on the table, or planning and bringing a snack to the park.

Keep a Journal

My clients sometimes forget how far they have come. Progress can feel painfully slow. Most selective eaters will not suddenly devour roasted peppers (though they are really sweet) and bean salad. In the meantime, write down your victories.

- You had a peaceful meal tonight.
- Your child calmly passed a bowl of a food that used to trigger tantrums and gagging.
- Your child served himself some pizza, even if he only ate the crust this time.

> One client called a few weeks after we started working together and complained that her daughter hadn't eaten anything new. "She put a blueberry in her mouth, but spit it out," Mom said, exasperated. When I reviewed the notes with her from our initial visit, she could indeed see huge improvements. Her daughter no longer cried every morning on waking, whining for pasta. She no longer begged for food after school, but seemed to enjoy the routine and schedule of snacks, and my goodness, she put a blueberry in her mouth. She had never done that before.

Sometimes looking back to where you have been helps you see progress more clearly.

Have a Book Club

These are difficult topics to work through. If you have a support group or an adoptive parents' group, consider having a book club. Read this book, *Child of Mine*, or *Secrets of Feeding a Healthy Family*. Take a few minutes to review some of the worksheet questions as a group. Tell stories about how you were fed and how it backfired, share your successes, and be open to sharing your "failures," or as I prefer to call them, "learning opportunities." It can feel vulnerable to cry in front of other moms (I've been there), but also incredibly supportive when you realize you are not the only mom who dreads dinner or serves chicken nuggets every night, and that you can improve things, little by little.

Lean on Your Partner

Hold hands under the table or grab the chair during those transition meals when you want to jump in with old patterns. Check in with each other about a situation that seems difficult. Celebrate your successes together.

> Anneliese shared that when her selective eater took a piece of chicken while no one was looking, she could tell her husband was about to praise him. She grabbed his hand, and shook her head to remind him. They shared their joy over his progress after the kids were in bed.

Let Go of Guilt

More than one mom has asked how to deal with the guilt of realizing that some of their feeding practices made matters worse. First off, I've been there. I get it. I made feeding "mistakes." But for myself and my clients, and pretty much every other parent out there, this I do know: We do the best we can. As Fred Rogers said, "Of course, there were times in our parenting that we wish we'd done something differently, but we've tried not to feel too guilty about that. One thing's sure is that we always cared and we always tried our best." [7]

Through no fault of your own, you may have even been given bad feeding advice from family, doctors, and other "experts." Most of my clients have tried for months and years to do as they were told, knowing all along that something wasn't right and that things were not getting better, but they didn't have the right support or information. So, find a way to move forward. Take that intense emotion and use it to energize the effort to feed with structure and not fall into old patterns.

You would probably not harshly judge another parent who did her best with what she knew at the time. Extend that same kindness to yourself. Pray, cry, talk to a friend, or even write a letter to your child that you may, or may not, ever share with her. Then slowly move on.

If You Feel Stuck

If you feel stuck in the process—for example, you still want to bribe with dessert or are still pushing protein—work through the following exercises to examine your feelings and motives.

Ask Yourself:
What am I afraid of? _____

What am I currently doing to try to get my child to:

- Eat more? _____
- Eat less? _____
- Eat different foods? _____
- Notes: _____
  _____

Do I look *forward* to meals and snacks, or would I rather be poked with sharp sticks?

_____

How does it *feel?* _____

Is it working? _____
(Feel free to say yes, and in what way? For example, does bribing with dessert get in a few more bites?)

My support systems are_____

My partner believes in the Trust Model—yes or no: _____

Am I "All-In" or Picking and Choosing?
When change is needed, it is pretty much a universal human response to pick and choose change that feels comfortable and resist what feels scary. That is normal, but won't help you make the shift in thinking that needs to happen.

Be sure to review the following list with your feeding partner(s) so that you are on the same page before you are all sitting down to a meal. This will be that much harder if one parent is sticking with the plan while the other is still using control methods.

**Remember, you are not giving up control,
but the illusion of control, or temporary control.**

Which of These Statements Makes You Uncomfortable or Doubtful?
_____ Serve a small, child-sized portion of dessert *with* the meal.
_____ I trust that my child has the ability to learn to know how much to eat.
_____ This can work for my child.
_____ Serving family style and letting my child serve herself will help her.

_____ If my child is offered a variety of foods within the context of structure, she will move herself along to increase variety.

_____ It is not about what my child eats at one meal, but how the meal *feels*.

_____ I will try this, and even though milk (or protein or vegetable) is so important to me, I will not encourage or pressure her to drink/eat more.

_____ I know that tactics like bribing with dessert, or a "no thank-you bite," are not helping him learn to like new foods.

The items that trouble you, or where you are resistant, may indicate where you need to read and learn more, where you might slip up with the DOR, or where there is an unaddressed worry.

When You Are Stuck: A Summary

Step back and observe. Start with a deep breath as you consider the following:

- What is that DOR again? Am I doing my son's job? Am I letting my daughter do mine? (Can you think of some examples of when that has happened to you?)
- If you haven't gotten your jobs mixed up:
  - · What am I worried about? _____
  - · Is it a valid worry that I need to look into? _____
  - · Am I falling into old traps? _____
- Ask yourself, "What is/was my motivation?" _____
- Do I have enough information to deal with my worry? _____
- Would I feed him differently if he was leaner or if he was plumper? _____

Examine Your Motivation

That question about motivation helps. Early on in the transition process, you might overcompensate a little. Maybe you don't say anything about food or don't offer to pass a bowl. No, it's not pressure if you ask your son if he wants you to pass the potatoes; however, it *is* pressure if you ask him 10 times or while pleading.

Your motivation is critical. Your child will get the difference. If I say, "No, you can't have any more shrimp, that's enough, you should be full," it's very different than saying, "That's your share of shrimp. It's such a treat and a little expensive, but if you're still hungry you can have more crackers and milk." Feel the difference? *Your child will.*

> Ask yourself, how would I feed my child if I wasn't worried about nutrition or her size? If she was thinner, or weighed more, how would I respond? That will usually give you some insights when you feel stuck.

Seeing It From the Child's Perspective

Earlier in the book, 16-year-old Yiseth advised parents to try to see if from *"the kid's point of view."* This exercise might help. If you have a partner, consider putting on a little play, or act it out with your book club.

"Pudding" on a Play

Props: two pudding cups

Put something in the cups that might be unexpected, like cinnamon, walnuts, or raisins, but don't tell your partner what it is—be kind here, no anchovies or hot sauce.

Ask the audience (or yourself) to focus on how it feels to be the child. Before the exercise, read these questions and ask the audience to pay attention to them as you role-play:

- How does each scenario feel? Comfortable, pleasant, stressful?
- What made me want to try the food?
- What turned me off or made me not want to try the food?
- Can you guess which of the scenes represents the Trust Model? (If you get this wrong, you may need to re-read this book from the beginning.)

Scene 1:

Parent: Standing, with phone in hand, hands the cup to the child and says, *"Here is your snack."*

Child: *"I don't want that, it's gross."*

Parent: *"It's not gross, you like it, and it's good for you. It's organic and has calcium for your bones and protein for your muscles."*

Child: *"But I don't want it. I've never had that kind before. I want graham crackers."*

Parent: *"You'll like it!"* (Phone rings, parent answers phone, *"Ok, just a minute, I'll call you right back, I'm giving Max his snack. I can't stand it, he's so picky!"*) To child: *"You need to eat at least half of this. If you eat half, I'll give you a graham cracker. I have to grab this call, and when I get back, you better have eaten half of this pudding."*

Child: *"I won't! It's slimy!"*

Parent: *"It's not slimy, it's good. If you don't eat it, I'll tell Dad, and he'll be really upset when he gets home. Think about all the kids who don't have enough food."* And parent leaves the room.

Curtain falls

Scene 2:

Parent: Has two pudding cups and spoons and napkins. Sits across from child. *"Thanks for washing your hands. Let's have snack now."* (Phone rings and Mom silences ringer.)

Child: *"What is that? I don't think I had it before. It looks gross."*

Parent: *"It's called rice pudding. I used to love this with frozen blueberries when I was little. It's got a vanilla flavor, like the pudding you like, but has a little chewiness to it."*

Child: *"I don't want any."*

Parent: Tries a bite and says, *"OK, you don't have to eat anything you don't want to. There's a napkin if you don't like it, you can spit it out.* * *I also put out graham crackers."*

Child: Takes bite of graham cracker.

Parent: Dips corner of graham cracker in rice pudding. *"I forgot to get a drink, would you like milk or water?"*

Child: *"Milk please."*

Parent: Gets milk, sits down. *"How did your play date go this morning? Did you like the new clay project?"* Takes a few more bites.

Child: Pokes corner of graham cracker into pudding and smells it.

Curtain falls

*Note that you don't have to tell her every time she can spit food out or explain that she doesn't have to eat what she doesn't want. That might be too much talking and can feel like pressure.

Review the questions from above. The following is usually how parents answer during workshops. See if your answers match up.

What made me not want to try the pudding?
- Being argued with, "It's not slimy" or "You'll like it"
- Being called "picky" made me mad
- Nutrition talk. If it's "healthy," I figure it won't taste good
- The pressure
- The threat felt scary
- Being left alone with the food
- Not having something that I wanted to eat

What made me want to try the pudding?
- Mom sitting with and eating the food
- Giving a flavor context, relating it to an accepted food
- Knowing I could spit it out
- Seeing Mom dip the graham cracker
- Relaxed atmosphere

The Foreign Country

If you're not a thespian at heart, simply imagine the following scenario. You are in a foreign country where you do not speak the language.

Scenario 1: You are alone at a restaurant. The owner comes and tells you in broken English, "This is house special. However, it is VERY rude in my country to spit out food, but this is very good for you, will make you very strong, and it is very cheap, too." He sets down a large bowl of lumpy gray food and walks away.

Scenario 2: Same country, same food. A friend gave you a recommendation of a well-respected chef and trusted member of the community. He sits with you, with a bowl of the same lumpy gray food in the middle of the table and a serving spoon. He says, "I am happy to share table with you. I made pudding that is a little sweet, with vanilla and dried grapes. I understand you don't like too much spice, so I hope you might enjoy this pudding with me." He sits, serves himself a small portion, and clearly savors his first bite. You have a paper napkin that you can spit your food into discreetly if you need to.

What Scenario 2 had was:
- Pleasant company
- Modeling
- Trust in the chef, by way of recommendation and his demeanor
- Enjoyment
- Context of flavor
- Permission to take a small portion and try at your own pace, knowing what to expect

In Scenario 1, you may have felt nervous, alone, and suspicious, with no context of whether it would be spicy or sweet, or what was in it—were those lumps mystery meat or fruit? You had very little control.

Which scenario felt safer and made you imagine taking a bite and enjoying it? This is what feeding feels like for small children who don't have a context, may have a language barrier, and other challenges. Try to put yourself in your child's shoes.

Let's consider these statements and how a child might feel:
- "You've had enough pork chops. Do you really need another one?"
- "We ran out of bread, but you can have more celery if you want to. You can eat as much celery as you want."
- "You don't know if you're full yet; you have to wait 20 minutes, then you can have more fruit if you are hungry."
- "You can't be full, you only ate two bites."

Notes: _____

_____

Can you think of other things that were said to you growing up, or that you say to your child, and think about how it feels? _____

_____

_____

Behavior During the Transition

Many parents worry so much about keeping the table pleasant as they make the transition that they second-guess themselves relative to managing behavior at the table. You can and should deal with disruptive, naughty, or mean behavior at the table. However, you should avoid discipline based on what or how much your child is eating.

The amazing thing is, once you employ the DOR, and they don't *have* to push back against all the pressure, meals are a lot more fun, and that transformation often happens pretty quickly. Remember it's the attitude that improves first. Enjoy it.

But some kids will continue to act out—because they are two or three years old, are tired or traumatized, or have a history of prenatal exposure, ADHD, or anxiety—or it's what they do. Parents occasionally note that behavior initially *worsens* at the table when they institute the DOR. They are often relieved to learn that it might be because as the conflict around food goes away, the child feels safe enough to experiment with limit setting in other ways. This child who felt anxious, cornered, and locked in a battle over food is now relaxing and experimenting with more typical toddler behaviors, like throwing her fork on the floor repeatedly or teasing the dog.

Annaliese recalls that only days into the transition, she found her two-year-old son, Adan, had dumped all the shampoo out on the floor. *"I was actually happy. This is normal two-year-old stuff, which when he was food obsessed and clinging to me, he never seemed to have the energy or interest to explore. Yesterday, he was standing on the table pretending to sword-fight with his brother and I clapped—I was so happy I couldn't help it, though of course I got them down. I can't believe how he has blossomed with just addressing his food worries."*

Use your typical techniques for addressing behavior. If Sandy hits her brother, redirect, or use your chosen consequence. If Betty is having a meltdown, you can leave the table with her and explain that you will go back when she is ready to be pleasant at the table. She might need a little help calming down if she is upset.

Let's Check In

"He was also prone to tantrums at every single meal. If he didn't like what he saw on his plate, he would scream and cry. If he finished the cheese on his plate and ate nothing else he would signal that he wanted more cheese. If we told him he needed to finish his other food and then he could have more cheese he would spiral into a tantrum with no ability to rebound from it. Meals were extremely stressful."— Sue, of Marcus' mealtime tantrums

Can you spot a few opportunities to avoid the power struggles in this scenario? Think for a minute and write down your answers. _____

_____

_____

If you noticed the phrase, ". . . he didn't like what was on his plate," good for you! This family is starting with conflict before the meal even begins. Rather than setting down a plate with foods that create anxiety, serve family style. Put all the choices in bowls on the table and let him pick and choose.

He likes his cheese. With the DOR, he gets to choose how much from what is on the table, and he should be allowed to eat as much cheese as he wants without having to eat or earn other foods. So go ahead, let him have more cheese. Eventually, he will tire of cheese, probably a lot sooner if he is not restricted. Here, too, you can head off a tantrum. He can learn to trust you, and when the tantrums and behaviors improve, he can pay attention and approach the other foods without pressure and is more apt to learn to like them.

But *I* Just Can't:

- *Have desserts or treats in the house. They are my trigger foods.* This is a problem. If you are really struggling with your own eating to the point where you can't eat with your child, or can't have carbs or other foods your child needs to be exposed to, then you may need to enlist your partner or another family member while you address your own eating issues. One client was in therapy for an eating disorder and was still bingeing on carbs, so she had her husband eat with her son so he could enjoy the foods he wanted to eat, like breakfast cereal, bagels, and bread. Dad was willing to take over to help normalize his son's eating.

- *Handle letting her eat as much cheese (or Rice Krispies treats, or...) as she wants.* This can be a hard one. It can be scary when you let your formerly restricted child have free reign at those "treat" snacks, or if your child has a history of severe restriction. If you are scared to do the "treat snack" where you let them have as much as they want once or twice a week, start with a less threatening food. Consider raisin-oatmeal cookies instead of Oreos, for example. It often helped clients to serve treat snacks with milk and fruit. Consider what her favorite fruits might be, and whether it is kiwis or pears, serve that along with the snack. Most of the time, clients share that their children eat some of the treat and some of the fruit and milk.

  When you are planning what to serve, you may be thinking something along the lines of, "Hmm, he ate a good amount of cheese at snack time, so I'd feel better if I offer his favorite squash for dinner and chicken," or, "Sam hasn't liked my chili before, so I will plan to round out his intake by making cornbread and a fruit he usually goes for so he can be satisfied." This is fine, but don't let your kids in on your thought process. For example, I won't say to my daughter what I am privately thinking: "We're having corn muffins because I know you probably won't eat much of the chili I made, but at least I know you will have something you like at the table."

- *Let him go to school without a good breakfast.* Many parents fret over breakfast. Some children aren't hungry early in the morning. Offer a balanced variety and trust your child. If you are transitioning a really selective eater who is eating something in the mornings and you are really worried, maybe leave breakfast alone for now. Let him eat his favored foods for breakfast so you can relax while you get settled in with structure and not pressuring. I talk a lot about helping your child be less anxious, but you also have to address your own anxieties. If you can't let your son go to bed without a good dinner, it might be harder to stand up to his whining for his favorite foods. Address your worry and perhaps plan for that "rescue snack" shortly before bed (see page 112).

- *Stop praising him when he tries new things, even if he asks for it.* Many parents have been told to clap, congratulate, and sing the praises of the "big boy" for trying a new food, or licking it, or whatever the goal is. When you initially make the transition, your child may continue to ask for praise if he tries something new. As Rachel, Mom of Andrew, says, *"He has never eaten a carrot before, and he was so excited and kept asking for us to acknowledge it. I know I'm not supposed to make it a big deal, but he was so happy, I didn't know what to do."*

  Again, following the child's lead will help. This little guy was excited and perhaps proud or looking for attention. All the praise in the world had not helped his eating for the last two years, but he was sensing that things were changing, was more open to explore foods, and was looking for feedback. There are ways that Mom could share his excitement without spoiling his sense of accomplishment. She could say, "I'm so happy that you are excited. I'm glad you liked that carrot. Mommy likes carrots, too." Focus on how he feels, not on the food. However, it's far too tempting to praise, which in and of itself can feel like pressure and lead to outright pushing. "What a big boy for trying that carrot. *Maybe you can try the tomato now?*"

This transition is not always easy, but many moms and dads share their relief with finally feeling that they are on the right track.

If You Need More Help

Some of you will read this book, perhaps with other resources such as a Webinar, DVD, or blog. Armed with new information, you will institute the changes necessary to establish a satisfying and healthy feeding relationship. You will be able to step back and observe your feeding behaviors, your child, and his responses, and then address any counterproductive feeding dynamics. Once you take the lead, assuming your child is capable of coming along with you, you will enjoy (mostly) pleasant family meals and, with time, a child who is capable with self-regulation and who enjoys a variety of foods.

Some of you will read this book and be confident that this is the right approach for you, but need a little more support. That is the kind of work I offer to clients, with consultations by phone and occasionally in person. There may be a few lingering questions, doubts, or scenarios not covered in the book. Many parents I have worked with needed help seeing progress and receiving encouragement and reassurance that what they are experiencing in the transition is normal.

And some families will simply need even more help. A hallmark of a loving parent is recognizing when things aren't going well and seeking help. If you think back to the worry cycle, most families who are deep into the cycle of pressure and resistance will need support turning things around. I see this most often when:

- Problems are more entrenched over the years, perhaps with several different therapeutic approaches attempted.
- Serious concerns about weight or nutrition continue.
- The parent is unable to observe and respond to feeding challenges due to her or his own mental health issues, including depression, anxiety, substance abuse, or eating disorder.
- The child has more severe behavioral, medical, nutritional, oral-motor, or sensory challenges.

These families will likely benefit from ongoing, intensive support. Often, families can't really work on feeding until other more pressing issues are addressed.

I have been surprised by some families who have suffered for years, sometimes even failing multiple therapeutic interventions, and have turned things around with a book and a few phone calls and emails for support. Other families, with neurotypical children and seemingly less severe concerns around selective eating or heightened interest in sweets, have been unable to trust the process and continue to engage in regular conflict with their children.

If you think you fall into this group of parents needing more support, read this book and others listed in the Resources section of www.thefeedingdoctor.com, and find the professionals who can support you through this process at the level you need. You may already be working with a pediatric RD, attachment therapist, couples counselor or family therapist, pediatric psychiatrist, or social worker. Your child may need support, but you, the parent, may also need help, particularly if you are unable or unwilling to make necessary changes on behalf of your child. For example, the father who says he knows it is wrong to force-feed his son but continues to do it, or the mother who is battling her own eating disorder and is unable to stock the home with foods to meet her child's nutritional needs.

Chapter 10
Trust Yourself, Trust Your Child

It really will get better…one meal at a time.

"It is amazing that already he seems happy again. He has come running to me saying, 'I am so happy, I love you Mommy!' And even, 'I am full Mommy!' followed by a full belly laugh. I know that it may seem impossible to see his happiness return already, but it has."
— Annaliese, mom to Adan, adopted from Ethiopia at 11 months and struggling with food obsession, now age two, written three days after reading a draft of this book

When I read Annaliese's words, I shed a joyful tear or two. I feel a deep satisfaction in accompanying parents on this journey of raising kids who are "healthy and happy." Adan and Annaliese are on their way. The idea that this book can touch and transform lives is my hope—and to make room for more "belly laughs."

Annaliese adds, *"We kept thinking, when will we start enjoying our family? We waited and worked so long to have our family, and for more than a year, there was no joy. We are finally enjoying our son, because he is thriving."*

I know this book will not be a perfect resource. The day after it heads to the printer, I'll find new stories and studies I want to include. You'll still have questions I haven't addressed, and I simply can't address every concern or scenario that might come up, but I want this information out there to help families, and the professionals who help them, to raise children who feel good about food and their bodies. The Trust Model, with its Division of Responsibility, should give you a secure grounding that you will grow more confident over time to address the scenarios that come up as you feed and parent your children.

This is a process, a journey you get to take with your family. Some things will improve right away, others won't. Some days you will see progress, and other days you might feel frustrated and stuck. Observe your child, compare him only to himself, and remain open and curious while you do your jobs with feeding. You know your child better than anyone else. Trust yourself and trust your child. And if you've lost your way, may you find *your* "return to happiness."

What Parents Who Have Been There Want You to Know

Your best support will come from:
- Friends and acquaintances
- Family
- Pediatrician
- Pediatric dietitian
- Pediatric specialists

The most judgment and hurt will come from:
- Friends and acquaintances
- Family
- Pediatrician
- Pediatric dietitian
- Pediatric specialists

About serving meals and snacks:
- Make one meal for the whole family, with choices for your child. Avoid making separate food for kids.
- The parent decides what, when, and where, and the child decides if and how much.
- Take a moment to chill before dinner (we pray).
- Serve a small dessert with meals (helped me too)!
- Let her eat until she is done and stops on her own, rather than stop her at what should be "correct" amounts.
- Make snacks more filling and hearty.
- Don't go "by the books" when it comes to amounts of formula or food.
- Don't try too hard to eat "healthy." My intense focus on "healthy" eating caused so many battles and didn't make him eat any better.

About developmental issues:
- Adopted kids have more developmental delays, and developmentally delayed children tend to have feeding issues.
- Check out services from your local school system. They have some amazing early intervention services.

About the process in general:
- This model exists and works.
- Even if it takes longer, involving children in cooking is worth it.

- One meal at a time. I know that mealtime needs to be pleasant and enjoyable. This was so incredibly difficult to do when I was in the midst of meal after meal after meal with a screaming child. But I would tell other parents that it really will get better... one meal at a time.
- The family meal is an adjustment, but now is something we really enjoy.
- Bad therapy is worse than no therapy.
- If it doesn't build your relationship, don't do it.
- Don't worry about hurting other people's feelings when it comes to doing the right thing for your child.

References

Introduction

1. Satter EM. The Feeding Relationship. *Journal of the American Dietetic Association.* 1986;86:352-56.
2. Rogers, Fred. *The Mister Rogers Parenting Book*: *Helping To Understand Your Young Child.* Philadelphia, PA: Running Press, 2002.
3. Perry B. "Bonding, Attachment and the Maltreated Child." PDF. Available at: www.ChildTraumaAcdemy.org (accessed 2012).
4. Minnesota International Adoption Project. *IADP Newsletter* (Fall 2003). Available at: http://www.cehd.umn.edu/icd/iap/Newsletters/default.html (accessed 2012).
5. Linscheid TR, Budd KS, Rasnake LK. "Pediatric Feeding Problems," edited by MC Roberts. *Handbook of Pediatric Psychology.* 3rd Edition. New York: Guilford Press. 2003:481-98.
6. Manikam R and Perman J. Clinical Reviews: Pediatric Feeding Disorders. *Journal of Clinical Gastroenterology.* 2000;30:34-6.
7. Bryant-Waugh R, Markham L. Feeding and Eating Disorders in Childhood. *International Journal of Eating Disorder.* 2010;43:98-111.
8. Lohse B, Psota T. Eating Competence of Elderly Spanish Adults Is Associated With a Healthy Diet and a Favorable Cardiovascular Disease Risk Profile. *Journal of Nutrition.* 2010;140:1322-7.
9. Lohse B, Bailey RL. Diet Quality Is Related to Eating Competence in Cross-Sectional Sample of Low-Income Females Surveyed In Pennsylvania. *Appetite.* 2012;58:645-50.
10. Psota TL, Lohse B. Associations Between Eating Competence and Cardiovascular Disease Biomarkers. *Journal of Nutrition Education and Behavior.* 2007;39:S171-8.
11. Lohse B, Satter E. Measuring Eating Competence: Psychometric Properties and Validity of the ecSatter Inventory. *Journal of Nutrition Education and Behavior.* 2007;39:S154-66.

Chapter 1

1. Faulkerson JA, Story M, Neumark-Sztainer D. Family Meals: Perception of Benefits and Challenges Among Parents of 8-10 Year-Old Children. *Journal of the American Dietetic Association.* 2008;108:706-9.

2. Linscheid TR, Budd KS, Rasnake LK. "Pediatric Feeding Problems," edited by MC Roberts. *Handbook of Pediatric Psychology.* 3rd edition. New York: Guilford Press, 2003:481-98.

3. Manikam R, Perman J. "Pediatric Feeding Disorders. *Journal of Clinical Gastroenterology.* 2000;30:34-46.

4. Crawford PB, Shapiro LR. How Obesity Develops: A New Look at Nature and Nurture. *Obesity & Health.* 1991;5:40-1.

5. Nicholls DE, Lynn R, Viner RM. Childhood Eating Disorders: British National Surveillance Study. *British Journal of Psychiatry.* 2011;198:295-301.

6. Mascola AJ, Bryson SW, Agras WS. Picky Eating During Childhood: A Longitudinal Study to Age 11 Years. *Eating Behaviors.* 2010;4:253-7.

7. Orrell-Valente JK, Hill LG, Brechwald WA, et al. "Just Three More Bites:" An Observational Analysis of Parents' Socialization of Children's Eating at Mealtime. *Appetite.* 2007;48:37-45.

8. Stanek K, Abbott D, Cramer S. Diet Quality and The Eating Environment of Preschool Children. *Journal of the American Dietetic Association.* 1990;90:1582-4.

9. Ventura A, Gromis J, Lohse B. Feeding Practices and Styles Used by Diverse Sample of Low-Income Parents of Preschool-aged Children. *Journal of Nutrition Education and Behavior.* 2010;42;242-9.

10. Pelchat ML, Pliner P. Antecedents and Correlates of Feeding Problems in Young Children. *Journal of Nutrition Education.* 1986;18:23-8.

11. Pinhas L, Morris A, Crosby RD, Katzman DK. Incidence and Age-Specific Presentation of Restrictive Eating Disorders in Children: A Canadian Pediatric Surveillance Program Study. *Archives of Pediatric Adolescent Medicine.* 2011;165:895-9.

12. Zhao Y, Encinosa W. Hospitalizations for Eating Disorders From 1999-2006, Statistical Brief #70. *The Healthcare Cost and Utilization Project.* April 2009.

13. May A, Dietz W. The Feeding Infants and Toddlers Study 2008: Opportunities to Assess Parental, Cultural, and Environmental Influences on Dietary Behaviors and Obesity Prevention Among Young Children. *Journal of the Academy of Nutrition and Dietetics.* 2010;110:11-15. *This supplement to the Journal of the American Dietetic Association includes several papers discussing the results of the most recent Feeding Infants and Toddlers Study (FITS) conducted in 2008.*

14. Neumark-Sztainer D, Hannan P, Story M, Perry C. Weight-Control Behaviors Among Adolescent Girls and Boy: Implications for Dietary Intake. *Journal of the American Dietetic Association.* 2004;104:913-20

15. Gustafson-Larson AM, Terry RD. Weight-Related Behaviors and Concerns of Fourth-Grade Children. *Journal of the American Dietetic Association.* 1992;92:818-22.

16. Adair LS. The Infant's Ability to Self-Regulate Caloric Intake: A Case Study. *Journal of the American Dietetic Association.* 1984;84:543-6.

17. Scaglioni S, Salvioni M, Galimberti C. Influence of Parental Attitudes in the Development of Children Eating Behavior. *The British Journal of Nutrition.* 2008;99:S22-S25.

18. Rolls BJ. Sensory Specific Satiety. *Nutrition Review.* 1986;44:93-101.

19. MyPlate USDA. Available at: www.choosemyplate.gov (accessed 2012).

20. Forestall CA, Mennella JA. Early Determinants of Fruit and Vegetable Acceptance. *Pediatrics.* 2007;120:1247-54.

21. Davis CM. Self-Selection of Diet by Newly Weaned Infants: An Experimental Study. *American Journal of Diseases in Childhood.* 1928;36:651-79.

22. Barlow S. "Beyond the Scale and Tape Measure: Measurement of Obesity." (September 2011). Available at: www.my.americanheart.org (accessed 2012).

23. Romero-Corral A, Somers VK, Sierra-Johnson J. Accuracy of Body Mass Index in Diagnosing Obesity in the Adult General Population. *International Journal of Obesity.* 2008;32:959-66.

24. Ashworth A, Millward DJ. Catch-up Growth in Children. *Nutrition Reviews.* 1986;44, 157-63.

25. Johnson D, Gunnar M. "Growth Failure in Institutionalized Children." Chapter IV: Growth. *Monographs of the Society for Research and Child Development.* 2011;76(4):92-116

26. Johnson D, Guthrie D, Smyke AT, et al. Growth and Association Between Auxology, Caregiving Environment, and Cognition in Socially Deprived Children Randomized to Foster vs. Ongoing Institutional Care. *Archives of Pediatric and Adolescent Medicine.* 2010;164:507-16.

27. Teilmann G, Boas M. Early Pituitary-Gonadal Activation Before Clinical Signs of Puberty in 5- To 8-Year-Old Adopted Girls: A Study Of 99 Foreign Adopted Girls and 93 Controls. *The Journal of Clinical Endocrinology and Metabolism.* 2007;92:2539-44.

28. Legler JD, Rose LC. Assessment of Abnormal Growth Curves. *American Family Physician.* 1998;58:158-68.

29. Brann, LS. Classifying Preadolescent Boys Based on Their Weight Status and Percent Body Fat Produces Different Groups. *Journal of the American Dietetic Association.* 2008;108: 1018-22.

30. Serdula MK, Ivery D, Coates RJ, et al. Do Obese Children Become Obese Adults? A Review of the Literature. *Preventive Medicine.* 1993;22:167-77.

31. Satter EM. Internal Regulation and The Evolution of Normal Growth as the Basis for Prevention of Obesity in Childhood. *Journal of the American Dietetic Association.* 1996;96:860-4.

32. Eisenmann JC, Katzmarzyk PT, Arnall DA, et al. Growth and Overweight of Navajo Youth: Secular Changes From 1955 to 1997. *International Journal of Obesity.* 2000;24:211-8.

33. Ryan A, Martinez G, Baumgartner R, et al. Median Skinfold Thickness Distributions and Fat-Wave Patterns in Mexican-American Children Form the Hispanic Health and Nutrition Examination Survey (HHANES 1982-84.) *The American Journal of Clinical Nutrition.*1990;51:925S-35S.

34. Ryan AS, Martinez GA, Roche AF. An Evaluation of the Association Between Socioeconomic Status and the Growth of American Children: Data from the Hispanic Health and Nutrition Examination Survey. (HHANES 1982-1984.) *American Journal of Clinical Nutrition.* 1990;51:944S-952S.

35. Haines K, Neumark-Sztainer D. Prevention of Obesity and Eating Disorders: A Consideration of Shared Risk Factors. *Health Education Resources.* 2006;21:770-82.

36. Scaglioni S, Salvioni M, Galimberti C. Influence of Parental Attitudes in the Development of Children's Eating Behavior. *The British Journal of Nutrition.* 2008;99:S22-S25.

37. Neumark-Sztainer D, Wall M, Story M, Fulkerson JA. Are Family Meal Patterns Associated With Disordered Eating Behaviors Among Adolescents? *Journal of Adolescent Health.* 2004;35:350-9.

38. von Kries R, Toschke AM, Wurmser H, et al. Reduced Risk of Overweight and Obesity in 5-and 6-Year-Old Children by Duration of Sleep—a Cross-Sectional Study. *International Journal of Obesity and Related Metabolic Disorders.* 2002;26:710-16.

39. Anderson S, Gooze R, Lemeshow S, Whitaker R. Quality of Early Maternal–Child Relationship and Risk of Adolescent Obesity. *Pediatrics.* 2012;129:132-40.

40. Hasler G, Buysse DJ, Klaghofer R, et al. The Association Between Short Sleep Duration and Obesity in Young Adults: A 13-Year Prospective Study. *Sleep.* 2004;27:661-6.

41. Taveras EM, Rifas-Shiman SL, Berkey CS, et al. Family Dinner and Adolescent Overweight. *Obesity Research.* 2005;13:900-06.

42. Rhee KE, Lumeng JC, Appugliese DP, et al. Parenting Styles and Overweight Status in First Grade. *Pediatrics.* 2006;117:2047-54.

43. Steel JS, Buchi KF. Medical and Mental Health of Children in the Utah Foster Care System. *Pediatrics.* 2008;122:703-9.

44. Orrell-Valente JK, Hill LG, Brechwald WA, et al. "Just Three More Bites:" An Observational Analysis of Parents' Socialization of Children's Eating at Mealtime. *Appetite*. 2007;48:37-45

45. Stanek K, Abbott D, Cramer S. Diet Quality and the Eating Environment of Preschool Children. *Journal of the American Dietetic Association*. 1990;90:1582-4.

46. Galloway AT, Fiorito LM, Francis LA, Birch LL. "Finish Your Soup:" Counterproductive Effects of Pressuring Children to Eat on Intake and Affect. *Appetite*. 2006;46:318-23.

47. Keck, Gregory and Kupecky, Regina. *Parenting the Hurt Child*: *Helping Adoptive Families Heal and Grow*. Colorado Springs, CO: Navpress, 2009.

48. Black M, Aboud F. Responsive Feeding—Promoting Healthy Growth and Development for Infants and Toddlers Responsive Feeding Is Embedded in a Theoretical Framework of Responsive Parenting. *The Journal of Nutrition*. 2011;141:490-4.

49. Rhodes-Courter, Ashley. *Three Little Words*: *A Memoir*. New York: Simon and Schuster, 2009.

Chapter 2

1. Position Statement: Nutrition Guidance for Healthy Children Ages 2 to 11 years. *Journal of the American Dietetic Association*. 2008;108:1038-47

2. Grey, Deborah. *Attaching in Adoption: Practical Tools for Today's Parents*. Indianapolis, IN: Perspectives Press, 2002.

3. CASA: The National Center on Addiction & Substance Abuse at Columbia University. *The Importance of Family Dinners IV*. 2007

4. Hofferth SL. How American Children Spend Their Time. *Journal of Marriage and the Family*. 2001;63:295- 308.

Chapter 3

1. Minnesota International Adoption Project. *IADP Newsletter* (Fall 2003). Available at: http://www.cehd.umn.edu/icd/iap/ (accessed 2012).

2. World Health Organization (WHO). "Complementary Feeding." Available at: http://www.who.int/nutrition/topics/complementary_feeding/en (accessed 2012).

3. Johnson D, Guthrie D, Smyke AT, et al. Growth and Association Between Auxology, Caregiving Environment, and Cognition in Socially Deprived Children Randomized to Foster vs. Ongoing Institutional Care. *Archives of Pediatric and Adolescent Medicine*. 2010;164:507-16.

4. Engle PL, Bentley M, Pelto G. The Role of Care in Nutrition Programmes: Current Research and a Research Agenda. *Proceedings of the Nutrition Society*. 2000;59:25–35.

5. Bryant-Waugh R, Markham L, Kreipe R, et al. Feeding and Eating Disorders in Childhood. *The International Journal of Eating Disorders*. 2010;43:98-111.

6. Horwitz S, Owens P, Simms M. Specialized Assessments for Children in Foster Care. *Pediatrics* 2000;106;59-66.

7. Steele JS, Buchi KF. Medical and Mental Health of Children in the Utah Foster Care System. *Pediatrics*. 2008;122:e703-9.

8. Forestall CA, Mennella JA. Early Determinants of Fruit and Vegetable Acceptance. *Pediatrics*. 2007;120:1247-54. Page 62

9. Satter, E. "The Picky Eater." Available at: http://www.ellynsatter.com/the-picky-eater-i-43.html (accessed 2012).

10. Wilbarger J, Gunnar M, Schneider M, Pollak S. Sensory Processing In Internationally Adopted, Post-Institutionalized Children. *Journal of Child Psychology and Psychiatry*. 2012;51:1105-14.

11. Zimmer M, Desch L, et al. Policy Statement: Sensory Integration Therapies for Children with Developmental and Behavioral Disorders. *Pediatrics*. 2012;129:1186-8.

12. Satter, Ellyn. *Child of Mine: Feeding With Love and Good Sense*. Boulder, CO: Bull Publishing, 2001.

13. Mascola AJ, Bryson SW, Agras WS. Picky Eating During Childhood: A Longitudinal Study to Age 11 Years. *Eating Behaviors*. 2010;4:253-7.

14. Scaglioni S, Salvioni M, Galimberti C. Influence of Parental Attitudes in the Development of Children Eating Behavior. *The British Journal of Nutrition*. 2008;99:S22-S25.

15. Engle PL, Pelto GH. Responsive Feeding: Implications for Policy and Program Implementation. *The Journal of Nutrition*. 2011;141:508-11.

16. Fraker C, Fishbein M, Cox S, Walbert L. *Food Chaining: The Proven 6-Step Plan to Stop Picky Eating, Solve Feeding Problems, and Expand Your Child's Die*. Cambridge, MA: Da Capo Press, 2007.

Chapter 4

1. Satter, EM. "Follow Growth at the Extremes With Z-Scores. Understanding and Using Z-Scores to Track Children's Growth." (Family Meals Focus #66). Available at: http://www.ellynsatter.com/february-2012-family-meals-focus-66-understanding-and-using-scores-to-track-childrens-growth-i-183.html (accessed 2012).

2. Legler JD, Rose LC. Assessment of Abnormal Growth Curves. *American Family Physician*. 1998;58:158-8.

3. Krugman S, Dubowitz H. Failure to Thrive. *Family Physician.* 2003;68:879-84.

4. World Health Organization. "Child Growth Standards." Available at: http://www.who.int/childgrowth/en (accessed 2012).

5. Keck, Gregory and Kupecky, Regina. *Parenting the Hurt Child*: *Helping Adoptive Families Heal and Grow.* Colorado Springs, CO: Navpress, 2009.

6. Scaglioni S, Salvioni M, Galimberti C. Influence of Parental Attitudes in the Development of Children Eating Behavior. *The British Journal of Nutrition.* 2008;99:S22-S25.

7. Mascola AJ, Bryson SW, Agras WS. Picky Eating During Childhood: A Longitudinal Study to Age 11 Years. *Eating Behaviors.* 2010;4:253-7.

8. Rogers, Fred. *The Mister Rogers Parenting Book*: *Helping To Understand Your Young Child.* Philadelphia, PA: Running Press, 2002.

9. Van der Horst K. Overcoming Picky Eating. Eating Enjoyment as a Central Aspect of Children's Eating Behaviors. *Appetite.* 2012;58:576-74.

10. Keck, Gregory and Kupecky, Regina. *Parenting the Hurt Child*: *Helping Adoptive Families Heal and Grow*, Colorado Springs, CO: Navpress, 2009.

11. Cline, Foster and Fay, Jim. *Parenting with Love and Logic.* Colorado Springs, CO: Piñon Press, 2006.

12. Fisher JO, Mitchell DC, Smiciklas-Wright H, Birch LL. Parental Influences on Young Girls' Fruit and Vegetable, Micronutrient, and Fat Intakes. *Journal of the American Dietetic Association.* 2002;1025:58-64.

13. Pliner P, Stallberg-White C. "Pass the Ketchup, Please:" Familiar Flavors Increase Children's Willingness to Taste Novel Foods. *Appetite.* 2000;34:95-103.

14. Havermans RC, Jansen A. Increasing Children's Liking of Vegetables Through Flavour-Learning. *Appetite.* 2007;48:259-62.

15. Galloway AT, Fiorito LM, Francis LA, Birch LL. "Finish Your Soup:" Counterproductive Effects of Pressuring Children to Eat on Intake and Affect. *Appetite.* 2006;46:318-23.

Chapter 5

1. Centers for Disease Control and Prevention. "Childhood Overweight and Obesity." Available at: http://www.cdc.gov/obesity/defining.html (accessed 2012)

2. Townsend E, Pitchford JN. Baby Knows Best? The Impact of Weaning Style on Food Preferences and Body Mass Index in Early Childhood in a Case-Controlled Sample. British Medical Journal Open. 2012;6;2(1):e000298.

3. Robison, GB. "The 'Childhood Obesity Epidemic:' What is the Real Problem, and What Can We Do About It?" PDF. www.no-obesity-epidemic.org (Accessed 2012).

4. Davison KK, Birch LL. Weight Status, Parent Reaction, and Self-Concept in Five-Year-Old Girls. *Pediatrics.* 2001;107:46-53.

5. Haines K, Neumark-Sztainer D. Prevention of Obesity and Eating Disorders: A Consideration of Shared Risk Factors. *Health Education Resources.* 2006;21:770-82.

6. Neumark-Sztainer D, Wall M, Story M, van den Berg P. Accurate Parental Classification of Overweight Adolescents' Weight Status: Does it Matter? *Pediatrics* 2008;121(6):e1495-502.

7. Centers for Disease Control. "About BMI For Children and Teens." Available at: http://www.cdc.gov/healthyweight/assessing/bmi/childrens_bmi/about_childrens_bmi.html (accessed 2012).

8. Brown L, and Weil J. "The Paradox of Hunger and Obesity in America." (July 2003). Food Research and Action Center. Available at: http://www.frac.org/html/news/071403hungerandObesity.htm. (accessed 2011).

9. Jones SJ, Jahns L, Laraia BA, Haughton B. Lower Risk of Overweight in School-aged Food Insecure Girls Who Participate in Food Assistance: Results From the Panel Study of Income Dynamics Child Development Supplement. *Archives of Pediatric and Adolescent Medicine.* 2003;157:780-4.

10. Eisenmann JC, Katzmarzyk PT, Arnall DA, et al. Growth and Overweight of Navajo Youth: Secular Changes From 1955 to 1997. *International Journal of Obesity.* 2000;24:211-18.

11. Ryan A, Martinez G, Baumgartner R, et al. Median Skinfold Thickness Distributions and Fat-Wave Patterns in Mexican-American Children Form the Hispanic Health and Nutrition Examination Survey (HHANES 1982-84). *The American Journal of Clinical Nutrition.*1990;51:925S-35S.

12. Ryan AS, Martinez GA, Roche AF. An Evaluation of the Association Between Socioeconomic Status and the Growth of American Children: Data from the Hispanic Health and Nutrition Examination Survey. (HHANES 1982-1984). *American Journal of Clinical Nutrition.* 1990;51:944S-952S.

13. Rosenbaum M, Hirsch J, Gallagher DA, Leibel RL. Long-term Persistence of Adaptive Thermogenesis in Subjects Who Have Maintained a Reduced Body Weight. *American Journal of Clinical Nutrition.* 2008;88:906-12.

14. Sumithran P, Prendergast LA, Delbridge E. Long-term Persistence of Hormonal Adaptations to Weight Loss. *New England Journal of Medicine.* 2011;365:1597-604.

15. Parker-Pope, Tara. "The Fat Trap." *The New York Times* (December 28, 2011). Available at: http://www.nytimes.com/2012/01/01/magazine/tara-parker-pope-fat-trap.html?pagewanted=all (accessed 2012).

16. Steele JS, Buchi KF. Medical and Mental Health of Children in the Utah Foster Care System. *Pediatrics.* 2008;122: e703-9.

17. Hadfield SC, Preece PM. Obesity in Looked After Children: Is Foster Care Protective From the Dangers of Obesity? *Child Care Health and Development.* 2008;34:710-12.

18. Satter, Ellyn. *Your Child's Weight: Helping Without Harming.* Madison, WI: Kelcy Press, 2005.

19. Shapiro LR, Crawford PB, Clark MJ, et al. Obesity Prognosis: A Longitudinal Study of Children From the Age of 6 Months to 9 Years. *American Journal of Public Health.* 1984;74:968-72.

20. Musher-Eizenman DR, Holub SC, Hauser JC, Young KM. The Relationship Between Parents' Anti-Fat Attitudes and Restrictive Feeding. *Obesity.* 2007;15:2095-2102.

21. Ventura A, Gromis J, Lohse B. Feeding Practices and Styles Used by Diverse Sample of Low-Income Parents of Preschool-aged Children. *Journal of Nutrition Education and Behavior.* 2010;42:242-9.

22. Birch LL, Davison KK. Family Environmental Factors Influencing the Developing Behavioral Controls of Food Intake and Childhood Overweight. *Pediatric Clinics of North America.* 2001; 48:893-907.

23. Fisher JO, Birch LL. Fat Preferences and Fat Consumption of 3-5 Year-Old Children are Related to Parental Adiposity. *Journal of the American Dietetic Association.* 1995;95:759-64.

24. Faith MS, Scanlon KS, Birch LL, et al. Parent-Child Feeding Strategies and Their Relationships to Child Eating and Weight Status. *Obesity Research.* 2004;12:1711-22.

25. Hurley K, Cross MB, Hughes SO. A Systematic Review of Responsive Feeding and Child Obesity in High-Income Countries. *The Journal of Nutrition.* 2011;141:496-501.

26. Birch LL, Davison KK. Family Environmental Factors Influencing the Developing Behavioral Controls of Food Intake and Childhood Overweight. *Pediatric Clinics of North America.* 2001;48:893-907.

27. Faith MS, Berkowitz RI, Stallings VA, et al. Parental Feeding Attitudes and Styles and Child Body Mass Index: Prospective Analysis of a Gene-Environment Interaction. *Pediatrics.* 2004;114:e429-36.

28. Rocandio AM, Ansotegui L, Arroyo M. Comparison of Dietary Intake Among Overweight and Non- Overweight Schoolchildren. *International Journal of Obesity and Related Metabolic Disorders.* 2001;25:1651-5.

29. Huh S, Rifas-Shiman S. Prospective Association Between Milk Intake and Adiposity in Preschool-Aged Children. *Journal of the American Dietetic Association.* 2010;110:563-70.

30. Rose HE, Mayer J. Activity, Calorie Intake, Fat Storage, and the Energy Balance of Infants. *Pediatrics.* 1968;41:18-29.

31. Rolland-Cachera MF, Bellisle F. No Correlation Between Adiposity and Food Intake: Why Are Working Class Children Fatter? *American Journal of Clinical Nutrition.* 1986;44:779-87.

32. Gunther AL, Stahl LJ, Buyken AE, Kroke, A. Association of Dietary Energy Density in Childhood With Age and Body Fatness at The Onset of the Pubertal Growth Spurt. *British Journal of Nutrition*. 2011;106:345-9.

33. Fernandes MM. The Effect of Soft Drink Availability in Elementary Schools on Consumption. *Journal of the American Dietetic Association*. 2008;108:1445-51.

34. Robison J, Putnam K, McKibbin L, et al. Health at Every Size: A Compassionate, Effective Approach for Helping Individuals with Weight-Related Concerns Part I and II. *American Association of Occupational Health Nurses*. 2007;55:185-92.

35. Hamer M, Stamatakis E. Metabolically Healthy Obesity and Risk of All-Cause and Cardiovascular Disease Mortality. *The Journal of Clinical Endocrinology & Metabolism*. April 2012. ePub; print forthcoming.

36. Wei M, Kampert JB, Barlow CE, et al. Relationship Between Low Cardiorespiratory Fitness and Mortality in Normal-Weight, Overweight, and Obese Men. *Journal of the American Medical Association*. 1999;282:1546-53.

37. Bacon L, Klein NL, Van Loan MD. et al. Evaluating a "Non-diet" Wellness Intervention for Improvement of Metabolic Fitness, Psychological Well-Being and Eating and Activity Behaviors. *International Journal of Obesity*. 2002;26:854-65.

38. Bacon L, Stern JS, Van Loan MD, Keim NL. Size Acceptance and Intuitive Eating Improve Health for Obese, Female Chronic Dieters. *Journal of the American Dietetic Association*. 2005;105:929-36.

39. Carroll S, Borkoles E, Polman R. Short-term Effects of a Non-Dieting Lifestyle Intervention Program on Weight Management, Fitness, Metabolic Risk, and Psychological Well-Being in Obese Premenopausal Females With the Metabolic Syndrome. *Applied Physiology, Nutrition and Metabolism*. 2007;32:125-42.

40. Allen DB, Nemeth BA, Clark RR, et al. Fitness is a Stronger Predictor of Fasting Insulin Levels Than Fatness in Overweight Male Middle-School Children. *Journal of Pediatrics*. 200;150:383-7.

41. Kulminski AM, Arbeev KG, Kulminskaya IV, et al. Body Mass Index and 9-Year Mortality in Disabled and Nondisabled Older U.S Individuals. *Journal of the American Geriatrics Society*. 2008;56:105-10.

42. Flegal KM, Graubard BI, Williamson DF, Gail MH. Excess Deaths Associated With Underweight, Overweight, and Obesity. *Journal of the American Medical Association*. 2005;293:1861-7.

43. Gruberg L, Mercado N, Milo S, et al. Impact of Body Mass Index on the Outcome of Patients with Multivessel Disease Randomized to Either Coronary Artery Bypass Grafting or Stenting in the Arts Trial—Truth or Paradox II? *American Journal of Cardiology*. 2005;4:439-44.

44. Howard BV, Manson JE, Stefanick ML, et al. Low-Fat Dietary Pattern and Weight Change over 7 Years: The Women's Health Initiative Dietary Modification Trial. *Journal of the American Medical Association*. 2006;295:39-49.

45. Bjorge T, Engeland A, Tverdal A, et al. Body Mass Index in Adolescence in Relation to Cause-Specific Mortality: A Follow-Up of 230,000 Norwegian Adolescents. *American Journal of Epidemiology.* 2008;168:30-7.

46. Bacon, Linda. *Health At Every Size.* Dallas, TX: Ben Bella, 2008.

47. Barlow S. "Beyond the Scale and Tape Measure: Measurement of Obesity." (Sept. 2011). Available at: www.my.americanheart.org (accessed 2012).

48. Serdula MK, Ivery D, Coates RJ, et al. Do Obese Children Become Obese Adults? A Review of the Literature. *Preventive Medicine.*1993;22:167-7.

49. Robison, GB. "The 'Childhood Obesity Epidemic:' What is the Real Problem, and What Can We Do About It?" PDF. www.no-obesity-epidemic.org (Accessed 2012).

50. Whitlock E, Williams S, Gold R, et al. Screening and Interventions for Childhood Overweight: Evidence Synthesis. United States Preventive Services Task Force: *Evidence Syntheses, No. 36:* Chapter 4. Discussion

51. Ogden CL, Carroll LR, Curtin LR, et al. Prevalence of High Body Mass Index in U.S. Children and Adolescents, 1999-2010. *Journal of the American Medical Association.* 2012;307:483-90.

52. Ueland O, Cardello AV, Merrill EP, Lesher LL. Effect of Portion Size Information on Food Intake. *Journal of the American Dietetic Association.* 2009;109:124-27.

53. Rolls B, Roe L, Halverson K, Meengs J. Using a Smaller Plate Did Not Reduce Energy Intake at Meals. *Appetite.* 2007;49:652-60.

54. McCormack LA, Laska MN, Gray C, et al. Weight-Related Teasing in a Racially Diverse Sample of Sixth-Grade Children. *Journal of the American Dietetic Association.* 2011;111(3):431-6.

55. Libbey HP, Story MT, Neumark-Sztainer DR, Boutelle KN. Teasing, Disordered Eating Behaviors, And Psychological Morbidities Among Overweight Adolescents. *Obesity.* 2008;16:S24-9.

56. Andreyeva T, Puhl RM, Brownell KD. Changes in Perceived Weight Discrimination Among Americans, 1995-1996 through 2004-2006. *Obesity.* 2008;16:1129-34.

57. Schwartz MB, Chambliss HO, Brownell KD, et al. Weight Bias Among Health Professionals Specializing in Obesity. *Obesity Research.* 2003;11:1033-9.

58. Rose HE, Mayer J. Activity, Calorie Intake, Fat Storage, and the Energy Balance of Infants. *Pediatrics.* 1968;41:18-29.

59. Mascola AJ, Bryson SW, Agras WS. Picky Eating During Childhood: A Longitudinal Study to Age 11 Years. *Eating Behaviors.* 2010;4:253-7.

60. Epstein LH, Saelens BE, Myers MD, Vito D. The Effects of Decreasing Sedentary Behaviors on Activity Choice in Obese Children. *Health Psychology.* 1997;16:107-13.

61. Teilmann G, Boas M. Early Pituitary-Gonadal Activation Before Clinical Signs of Puberty in 5- To 8-Year-Old Adopted Girls: A Study of 99 Foreign Adopted Girls and 93 Controls. *The Journal of Clinical Endocrinology and Metabolism.* 2007;92:2539-44 .

Chapter 6

1. Lohse B, Psota T. Eating Competence of Elderly Spanish Adults is Associated With a Healthy Diet and a Favorable Cardiovascular Disease Risk Profile. *Journal of Nutrition*. 2010;140:1322-7.
2. Lohse B, Satter E. Measuring Eating Competence: Psychometric Properties and Validity of the ecSatter Inventory. *Journal of Nutrition Education and Behavior*. 2007;39:S154-66.
3. Van der Horst K. Overcoming Picky Eating. Eating Enjoyment as a Central Aspect of Children's Eating Behaviors. *Appetite*. 2012;58:576-74.
4. Crum AJ, Corbin WR, Brownell KD, Salovey P. "Mind Over Milkshakes:" Mindsets, Not Just Nutrients, Determine Ghrelin Response. *Health Psychology*. 201;30:424-9.
5. Neumark-Sztainer D, Wall M, Guo J, et al. Obesity, Disordered Eating, and Eating Disorders in a Longitudinal Study of Adolescents: How Do Dieters Fare Five Years Later? *Journal of the American Dietetic Association*. 2006;106:559-68.
6. Hallberg L, Bjorn-Rasmussen E, Rosander L, Suwanik R. Iron Absorption from Southeast Asian Diets. *American Journal of Clinical Nutrition*.1977;30:539-48.
7. Barclay GR, Turnberg LA. Effect of Psychosocial Stress on Salt and Water Transport in the Human Jejunum. *Gastroenterology*. 1987;93:91-7.
8. Zellner DA, Loaiza S, Gonzalez Z, et al. Food Selection Changes Under Stress. *Physiology and Behavior*. 2006;87(4):789-93.
9. Herman CP, Polivy J, Esses VM. The Illusion of Counter-Regulation. *Appetite*. 1987;9:161-169.
10. Roemmich JN, Wright SM, Epstein LH. Dietary Restraint and Stress-Induced Snacking in Youth. *Obesity Research*. 2002;10:1120-6.
11. Science Daily. "Organic Snackers Underestimate Calories, Study Shows." (April 28, 2010). Available at: http://www.sciencedaily.com/releases/2010/04/1004281 73344.htm (accessed April 2012).
12. O'dea, J. School-Based Interventions to Prevent Eating Problems: First Do No Harm. *Eating Disorders*. 2000;8:123-30.
13. Neumark-Sztainer D. Preventing Obesity and Eating Disorders in Adolescents: What Can Health Care Providers Do? *Journal of Adolescent Health*. 2009;44:206-13.
14. Burney J, Irwin HJ. Shame and Guilt in Women With Eating-Disorder Symptomatology. *Journal of Clinical Psychology*. 2000;56:51-61.
15. Sabiston CM, Brunet J, Kowalski KC, et al. The Role of Body-Related Self-Conscious Emotions in Motivating Women's Physical Activity. *Journal of Sports & Exercise Psychology*. 2010;32:417-37.

16. Satter EM. "Children and Their Eating—Ellyn Satter's Guidelines for the School Nutrition Staff." PDF. Available at: http://www.ellynsatter.com/links-i-82.html (accessed 2012).

17. Perry B. "Bonding, Attachment and the Maltreated Child." PDF. Available at: www.ChildTraumaAcdemy.org (accessed 2012).

18. Pepino MY, Mennella JA. Sucrose-Induced Analgesia is Related to Sweet Preferences in Children But Not Adults. *Pain.* 2005;119:210-18.

19. Crow SJ, Peterson CB, Swanson SA, et al. Increased Mortality in Bulimia Nervosa and Other Eating Disorders. *American Journal of Psychiatry.* 2009;166:1342-6.

20. Pinhas L, Morris A, Crosby RD, Katzman DK. Incidence and Age-Specific Presentation of Restrictive Eating Disorders in Children: A Canadian Pediatric Surveillance Program study. *Archives of Pediatric Adolescent Medicine.* 2011;165:895-9.

21. Zhao Y, Encinosa W. "Hospitalizations for Eating Disorders from 1999-2006, Statistical Brief #70." *The Healthcare Cost and Utilization Project* (2009).

22. Dingemans AE, van Furth EF. Binge Eating Disorder Psychopathology in Normal Weight and Obese Individuals. *International Journal Eating Disorders.* 2012;45:135-8.

23. Fisher JO, Birch LL. Parents' Restrictive Feeding Practices are Associated with Young Girls' Negative Self-Evaluation of Eating. *Journal of the American Dietetic Association.* 2000;100:1341-46.

24. Roemmich JN, Wright SM, Epstein LH. Dietary Restraint and Stress-Induced Snacking in Youth. *Obesity Research.* 2002;10:1120-6.

25. Fisher JO, Birch LL. Fat Preferences and Fat Consumption of 3-5 Year-Old Children are Related to Parental Adiposity. *Journal of the American Dietetic Association.*1995;95:759-64.

26. Fisher JO, Birch LL. Eating in the Absence Of Hunger and Overweight in Girls from 5 to 7 Years of Age. *American Journal of Clinical Nutrition.* 2002;76:226-31.

27. Neumark-Sztainer D, Wall M, Story M, Fulkerson JA. Are Family Meal Patterns Associated with Disordered Eating Behaviors Among Adolescents? *Journal of Adolescent Health.* 2004;35:350-9.

28. Neumark-Sztainer D, Bauer KW. Family Weight Talk and Dieting: How Much Do They Matter for Body Dissatisfaction and Disordered Eating Behaviors in Adolescent Girls? *Journal of Adolescent Health.* 2010 Sep;47(3):270-6.

29. Reba-Harrelson L, Von Holle A, Hamer RM, et al. Patterns and Prevalence of Disordered Eating and Weight Control Behaviors in Women Ages 25-45. *Eating and Weight Disorders.* 2009;12:190-8.

30. Marcus MD, Bromberger JT, Wei HL, et al. Prevalence and Selected Correlates of Eating Disorder Symptoms Among a Multiethnic Community Sample of Midlife Women. *Annals of Behavioral Medicine.* 2007;33:269-77.
31. Davison KK, Earnest MB, Birch LL. Participation in Aesthetic Sports and Girls' Weight Concerns at Ages 5 and 7 Years. *International Journal of Eating Disorders.* 2002;31:312-7.

Chapter 7

1. Rapley, Gill and Murkett, Tracey. *Baby Led Weaning: The Essential Guide to Introducing Solid Foods and Helping Your Baby to Grow Up a Happy and Confident Eater.* New York: The Experiment, 2010.
2. Wright CM, Cameron K, Tsiaka M, Parkinson KN. Is Baby-Led Weaning Feasible? When Do Babies First Reach Out for and Eat Finger Foods? *Maternal Child Nutrition.* 2011;7:27-33.
3. Davis CM. Self-Selection of Diet by Newly Weaned Infants: An Experimental Study. *American Journal of Diseases in Childhood.* 1928;36:651-79.
4. Satter, EM. "12-17 Years: Feeding Your Adolescent." (2012). Available at: http://www.ellynsatter.com/12-to-17-years-feeding-your-adolescent-i-34.html (accessed 2012).

Chapter 8

1. Rangel C, Dukeshire S, MacDonald L. Diet and Anxiety. An Exploration Into the Orthorexic Society. *Appetite.* 2012;58:124-32.
2. Venter C, Pereira B, Voigt K, Grundy J. Prevalence and Cumulative Incidence of Food Hypersensitivity in the First 3 Years of Life. *Allergy.* 2008;63:354-9.
3. National Institute of Allergy and Infectious Diseases. "Guidelines for the Diagnosis and Management of Food Allergy in the United States, Summary for Patients, Families, and Caregivers." (2011). Available at: http://www.niaid.nih.gov/topics/foodallergy/clinical/Pages/default.aspx (accessed online 2012).
4. Millward C, Ferriter M, Calver SJ, et al. "Gluten and Casein-Free Diets for Autism Spectrum Disorder." (January 2009). Available at: http://summaries.cochrane.org/CD003498/gluten-and-casein-free-diets-for-autism-spectrum-disorder (accessed 2012).
5. de Magistris L, Familiari V, Pascotto A, et al. Alterations of the Intestinal Barrier in Patients with Autism Spectrum Disorders and in Their First-Degree Relatives. *Journal of Pediatric Gastroenterology and Nutrition.* 2010;51:418-24.

6. Black, D. "Nutritional Interventions for Children with FASD." (2002). Available at: www.come-over.to/FAS/FASDnutrition.htm (accessed 2012).

7. Taubes, G. "Salt, We Misjudged You." *The New York Times* (June 2, 2012). Available at: http://www.nytimes.com/2012/06/03/opinion/sunday/we-only-think-we-know-the-truth-about-salt.html?pagewanted=all (accessed 2012).

8. Hooper L, Bartlett C, Davey-Smith G, Ebrahim S. "The Long Term Effects of Advice to Cut Down on Salt in Food on Deaths, Cardiovascular Disease and Blood Pressure in Adults." (January 2009). Available at: http://summaries.cochrane.org/CD003656/the-long-term-effects-of-advice-to-cut-down-on-salt-in-food-on-deaths-cardiovascular-disease-and-blood-pressure-in-adults (accessed 2012).

9. Stolarz-Skrzypek K, Kuznetsova T, Thijs L. Fatal and Nonfatal Outcomes, Incidence of Hypertension, and Blood Pressure Changes in Relation to Urinary Sodium Excretion. *Journal of the American Medical Association.* 2011;305:1777-85.

10. Coldwell SE, Oswald TK, Reed DR. Biological Drive For Sugar as Marker of Growth Differs Between Adolescents with High Versus Low Sugar Preference. *Clinical Nutrition.* 2010;29:288–303.

11. Mayo Clinic. "Artificial Sweeteners: Understanding These and Other Sugar Substitutes." Available at: http://www.mayoclinic.com/health/artificial-sweeteners/MY00073 (accessed 2012).

12. Benton D. Plausibility of Sugar Addiction and Its Role in Obesity and Eating Disorders. *Journal of Clinical Nutrition.* 2010;29:288-303.

13. Newman J, Taylor A. Effect of a Means-End Contingency on Young Children's Food Preferences. *Journal of Experimental Child Psychology.* 1992;53:200-16.

14. Wardle J, Herrera MLCooke L, Gibson EL Modifying Children's Food Preferences: The Effects of Exposure and Reward on Acceptance of an Unfamiliar Vegetable. *European Journal of Clinical Nutrition.* 2003;57:341-8.

15. Lomer MC, Parker GC, Sanderson JD. Review Article: Lactose Intolerance in Clinical Practice-Myths and Realities. *Alimental Pharmacology and Therapeutics.* 2008;27:93-103.

16. Järvinen RM, Loukaskorpi M, Uusitupa. Tolerance of Symptomatic Lactose Malabsorbers to Lactose in Milk Chocolate. *European Journal of Clinical Nutrition.* 57: 701-705;

17. Academy of Nutrition and Dietetics. "Focusing on America's Children: The 2010 Dietary Guidelines for Americans." Available at: http://www.eatright.org/WorkArea/showcontent.aspx?id=6442464725 (accessed 2012).

18. Satter EM. A Moderate View of Fat Restriction. *Journal of the American Dietetic Association.* 2000;100:32-36

19. Huh S, Rifas-Shiman S. Prospective Association Between Milk Intake and Adiposity in Preschool-Aged Children. *Journal of the American Dietetic Association.* 2010;110:563-70.

20. Taubes G. The Soft Science of Dietary Fat. *Science*. 2001;291:2536-45.
21. Mozaffrian D, Aro A, Willett WC. Health Effects of Trans-Fatty Acids: Experimental and Observational Evidence. *European Journal of Clinical Nutrition*. 2009;63 Suppl2:S5.
22. Vicini J, Etherton T, Kris-Etherton P, et al. Survey of Retail Milk Composition as Affected by Label Claims Regarding Farm-Management Practices. *Journal of the American Dietetic Association*.

Chapter 9

1. Satter, Ellyn. *Child of Mine: Feeding With Love and Good Sense*. Boulder, CO: Bull Publishing, 2001.
2. Bentley B, Ritz S, Thopmson M. Practice Roundtable, Eosinophilic Esophagitis in Young Children: A comprehensive Approach. *Infant, Child and Adolescent Nutrition*. 2011;3:332-35.
3. Boorstein, Sylvia. *It's Easier Than You Think: The Buddhist Way to Happiness*. New York: Harper Collins, 1997.
4. Psych Central Weightless Blog. "How to Have a Fat-Talk Free Holiday Season." (November 2010). Available at: www.psychcentral.com/weightless (accessed 2012)
5. Ramsey SA, Branen LJ, Fletcher J, et al. "Are You Done?" Child Care Providers' Verbal Communication at Mealtimes That Reinforce or Hinder Children's Internal Cues of Hunger and Satiation. *Journal of Nutrition Education and Behavior*. 2010;42:265-70.
6. Ramsey, Jason. "Doctors Warn: Generation of Children Could Die Before Their Parents Due to Unhealthy Lifestyle." *Top News* (April 14, 2010). Available at: http://topnews.us/content/216676-doctors-warn-generation-children-could-die-their-parents-due-unhealthy-lifestyle (accessed 2012).
7. Rogers, Fred. *The Mister Rogers Parenting Book: Helping To Understand Your Young Child*. Philadelphia, PA: Running Press, 2002.
8. Keck, Gregory and Kupecky, Regina. *Parenting the Hurt Child: Helping Adoptive Families Heal and Grow*. Colorado Springs, CO: Navpress, 2009.
9. Eisenberg ME, Olson RE, Neumark-Sztainer D, et al. Correlations Between Family Meals and Psychosocial Well-being Among Adolescents. *Archives of Pediatric Adolescent Medicine*. 2004;158:792-6.
10. Neumark-Sztainer D, Wall M, Story M, Fulkerson JA. Are Family Meal Patterns Associated with Disordered Eating Behaviors Among Adolescents? *Journal of Adolescent Health*. 2004;35:350-9.
11. The National Center on Addiction and Substance Abuse at Columbia University. "The Importance of Family Dinners IV." (September 2007). Available at: http://www.casacolumbia.org/templates/publications_reports.aspx (accessed 2012).

Appendix I
Fact or Fiction:
Challenging Your Biases

Challenge yourself with this true/false quiz and learn where you may benefit from more information. Included are some of the most common "truths" and misperceptions I encounter in my work. Throughout this book, we have addressed all of these "myths." The truth will set you free.

Ninety-five percent of "overweight" and "obese" two-year-olds will be obese adults.
False: According to one study, about two-thirds of "overweight" (BMI at or above the 85th percentile) preschoolers will grow up to be in the "normal" range.

Making my child try two bites of something will help her learn to like it.
False: Pressure with feeding most often backfires. Children who are pressured to like a new food tend to like it less well.

Offering food and having it available all day long will help my small child grow.
False: Grazing, or pushing food on a child all day, generally worsens nutrition and makes her grow less well.

Taking soda out of schools makes kids lose weight.
False: Studies that took soda out of schools, and otherwise decreased calories and fat in school foods, did not make a difference in body mass index (BMI) in students.

BMI is a reliable indicator of health risks.
False: Fitness level is a more reliable health indicator.

If parents only knew their child's BMI, they could help the child lose weight.
False: Studies suggest that labeling a child as "overweight" or "obese" does not improve health, and might actually promote worse health behaviors such as dieting and disordered eating.

Limiting portions and forbidding high-fat and sugary treats is a good way to help a child lose weight.
False: The more restricted the child is, the more liable she is to eat in the absence of hunger and weigh more, not less.

Infants and young toddlers should only have plain vegetables and fruits so they learn to like them without sauces or cheese.
False: There is no evidence to support this. Studies support that a little sweetness, or condiments, help children like a greater variety of foods.

Pushing my child to eat the food pyramid every day, including five servings of fruits and veggies, will ensure good nutrition.
False: Pressure will make him less likely to eat well. If children are offered a variety of foods, their nutrition tends to even out over several days.

Kids will more often try a food they helped prepare or grow.
True: But it's no guarantee.

Food messages to children should be positive.
True: Messages that focus on avoidance, or create anxiety around certain foods, increase anxiety and do not help raise a competent eater.

If I encourage my child to control her weight in healthy ways like watching portions or limiting sweets, she will not become obese.
False: Even "healthy" weight control measures in teens resulted in teens who weighed more and had more disordered behaviors than their nondieting counterparts.

How did you do? If you got most of them wrong, don't despair. Ten years ago, I would have too. I included this quiz to show you how many of our commonly accepted "truths" around kids, weight, and food are simply wrong.

Appendix II
Medical Issues That Can Affect Feeding

This is by no means an exhaustive list, but is an overview of some of the more common medical issues that may affect eating (and a few uncommon ones you might want to know about). Remember, if there are changes or concerning symptoms, it's always safest to check with your child's doctor.

> A "differential" is a list of possible diagnoses that a health care provider must consider based on symptoms and history.

Anal Fissures
Painful tiny tears in the anal tissue associated with firm stool, withholding, and constipation (see Constipation). Treatment is same as for constipation, but additionally, some prescription creams may be helpful. Constipation can lead to stomach upset and decreased appetite. In addition to painful bowel movements (BMs), you may see small amounts of bright red blood when wiping with toilet paper.

Anatomical Abnormalities
Such as cleft palate, cleft lip, and malformations of the breathing and swallowing tubes make the mechanics of feeding more difficult (oral-motor challenges).

Anemia
Not enough oxygen-carrying and energy-carrying capacity in the blood (low hemoglobin, which binds to the oxygen). Usually due to iron deficiency, the greatest risk is during and after catch-up growth or growth spurts, and the first several months a child is with you. (See Iron Deficiency below.) Very rarely, anemia can be due to a blood disorder. Follow-up lab tests after iron supplementation (to confirm improvement) is critical.

Behavioral Concerns
There is a long list of issues that manifest with behavior problems or have a behavioral or judgment component: grief, attachment problems, post-traumatic stress, prenatal exposures (FASD), temperament, anxiety, depression, learning disabilities, verbal and

auditory processing challenges, ADD/ADHD, and others. All play a role in the feeding relationship.

Constipation

Sometimes a painful diaper rash or other issue can set up the cycle of withholding stool that the child can simply "out-clench," in spite of a diet full of fruits and fiber. Other times, low fiber or fluid intake can contribute. In addition, some children with food intolerances may experience constipation.

For some reason, more often than not I see constipation and later toilet training in children who are also selective eaters where there are significant feeding battles. I don't understand the connection, but I have theories: A medical issue, pain from constipation is decreasing the child's appetite, or the child is very intent on doing things on his or her own time frame and is still working for control.

If your child is FOS (full of sh... is the unofficial medical term) she is probably not very comfortable. It can also lead to decreased appetite and, at times, intense abdominal cramping and even vomiting—not to mention pain with BMs and, rarely, anal fissures, which are very painful and make matters worse (see Anal Fissures). A fissure is like a paper cut on the sensitive anal tissue, and it hurts as badly as it sounds. Some children can have a BM most days and still have significant constipation. If your child has unexplained abdominal pain, soiling of the underpants (encopresis, which happens when stool leaks around a firm ball of stool), or a distended abdomen, then impaction and constipation need to be ruled out. A simple X-ray can be diagnostic if the history is not clear-cut. Very rarely, there are anatomical reasons for chronic constipation, but most often it is a "functional" problem that can be corrected without surgery.

> If you are seeing your child's provider for constipation or other gut issues, s/he may want to do a rectal exam, where a gloved finger is put in the child's bottom. If your child has a history of past abuse or extreme anxiety, please discuss this with your child's social worker and doctor before the visit. Often, a trial of treatment can be done without the need for a rectal exam at the initial visit. Just be aware.

Toileting is a whole other area of consternation for some families of adopted and foster children who may have experienced abuse, punishment around accidents, or early sexualization. Therapists trained in working with hurt children can be very helpful with this issue.

Once a child is significantly constipated for weeks or months, the colon stretches, and this becomes a "chronic" condition. The colon is made of smooth muscle, and like any other muscle, it can get out of shape. There is no quick fix. It takes up to six months for a dilated colon to heal and get back into "shape" and proper function. Many families will try medication for a few days or even a week, thinking things are better and stopping treatment only to have the problem resume almost immediately. Parents often get angry with the child and think they are being naughty. Truth is, if a child has had significant constipation or pain, the body's natural reflex is to hold the BM in. Over time, it can be hard for them to understand and pick up on what their bodies are telling them. As parents stand over the sweating, purple-faced withholder shouting, "Let it out of your body, you will feel better!" the child simply can't comply.

In general, I recommend optimizing intake of liquids, fruits, and vegetables. However, chances are if you are reading this book, this is already a challenge! So, when that fails in the short term, MiraLAX laxative, which is flavorless and disappears when stirred into liquids, is an amazing tool to use while you work on feeding. The goal is to help your child have a daily, soft, pain-free BM for *months*. And by soft, I mean the consistency of toothpaste. Sorry for that image, but it helps define "soft." If you find a fiber product, or something else that works for your child, you and your doctor can go with that. My main point is that it takes *lots and lots of time*. You basically need to overpower the child's ability to hold in the BM. Keep up the beginning dose, and decrease the dose over a period time as long as symptoms don't return.

> You should be working with your child's health care provider to monitor symptoms and rule out any other causes for the constipation.

Stay home when you start this process and expect soiling and accidents initially, but every few months wean the dose down and see what happens. Your child might be on MiraLAX for 18 months or more, but hopefully by then she will have learned to respond to her body's cues. Oh, and don't forget to relax yourself, don't pressure, stay emotionally neutral, and don't stop too soon.

New-onset constipation with other concerning signs could mean that sexual abuse is on the list of things to consider. Older children may also regress with toileting in times of upheaval.

Dental Health

Some sources estimate that up to 20 percent of children adopted internationally have dental problems, from cavities to tooth enamel defects. For example, Katherine's daughter Kaia had a cavity in every single tooth when she came home at age five.

Even children adopted as infants, and with impeccable oral hygiene habits, may have frequent cavities due to poor early or in-utero nutrition. Similarly, children who have been living in poverty or in the foster-care system in the United States, with poor access to dental care, more commonly have problems with decay.

If a child is having problems chewing or eating, a dental evaluation is in order. Aside from lack of hygiene and poor early nutrition, a critical factor in developing tooth decay is the *frequency* of snacking or drinking. A child who was pacified with a bottle of juice or a sippy cup of sweetened beverages all day, or put to bed with a bottle, may also have dental issues as well as a higher risk of unhealthy weight gain. Structured meals and snacks with no grazing, and only water in between, promotes good dental health.

Diabetes

Diabetes occurs when there is a problem with the hormone insulin or the insulin receptors. Insulin gets energy (glucose) into the cells where it can fuel the body or be stored for energy.

Type I diabetes occurs when the pancreas does not make enough insulin. It is rare, but should be considered if there is weight loss, decreased energy, increased thirst and urination, extreme hunger, and sometimes bedwetting. It is diagnosed most frequently in children and used to be called "juvenile" diabetes. See your doctor if you are concerned. If a child has type I diabetes, that complicates the feeding relationship greatly as there is a real risk of blood sugar being too high or too low, and intense attention must be paid to how much and what the child is eating in order to dose insulin injections. The Trust Model *can* be used successfully with these children, however. (Visit the Ellyn Satter Institute at http://www.ellynsatter.com; click on "Resources," then "ESI Child Diabetes Position Statement.")

Type II diabetes occurs when the body isn't able to use insulin effectively. It is also exceedingly rare in children, but pre-diabetes or Type II diabetes can be considered in the older child or teen, particularly if the child has experienced weight acceleration and has a very high BMI, which is correlated with an increased risk of type II diabetes. It is often without symptoms. Doctors can screen for this relatively easily.

Diarrhea

Diarrhea can be complex to diagnose. There may be infectious causes like parasites, bacteria, or viral infections that are common. There can also be diarrhea associated with antibiotics. Loose stools may result from excess fiber, such as when a child consumes large amounts of fruit, and may not be problematic. Food intolerance or allergies should be considered in the differential. Changes in stool or concerns over stool pattern or consistency, particularly in internationally adopted children, or with other symptoms like fever or pain, should be discussed with your doctor. Bright red blood or very dark or black stools (which may indicate blood from higher in the digestive tract) are worrisome and must be looked into immediately.

Eczema

Also known as atopic dermatitis, eczema can start in infancy. This condition presents often with dry, bumpy, red and itchy patches. Itching may develop before the rash. The skin may also be darker than usual. It is associated with asthma and other allergic conditions, including food allergies, which should be considered. It is often triggered by dryness or too much water exposure, such as swimming or frequent bathing. In addition to skin care, topical (applied to the skin) steroid medications can help with flares and prevention, and oral anti-histamines like Benadryl can help with the itching. Keep your child's fingernails short to minimize trauma from scratching.

Skin Care

Some theories state that skin rashes and a breakdown of the skin's protective barrier play a role in the increasing rates of allergic illnesses and food allergies. To keep skin healthy, the following tips might help, and don't hurt.

- Avoid using soaps often on infants or small children. You don't need to bathe a child daily or wash hair unless they have been out playing in the mud or had a leaky diaper.
- You can use oils in bathwater or for massage, like grape seed oil or even olive oil. Massaging an infant or small child with all-natural oils can soothe skin, help with bonding, and be a nice bedtime ritual. With an older or traumatized child, follow her lead with touch. She may allow and even enjoy having lotion rubbed into hands and feet.
- Vanicream is a line of soaps and creams that are free from irritants. If you see red or rough spots, moisturize twice daily. Even many "baby" products are full of perfumes and skin irritants.
- Wash clothes in detergents formulated for sensitive skin. Avoid fabric softeners.
- Double-rinse clothing in the wash cycle to remove excess irritants.

Eosinophilic Esophagitis

Eosinophilic esophagitis (EoE) is an inflammation of the esophagus, or swallowing tube, associated with food allergies and more common in children with an atopic (eczema) or allergic history. It is associated with food refusal due to severe pain and can distort feeding. If a child presents with "reflux" symptoms that don't resolve with treatment, EoE should be on the differential list. It may present with poor weight gain, weight loss, unusual vomiting or gagging, or history of foods getting stuck. It is not common.

Fetal Alcohol Spectrum Disorder

Fetal alcohol spectrum disorder (FASD) occurs when the mother consumed alcohol during pregnancy. Fetal alcohol *syndrome* (FAS) has the hallmark of the characteristic facial features, although it is thought that many times more children are affected by alcohol exposure who do not have the facial features. This in part is why the term "spectrum" was added to the definition, to indicate that there is a range of expressions of the exposure. Children with FAS are often shorter than average height and weight (and have higher rates of microcephaly or smaller head size), which affects growth measures, interpretation, and ultimately feeding, since there is often pressure put on the parent from size worries. Children with FASD may have sleep and sucking problems as babies and have higher rates of sensory integration issues, which also affect eating. Behavior also affects the feeding relationship with difficulty concentrating and with judgment. There is no blood test to confirm diagnosis, and there is overlap with other conditions, like ADHD, autistic spectrum disorders, nonverbal learning disorders, and the effects of past institutional care. If you are concerned, pediatric developmental specialists and psychologists can help with diagnosis and treatment.

Hemorrhoids

Hemorrhoids are often painful or itchy swellings of tissue in the rectal area, which sometimes protrude from the anus. These are usually associated with constipation, so treatment of constipation is key, although some prescription creams, wipes, or suppositories, may help. Good hygiene is critical.

Iron Deficiency

Iron deficiency (ID) is most common in the first several months due to poor nutrition or care, as well as after catch-up growth. It must be considered and should be routinely checked. (See Anemia for iron-deficiency anemia.) ID is characterized by:

- Fatigue and weakness
- Shortness of breath
- Headache
- Lightheadedness
- Cold hands and feet
- Inflammation or soreness of tongue
- Brittle or spoon-shaped nails
- Unusual cravings for non-nutritive substances, such as ice or dirt (a condition known as "pica")
- Poor appetite (especially in infants and children)
- Irritability
- Difficulty concentrating
- Rapid pulse
- Hair loss

Iron deficiency must be treated with iron supplementation. Talk to your provider for the dose and follow-up testing. (See www.adoptionnutrition.org or www.adoptmed.org for more information.)

Lead Poisoning

Lead levels should be screened in all children, but children in foster care and adopted children, including internationally, may be at higher risk. Have your child screened at the earliest possible opportunity if there hasn't been a recent test. High lead levels often have no clear symptoms, but can present with irritability, GI symptoms, loss of appetite, decreased energy, weight loss, and learning difficulties—which may be irreversible. Lead exposure is primarily from environmental sources like paint, toys with lead, and contaminated dirt and dust. Treatment is to first remove any sources of exposure, and medication that binds with and excretes the lead. (Visit the Centers for Disease Control and Prevention (CDC) Website at www.cdc.gov for prevention information.)

Feeding During the Flu or Short-Term Illness Like Gastroenteritis or Colds

When kids are sick, all bets are off, especially with infants and pre-verbal kids who may have trouble reading their own appetite and hunger signals. It's just hard to know what is going on, and they may be more whiney or clingy. Are they crying because their ears or throat hurt, or are they hungry?

Taking care of sick kids is scary and confusing for everyone, but especially for parents who already worry about a child's intake or size. In general, sick infants and children eat less. When you are cued in to your child's appetite, it can be an early sign that something is going on. My own daughter seemed to lose her appetite a few days before the runny nose or the vomiting (yuck) would start.

It can take more than a week for appetite to return to normal, and if your child is on any medicines, particularly antibiotics, that can make it even worse. Antibiotics taste bad and can interfere with normal bacteria in the gut and cause diarrhea.

Support your child by offering foods and drink often when they are ill. Throw away the usual schedule when your toddler is sick and let them nibble and sip throughout the day. The infant who normally finishes a bottle in 20 minutes might only suck for five, or for 40, or intake might drop in terms of quantity too. Kids don't have to eat much when they are ill for a few days. Even a few bites might be all they take. (However, if your child is medically fragile or his nutritional status is already compromised, monitor him closely and keep your doctor informed. Even a limited illness in some children is poorly tolerated.) When kids are sick, consider giving Popsicles, Jell-O, or watered-down juice as appropriate to boost fluid intake. If there is severe vomiting or diarrhea, you may need to talk to your doctor about rehydration or use a commercial product for rehydration.

Have faith that their appetites will return when they feel better, and see your doctor if it doesn't. Know that the Trust Model of feeding is flexible and that you can get back to regular feeding and schedules when your child is better. There might be a little whining for Jell-O when they feel better, but you'll know how to handle that too! You may also serve yogurt or other foods or supplements with probiotics if your child has a diarrhea or is on antibiotics.

If you have any questions or concerns, be sure to see your child's health care provider. If your child is listless or acting "off," don't hesitate to ask questions. Kids can get dehydrated with diarrheal or vomiting illnesses, so be sure to check in with your doctor.

Mouth Breathing and Eating With Mouth Open

A complaint I commonly hear is about the child with "bad manners" who eats with his mouth open. Aside from the battle over manners, which often actually promotes the behavior, there are medical reasons why a child might chew with his mouth open or mouth-breathe. Snoring may also be another clue. Some kids have nasal allergies or inflammation from infection that can make it hard to breathe through the nose. Think about a time when you had a cold and were stuffed up, and you had to open your mouth to breathe.

Another possibility is enlarged adenoids. This can also cause obstruction or blocking of the airway and difficulty with nose breathing. I'm not saying you have to have adenoids removed, but be aware that there may be a real reason why your child chews with his mouth open.

Children who chew with their mouths open may also have oral-motor or sensory delay (see Chapter 3).

PANDAS

Rare at any age, but especially after age 12, pediatric autoimmune neuropsychiatric disorders associated with streptococcal infections (PANDAS) is a neuropsychiatric (brain and behavior) reaction to strep infections. There is often sudden onset or worsening of symptoms of obsessive-compulsive disorder (OCD) and a combination of other associated symptoms that all start around the same time. PANDAS might be more common with FASD. Some common accompanying symptoms can be:

- Severe separation anxiety
- Generalized anxiety, which may become outright panic
- Hyperactivity, abnormal movements, and restlessness
- Sensory abnormalities, including hypersensitivity to light or sounds, distortions of visual perceptions, and occasionally, visual or auditory hallucinations
- Concentration difficulties and loss of academic abilities, particularly in math and visual-spatial areas
- Increased urinary frequency and new-onset bedwetting
- Irritability (sometimes with aggression) and mood swings. Abrupt onset of depression can also occur, with thoughts about suicide
- Developmental regression, including temper tantrums, "baby talk," and handwriting deterioration (also related to motor symptoms)

PANDAS is a subcategory of the recently described PANS (pediatric acute-onset neuropsychiatric syndrome), which is similar but is not proven to be related to a strep infection. (Visit the National Institutes of Mental Health Website at www.nimh.nih.gov for more information.)

Think of the seven-year-old, who has been happily bumping along, when suddenly she stops eating and develops severe anxiety and mood swings. She rapidly loses weight with no other explanation. There may or may not be a recent history of a sore throat, but PANS must be on the differential diagnosis.

Parasites

Up to 35 percent of internationally adopted children have intestinal parasites. The range is seven to 50 percent, depending on country. It should be considered and tested for at initial physical. (Visit www.adoptmed.org for more information.)

Pica

Pica is when an individual eats nonfood items. The condition may be behavioral or linked with certain nutritional deficiencies. You may need to ask your doctor if checking a lead level is in order if pica is a concern (eating dirt, for example).

"I want to say that her pica has resolved, but last time I said that we got a call from the school that she'd eaten half a plant and was sobbing because the preschool director yelled at Kassa! The pica is much better, but she'll definitely have no problem eating a box of raisins and the actual box, unless we stop her. She's pretty reliable on the whole but it requires a lot of vigilance because even if she knows she's not supposed to eat something, she either just wants to keep chewing (and I think she likes the chewing part more than the actual eating) or has some actual interest in the item. I don't think she's trying to be disobedient and I don't think it's the kind of pica that's related to nutritional deficits or anything, more like a form of OCD." — Amy, Mom to Kassa, age three

Prematurity

Even in the best medical centers in the United States, with "standard" care and committed parents, prematurity is a major risk factor for feeding problems. Guess why? It's worry.

Premature infants tire quickly and may be weak, but as they get more capable with sucking, swallowing, and the mechanics of eating, they too can self-regulate. There is a great feeding resource know as Support of Oral Feedings for Fragile Infants (SOFFI). Ask your health care professional to look into it if you are having trouble with feeding. As of now, there seem to be no direct-to-consumer resources. (See "The SOFFI Reference Guide: Text, Algorithms, and Appendices: A Manualized Method for Quality Bottle-Feedings" by Kathleen Philbin and Erin Ross in the *Journal of Perinatal and Neonatal Nursing*, October/December 2011.)

Reflux Is Confusing

Over dinner with my mommy's group one night, it come up that five of the seven kids had been on Prevacid (a proton pump inhibitor that lowers the acidity) for reflux. It struck me as a very high number. Similarly, when polling the staff of a local center for baby classes where I give workshops, the staff remarked on the surprisingly large proportion of infants they see with the reflux diagnosis and prescription.

Less than 10 years earlier, during my clinical years, infants were not routinely treated with strong proton-pump inhibitors (PPIs). Diagnoses of colic, a hug, and a "hang in there" were common; PPIs were not. Were some cases of reflux missed? Probably, but what I fear is happening now is that many more cases are "diagnosed" that may not be significant reflux, or reflux at all, and the PPIs are prescribed with little concern for possible effects. There simply have not been long-term studies on the safety in infants to warrant indiscriminant use. (In fact, the use of these medications is "off-label," meaning it is not an indicated use and that safety testing has not been done.)

How Is Reflux Diagnosed?

Mostly, this is a diagnosis that clinicians make by history and symptoms. Does the baby scream with feeding, or does he arch his back and appear to be in pain? That is often enough to earn you a quick prescription and diagnosis.

Let me tell you about a little baby with the diagnosis. Mom was scared from day one that her little boy was not eating enough. The nurses stressed that he was "small" and encouraged feeding a certain amount every few hours, waking him from sleep to do so. It wasn't long before things were going downhill. He didn't seem to want the breast or pumped milk from a bottle. He was diagnosed with reflux and started on Prevacid. However, no one asked HOW this mom was feeding her little boy. When she was told by the specialist to "get food into that kid," she took to forceful feeding. Now, how might you react if someone was forcing a bottle into your mouth? Might you scream? Arch your back and turn your head away?

The child had a normal pH probe test (where a small probe is placed through the nose into the esophagus for 24 hours to detect acid levels—the gold standard for diagnosis), and the Prevacid did not help the concerns. Did he have reflux? I doubt it. The point is: doctors need to be asking more questions. I am concerned that this has become another "quick fix" for too many children. Are some children in pain and need medication and benefit from it? Absolutely. But perhaps a thorough history and exam and a few more "hang in there's," along with some feeding support, would also be in order. Reflux is something to have on a list of possible diagnoses, but should not be diagnosed in a five-minute office visit, sending you out the door with a prescription.

Reflux

Reflux is a condition where the stomach contents slip up into the esophagus or swallowing tube. The lower esophageal sphincter (the muscle between the stomach and the esophagus) is relatively underdeveloped in infants, which is part of why they spit up so easily. Infants spit up often, and if they are not bothered by it and are gaining weight, it is almost always nothing to worry about (other than the laundry burden). Clinical reflux is when the acidic stomach contents irritate and erode the esophagus lining, causing pain and affecting eating. Reflux is associated with signs of pain and decreased appetite, perhaps to the point of affecting weight gain and growth. The baby may arch or scream with feeding. Coughing or lung infections can occur with aspiration if the stomach contents make it into the lungs. Most infants outgrow spitting up and mild reflux. More serious reflux that effects weight gain and is accompanied by pain should be addressed with your doctor and may warrant a trial of treatment.

Thyroid Abnormalities

Thyroid hormones help regulate metabolism, energy, and weight. If your child has either high or low weight, or there are concerns about energy or listlessness, a thyroid test is reasonable to rule out hypo- or hyperthyroid (under- or overactive thyroid).

Urinary Tract Infection

A urinary tract infection (UTI) happens when the otherwise sterile bladder gets infected. The bacteria irritate the bladder, leading to the usual symptoms of pain, urgency (the need to urinate that comes on fast), and frequency of urination. Unexplained fevers in infants and preverbal children can indicate a UTI and should be considered. Children with severe constipation may also be more prone to UTIs with incomplete bladder emptying if there is stool impaction. UTIs are far more common in girls. Depending on the age of onset and the number of infections, more testing to look at the urinary tract, ureters (tubes to the kidneys), and kidneys may be in order. Always teach girls proper toilet hygiene and wiping, avoid bubble baths, take off swimsuits after swimming, and use the skin care advice under the eczema section above in terms of soaps and detergents. If there are other symptoms or any concerns, sexual abuse may need to be considered.

Vitamin Deficiencies

Please visit the Adoption Nutrition Website at www.adoptionnutrition.org for a complete discussion of vitamin and nutrient deficiencies. Nutrients to consider are iron, Vitamin D, and Vitamin C.

*For more information about medical issues that are more common in internationally adopted children, see www.adoptmed.org, www.adoptionnutrition.org, and www.peds .umn.edu/iac

Appendix III
Tips for Dealing With Health Care Providers

Some families dealing with feeding and weight worries or a child with health or developmental issues will have ongoing care with multiple providers. The reality is, you are your child's "care coordinator." Keep copies of medical records starting on day one. Danny's mother Beverly shared that she often picked up on things, including a potential drug interaction, before the doctors did. Here are some tips for navigating the health care system, which can be a major burden of its own.

Find Your Partners in Care
- Ask other families for recommendations, try a local online forum, or contact your state agency for a list of providers.
- Consider a female provider. I hear from parents that female providers tend to be better listeners, though I know many excellent male doctors.
- Consider an "allied" health professional, like a nurse practitioner or a physician's assistant. Adoptive mom Camille found her best partner in a nurse practitioner, who listened, researched, and advocated.
- Ask for a point person at the doctor's office if your child has complex needs. Someone should be familiar with your child if you have questions and your doctor is unavailable.

Stay Organized
- If you have a friend or a family member who is a doctor or nurse, ask him or her to review and explain any medications or conditions if you still have questions.
- Keep an updated medical history with current medications, conditions, surgeries, etc. Keep a printout in a known place in case you or a sitter has to make an urgent-care or E.R. visit. There are also smartphone apps for this.
- Start binders and folders now. Document every phone call, time, date, and who you spoke with if you are dealing with insurance or billing issues.
- Write letters or emails and keep copies.

Make the Most of Your Visit

- If your child is being sedated for any reason, call the other doctors involved in your child's care to ask if there are any other necessary procedures that can be done at the same time to avoid additional sedation.
- Take your partner or another family member with you to critical appointments. Have one person take notes.
- Follow up and give medications as instructed.
- Have growth data and plot it yourself if you have to, including Z-scores (see pages 20 and 77–78).
- If your child has concerning symptoms, write down:
  - · When did it start?
  - · Was it related to an event, travel, food, or medications?
  - · How has this impacted your child? Is it interrupting sleep, appetite, any other details like bowel changes, rashes, etc.?
  - · What have you already tried?
  - · What are you worried it might be? (Bring in your Internet search if you have to. You need to have your questions answered; even if your suspicions aren't the answer, you won't worry about it any more.)

Don't be afraid to ask for the reasoning behind invasive testing and what the plan is for follow-up Doing this helped Sue postpone and eventually avoid a swallow study while her daughter progressed. Avoiding *necessary* tests is not the goal, but it is helpful to be clear about what you want to learn from a test, if it is safe to wait and see, and if there are other options.

This final tip seems out of place in the 21st century, but sadly, I have found that some mothers still find it necessary. If you are a mother and sense you are having trouble getting your health care providers to listen to your concerns, take your husband, or other man close to the family, along to appointments. I have simply heard from too many mothers who sought help and perhaps even a second opinion (woe if you seek a third opinion) who felt their concerns were ignored. I have also experienced how differently I have been treated with a complex and confusing medical issue when I brought my husband with me—and I'm a physician myself! The three-minute visit with antibiotics and a boot out the door became a thoughtful, 20-minute discussion of treatment options. My husband didn't even have to say a word. He just sat in the room. Go figure.

"The first two doctors kept blowing me off, and only wanted to talk about Adina's weight. I have two other children; I knew something was wrong. I'm not unreasonable, but I needed an explanation for what I was observing. When I sought out a third doctor, he was rolling his eyes as he entered the room, and said, 'Well, she's already seen two doctors for this, obviously she's fine.'"
— Rebecca, mother of Adina, age 2½, adopted from Ethiopia at 8 months

It turns out Adina (who was food-preoccupied) had blood in her stool and was not progressing with her physical therapy as expected. While the doctors all focused on her weight, several red flags were ignored and indicated tests were not done—including basic blood work like iron levels to rule out anemia, which is common in IA children who have experienced catch-up growth. Rebecca felt that she was written off as a "hysterical" mother. (Adina's experience is also an example of how medical weight bias, discussed in Chapter 5, can negatively impact care.)

Another dad explained that his daughter was quickly dismissed as having "psychological" problems, when a GI evaluation had not yet been pursued for new and rapidly increasing vomiting episodes. Even if it turns out that there are no underlying medical concerns, it is imperative that you find a health care provider who will listen to and address your concerns.

Too many mothers get labeled as irrational or hysterical when they are desperately scared. Becky Henry, author of *Just Tell Her to Stop,* explains that this is a common scenario for parents seeking help for a child's eating disorder. *"When we've been fighting for our child's life and getting nowhere and show up crying, it is assumed we are controlling and hysterical so we're not taken seriously. I wish I had said, 'I'm crying because my child is seriously ill and I feel helpless but I still need to be treated respectfully.'"*

Adina's mother Rebecca adds, *"I should have brought my husband. I could tell the doctor had no patience for me. He told me Adina was fine before he even examined her or asked a single question."* You may find the idea offensive that a mother needs to be accompanied by a male in order to be taken seriously, but when you want answers, you might be willing to do anything it takes. It's all part of advocating for your child—doing what has to be done. imperative that you find a health care provider who will listen to and address your concerns.

Appendix IV
Feeding Your Baby

In making feeding decisions for your baby, go by what he can do, not by how old he is. The ages in this figure are given in ranges, and even then they are ball-park estimates. Your baby is the only one who can really say when he's ready!

What Your Baby Can Do and How and What to Feed Him

Age	Feeding Capabilities	Manner of Feeding	Suggested Foods
Birth to 6 months	Cuddles Roots for nipple Sucks Swallows liquids	Cuddling and nipple-feeding from breast or bottle	Breastmilk and/or iron-fortified infant formula
5 to 7 months	Sits supported or alone Keeps head straight when sitting Follows food with eyes Opens for spoon Closes lips over spoon Moves semisolid food to back of tongue Swallows semisolids	Spoon-feeding of smooth semisolid food Cuddling and nipple-feeding from breast or bottle	Iron-fortified rice or barley cereal mixed with breastmilk or iron-fortified formula Breastmilk and/or iron-fortified formula
6 to 8 months	Sits alone Keeps food in mouth to munch Pushes food to jaws with tongue Munches, mashes food with up-and-down movement Palms food (palmar grasp) Scrapes food from hand into mouth Drinks from a cup but loses a lot	Spoon-feeding of thicker and lumpier food Finger-feeding of thicker, lumpier food: "If it hangs together, it's a finger food." Cup drinking Cuddling and nipple-feeding from breast or bottle	Well-cooked, mashed, or milled vegetables and fruits Mashed potatoes Sticky rice Wheat-free dry cereal like Cheerios or Corn Chex Breastmilk and/or iron-fortified formula

Source: Figure 7.1 from *Child of Mine,* copyright © 2012 by Ellyn Satter. Reprinted with permission.

What Your Baby Can Do and How and What to Feed Him

Age	Feeding Capabilities	Manner of Feeding	Suggested Foods
7 to 10 months	Sits alone easily Bites off food Chews with rotary motion Moves food side-to-side in mouth, pausing with food on the center of the tongue Begins curving lip around cup Palmar changing to pincer grasp (thumb and forefinger)	Finger-feeding of lumpy food and pieces of soft food Cup drinking Cuddling and nipple-feeding from breast or bottle	Chopped cooked vegetables Chopped canned or cooked fruits Cheese Mashed cooked dried beans Strips of bread, toast, tortilla Crackers and dry cereals containing wheat Breastmilk and/or iron-fortified formula
9 to 12 months	Getting better at picking up small pieces of food (pincer grasp) Curves lip around cup Getting better at controlling food in mouth Getting better at chewing	Finger-feeding soft table foods Drinking by himself from a covered toddler cup Cuddling and nipple-feeding, away from mealtime	Cut-up soft cooked foods Cut-up soft raw food (like bananas or peaches) Tender chopped meats Casseroles with noodles cut up Dry cereal Toast and crackers Eggs and cheese Breastmilk and/or iron-fortified formula
12 months and beyond	Becomes more skillful with hands Finger-feeds Improves chewing Improves cup-drinking Is interested in food Becomes a part of the family with respect to eating	Finger-feeding soft table foods Cup-drinking by himself Nipple-feeding only at snack time, not at mealtime Begins to use spoon	Everything from the family table that is soft Avoid smooth pieces that can choke: whole grapes, hot dog rounds Cut up meat finely All right to change to whole pasteurized milk

Snack and Meal Ideas

All snacks and meals should *offer* a carb, protein, and fat, even if children don't eat from each category. If it's easier, you can plan in terms of the food groups. Look for a starch or grain, add a fruit and/or veggie, some fat source, and you should be covered. It takes a lot of planning, but your kids can learn to enjoy a variety of foods if given the opportunity, without pressure. Choose and prepare foods (such as grapes and meats) based on your child's ability to chew and swallow. Address any allergy concerns with your child's health care provider. I am hoping this list will give you a few ideas as you stare into your pantry. There is a mix of convenience and from-scratch items to get you thinking. Plan for sit-down snacks and meals every 2 to 3 hours for younger children, and every 3 to 4 hours for older children. You will notice many of the snacks could be meals too. Good luck!

In General for Snacks

Aim for two to three items from various groups:

Grains (carbohydrates): pita bread, bread, rice, cereal, crackers, graham crackers, whole-wheat crackers, pasta, tortillas, bagels, English muffins, popcorn, rice cakes, and crackers.

Fruits (fresh, frozen, dried, or canned): banana, apple, pineapple, pear, melons, applesauce, grapes cut in half, mangos, kiwis, strawberries, berries, dried fruits like prunes (cut up,) raisins, Craisins, and 100% fruit nectars or 100% juices (not sugar-added drinks).

Veggies: carrots, peas, corn, peppers, cucumbers, pickles, cherry tomatoes, beets, squash, edamame (green soybeans), sweet potato, potato, lettuce, avocado, celery, and beans.

Meats and protein: lunch meats, chicken, pork, beef, turkey, hummus (chick pea dip), baked beans, peanut or other nut butters, refried beans, milk, cheese, Greek yogurts, soy products like edamame or tofu, shrimp, and fish. (Try ground meats or prepare them in the slow cooker. Add sauces and gravies to make them easier to chew.)

Dairy: two to three servings a day (milk, cheese, yogurt, cottage cheese, puddings, and smoothies).

Fats: often included with dairy (butter, milk, yogurt, cheese, and cream cheese) and meats and some crackers like Ritz. In addition, sauces and dips (ranch, thousand island, etc.) oils, avocados, olives, homemade dressings, nuts and nut butters, ice cream, cookies, fried foods.

Sample Snacks

Serve with milk or water, or watered-down fruit juice on occasion.
- Baked beans, crackers
- Small muffin with butter, carrot sticks
- Scrambled egg with grated cheese, apple slices
- Leftover pizza, raisins, cherry or grape tomatoes cut in half
- Ham sandwich (whole-wheat bread, ham, cheese or mayo) leftover veggie like carrots and peas, cut-up pineapple
- Leftover mac-n-cheese with tuna, pickles (spears or rounds)
- English muffin with flavored cream cheese, sliced red peppers
- Leftover spaghetti with marinara or meat sauce, yogurt, Clementine
- Rolled-up lunch meat with cream cheese or Miracle Whip, applesauce
- Whole-wheat bread with turkey and hummus, cut-up grapes
- Soft mini-bagel with cream cheese, sliced strawberries
- Cooked shrimp with cocktail sauce, whole-grain crackers, cucumbers
- Whole-grain crackers, cheese stick(s)
- Apples with nut butter, dry cereal (like Chex or other with <6 g. sugar per serving)
- Oatmeal and raisin cookies
- Ants on a log (celery with peanut butter or cream cheese with raisins)
- Tortilla chips with melted cheese (and salsa), canned mandarin oranges
- Baked pita chips with hummus, baby carrots
- Quesadilla (tortilla with refried beans and melted cheese), pickles
- Tuna salad (tuna with Miracle Whip or mayo and sweet pickle relish), crackers
- Cut-up grapes, fig cookies
- Cucumber strips, ranch dip or hummus, pita bread
- Banana smoothie with yogurt and berries, graham crackers
- Cinnamon-raisin toast with butter, fruit yogurt
- Waffles or pancakes (freeze well and toast) with syrup or jam, applesauce
- Frozen mixed veggies (some kids like it frozen!), crackers
- Cottage cheese, berries, crackers
- A few slices of shredded lunch meat (or rolled with cream cheese), toast, pineapple
- Carrots and ranch dressing, raisins
- Rice Krispies treats, banana
- Tortilla rolled with cream cheese or butter, apple slices
- Tortilla with melted cheese, orange slices
- Popcorn with butter and a sprinkling of salt and/or sugar, dried fruit

Visit www.thefeedingdoctor.com for updated snack and meal ideas!

Feeding and Intake Journal

"We did a food diary before. How is this different?" A standard nutrition intake form offers only a small part of the picture. It reflects WHAT and usually ignores HOW you feed. The Feeding Doctor Feeding and Intake Journal on the following page *asks for far more detail, including when and where are you offering foods. What are you offering, how is the interaction going? How does it feel? What is the context for the intake?* This is often a great starting point for my sessions with clients and will provide an invaluable tool as you work on your feeding relationship and see patterns with structure, what you are offering, and interactions. It can also give your registered dietician (RD) or pediatrician a better picture of what is going on.

Instructions

Record what your child has eaten or drunk immediately after the meal or snack. List each food on a separate line. Don't forget to include condiments. When possible, state the brand name, type of milk (whole, 2%, 1% or skim), and whether the food was fresh, frozen, or canned. Specify amounts in terms of cups, tablespoons, teaspoons, and dimensions of a piece of pizza or serving of lasagna. Be sure to include everything, even liquids and candy. Include at least two consecutive weekdays and one weekend day. In the notes you may wish to write where or how your child was fed or anything else you feel may be helpful for the provider to know.

FEEDING AND INTAKE JOURNAL

Name: _____

Date of Birth: _____　**Ht:** _____　**Wt:** _____　**Day 1 Day & Date:** _____

Meal/Snack	Time of day	Food(s) and/or beverage(s) offered	Amount(s) consumed	Notes

Lunch Box Card

Copy, fill in, and laminate this "lunch box card" (also available online at The Feeding Doctor under "Resources"). Place it in your child's lunch box and tell him that if an adult asks him to eat certain foods, he should hand over the card. This is hard to ask a child to do, but it may work for some.

Dear Friend of_____,
Please allow _____ to decide how
much to eat, and in what order, from what
I have packed. Even if that means all
_____ eats for lunch is "dessert," or if
_____ starts with dessert. I trust that
_____ can rely on hunger and
fullness signals to know how much to eat.
Please call my cell _____ if you
have any questions. The nice thing is,
this should be less work for you. If _____
needs help opening containers, I thank
you for that help, otherwise,
_____ should be good to go.
Thank you for all you do for our children.

Index

Made in the USA
Middletown, DE
16 June 2015